Atlas of Dentomaxillofacial Anatomical Imaging

Antigoni Delantoni • Kaan Orhan
Editors

Atlas of Dentomaxillofacial Anatomical Imaging

Springer

Editors
Antigoni Delantoni
Faculty of Dentistry
Aristotle University of Thessaloniki
Thessaloniki, Greece

Kaan Orhan
DentoMaxillofacial Radiology
Ankara University
Ankara, Turkey

ISBN 978-3-030-96839-7 ISBN 978-3-030-96840-3 (eBook)
https://doi.org/10.1007/978-3-030-96840-3

This Springer imprint is published by the registered company Springer Nature Switzerland AG
The registered company address is: Gewerbestrasse 11, 6330 Cham, Switzerland

To my family and students,

And to my mentor from whom I learned Anatomy,

Prof. Dr. Bayram Ufuk Şakul

To my family from who I learn daily,

And to my teachers who made me love anatomy

Preface

Accurate interpretation of indications for treatment is the cornerstone of success in medicine. The book examines the relation between clinical features, diagnosis, and choice of minimally invasive technique for a range of dentomaxillofacial anatomy and disorders. It explains how selection of imaging technique is intimately related to clinical and diagnostic aspects and how recognition of this relation forms the foundation for an optimal outcome. In addition to examining the various modalities, careful attention is paid to the role of including the latest imaging techniques. The book will provide detailed discussion of the pathology, treatment, and prognosis of common and rare diseases, congenital/developmental malformations, and more in dentomaxillofacial area which is underestimated and also not well known by radiologists. This comprehensive imaging book will help radiologists and dentists in their training and daily practice. Pathological descriptions of radiologic diagnoses help clarify the pathophysiology of the disease. Pearls and pitfalls of imaging interpretation are presented for quick reference. Authors are world-renowned dentomaxillofacial radiology experts.

In this book, the chapters fall into several categories: The anatomy, technique, and fundamentals of 2D modality are discussed in Chapters 1–6. Chapters 7 to 9 briefly review general considerations for 3D CBCT/MDCT in head and neck as well as its anatomy, Chapter 10 physical principles of ultrasound as well as finally, advanced MRI, angiography and micro-CT imaging in Chapters 11–15.

This is an outstanding book for learning and understanding the DMFR imaging in dentomaxillofacial radiology that will stimulate both radiologists and students to seek a more in-depth appreciation of the subject and its contribution to the scientific community of radiology. As a result, this book offers a comprehensive review of the state of the art in dentomaxillofacial imaging.

Thessaloniki, Greece
Ankara, Turkey
July 2021

Antigoni Delantoni
Kaan Orhan

Contents

Introduction to Dentomaxillofacial Imaging

1

Kaan Orhan and Antigoni Delantoni

1.1 Introduction

The correct diagnosis for the treatment of oral and maxillofacial pathologies has an important place for accurate treatment. Radiographic imaging is an important element in the diagnosis. Because of the anatomic complexity of the dento-maxillofacial region and wide variety of diseases, the diagnosis can be problematic. Radiographs are an essential part of proper diagnosis. From the early days of dental radiography, the clinical objective has been to produce accurate images of dental structures that are normally visually obscured and not always readily visualized. An early method for aligning the X-ray beam and image receptor with the teeth and jaws was the bisecting-angle technique.

Dentists, should make sure that operators do not take for granted the impact of their actions when they take X-rays. Radiographs which are based on the patient's intraoral examination are taken and always following a review of the patient's medical history. A proper radiograph will ensure a good diagnosis and thus proper treatment of the patient. Taking dental radiographs correctly the first time saves the patient unnecessary radiation exposure and the practice time and expense. There are several methods that can be used in dental radiology from conventional to 3D contemporary advanced techniques. Depending on the pathology one should know about the proper indication and also the use of radiology technique esp. dose concentrations.

The objective of this textbook is to offer the reader a concise summary of the fundamentals and principles of dental radiology. In addition, the more common osseous pathologic lesions will be given along the chapters. This book is intended to be a handy resource for the student and the practicing clinicians.

1.2 What Does the Clinician Need in Terms of Imaging?

In today's dental practice, one should only use a well-designed X-ray machine where the time exposure controls are electronic and thus accurately deliver the proper exposure to patients. In most countries, these are the only types of controls that pass inspection. If one is not using a machine that uses electronic controls, they should replace it as soon as possible. To obtain proper images of the oral cavity and dental tissues, one must at all times be aware of the basic rule of radiology:

K. Orhan (✉)
Department of DentoMaxillofacial Radiology, Faculty of Dentistry, Ankara University, Ankara, Turkey
e-mail: knorhan@dentistry.ankara.edu.tr

A. Delantoni
Department of Dentoalveolar Surgery, Implant Surgery and Radiology, Faculty of Dentistry, Aristotle University of Thessaloniki, Thessaloniki, Greece
e-mail: andelant@dent.auth.gr

A. Delantoni, K. Orhan (eds.), *Atlas of Dentomaxillofacial Anatomical Imaging*,
https://doi.org/10.1007/978-3-030-96840-3_1

ALARA (as low as reasonablyAttainable). This means dentists are taking images using As-Low-As-Reasonably-Achievable doses of radiation. In order to be protected from the biological effects of radiation, some precautions must be taken and also proper use of radiographs should be known by the professions. Dose limitations are at the forefront of these measures:

1. Necessity of applications: Radiation applications that will not provide a clear benefit should be avoided. (Justification: justification-necessity).
2. Optimization (Best of the Alternatives): Considering the economic and social factors, all irradiation should be kept at the lowest level possible.
3. Dose limitation: the maximum permissible doses (MPD: maximum permissible dose) should not be exceeded. The exposure and dose reduction, as well as clinical indications must be established after careful clinical examination.

Maximum patient benefit should be targeted, with minimum patient and operator dose. Considering the presence of risk, although it is minimal in all individuals, efforts should be made to use as low as possible doses, and all unnecessary exposures should be avoided. When following these basic rules, the amount of radiation to which both the patient, the practitioner and the environment will be exposed can be minimized in occupational radiation applications.

Moreover, the clinician should take care all precautious; before irradiation, during irradiation, and after irradiation.

Precautions before irradiation: Determining the appropriate indication and technique for the patient, after the anamnesis and clinical examination. It should be noted whether there is a systemic condition (such as pregnancy in female patients), the use of Pb aprons, reducing the number of films and exposure time should be taken into consideration. The indication for taking radiographs in children and young people should be reduced as much as possible. The X-ray equipment should be safe, well-calibrated, and periodically maintained and checked.

Precautions during irradiation: For radiation control reasons, lead aprons and collars should be applied to all patients, regardless of patient age or the number of films to be taken, to protect the thyroid and gonad areas. Appropriate kVp should be selected for diagnostic purposes. Generally 70–100 kVp is a suitable range for various purposes in dentistry. When kVp decreases, the energy of the beam decreases, the image contrast increases, when kVp increases, the energy of the beam increases and the image contrast decreases. High-contrast images are useful in monitoring very different densities within a structure, such as caries or soft tissue calcifications, while low-contrast images are useful in identifying dissimilar densities, such as early and minor bone changes in periodontal disease. The films should be placed correctly in the mouth and moving of the films should be avoided. This minimizes distortion and prevents unnecessary radiation of the patient's hand when using bi-secting technique. However, the use of the parallel technique should be performed with the proper film holders. This prevents possible exposure to patient's hand and provides proper placement of the film with a reduction of patient's exposure dose. The parallel technique is a more suitable technique in terms of protection because it allows the closest image to its real size with more parallel rays.

Precautions after irradiation: The proper selection of the appropriate technique, its correct application of the chosen technique, the prevention of film repetitions, and the obtaining of high quality radiographs with minimal radiation are important. The radiographs should be evaluated with a proper display (preferably dedicated medical displays). The environment in which the assessment takes place should be semi-dark. Window light or unit light are not suitable for examining films. Quality assurance programs: Every clinic should have a quality assurance protocol in order to consistently obtain high quality images with minimal exposure. Continuous education programs should be followed in order to follow the innovations in imaging technology and new information on radiation safety. Dental clinicians should combine the clinical examination to possible diagnosis, and then refer for imaging to the radiologists. The most important part while sending the patient to a radiologist for a radiograph, is to provide as much clinical information to the radiologists allowing for both sides (dentists and radiologists) to have a proposer diagnosis in a realistic way and also avoid any medico-legal implications.

1.3 How Does the Clinician Decide What Kind of Imaging?

Few diagnostic tests provide as much useful information as dental radiography. This is the reason why, the clinician is sometimes tempted to prematurely make a definitive diagnosis based solely on radiographic interpretation. However, the image should be used only as a preliminary tool, providing important clues to set the diagnostic investigation. When not combined with a proper history and clinical examination, the radiograph alone can lead to a misinterpretation of normality and pathosis. Since treatment planning is ultimately based on this diagnosis, the potential for non proper treatment may be higher, if the radiograph is used alone for setting the final diagnosis. The clinician should not subject the patient to unnecessary multiple radiation exposures; often two pretreatment images from different angulations are sufficient. But in extenuating circumstances, especially when the diagnosis is difficult, multiple exposures may be necessary in order to determine the presence of multiple roots, multiple canals, resorptive defects, caries, restoration defects, root fractures, and the extent of root maturation and apical development.

As stated above, there are several guidelines for the evaluation of clinical history and examination for diagnosis. However, the methods of diagnostic imaging of the temporomandibular joint in the dentoalveolar structures, measure the degree of integrity of its components and should be done along with the clinical findings for evaluation in cases of different pathologies such as trauma, occlusal changes, limited mouth opening, systemic diseases, infections etc.

The conventional diagnostic tools of two-dimensional radiographs have shown various advantages such as low amount of radiation doses, simple and quick, non-invasive, and low-cost advantages. The appearance of new digital two-dimensional systems with numerous features of image enhancement, in addition to the mentioned advantages, might represent digital two-dimensional radiography as a simple and acceptable modality in this field as well.

However, 2D radiographs have several drawbacks, including errors that are classified as "errors of projection" and "errors of identification." Errors of projection are due to the two-dimensional (2D) which causes a shadow of the three-dimensional (3D) object. As a result this distorion together with differential magnification which may lead to errors of identification and reduced accuracy in the diagnosis.

New technological advances in dentomaxillofacial imaging were started to resolve these errors and are becoming increasingly popular for orthodontic diagnosis and treatment assessment. 3D computed tomography (CT) avoids the superimposition of tissues and problems due to magnification and offers the ability to visualize the craniofacial structures with more precision than the 2D method. Along with 3D CT, the effective dose of MDCT is much higher than the conventional radiographs and also expensive procedure and scanners are not easily accessible by dentists. In the last decades, a technique called as cone beam computed tomography (CBCT) was proposed for the maxillofacial imaging and started using routinely. The major advantages of this imaging modality are; lower radiation dose than MDCT, the possibility of individualized overlap-free reconstructions and DICOM data that can be in-and exported for other applications which started to use routine imaging. A low-dose high-resolution three-dimensional scans such as CBCT images might be given more accurate diagnostic data for certain conditions such as surgical intervention, anatomic variations, etc. MRI and USG

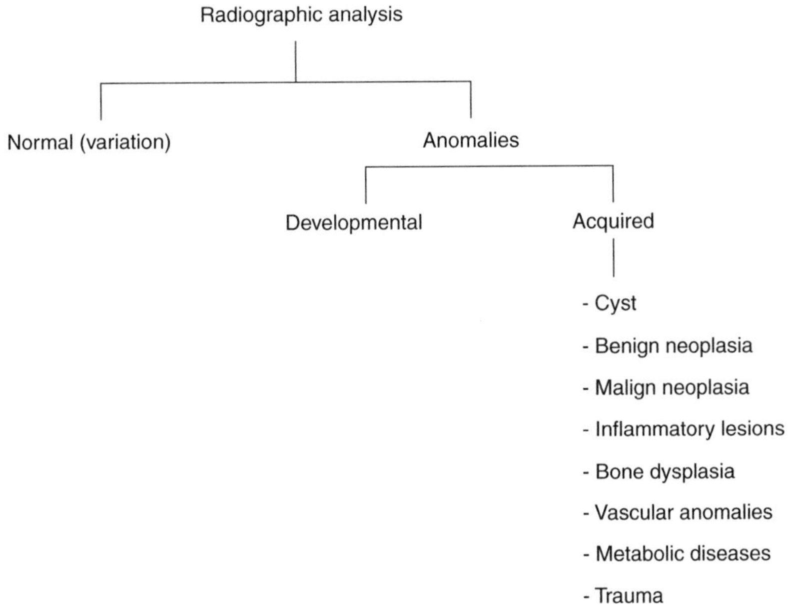

Fig. 1.1 Flowchart showing the radiographic analysis of the DMFR regions

are also other contemporary techniques which can be used for visualization of the soft tissues.

While evaluating various pathological lesions clinically and radiographically, the rules regarding the creation of the radiographic image should be considered. First of all, the radiographic examination decision must be made at the end of the clinical examination. The resulting radiographs produced, should be of sufficient diagnostic quality, sufficient quantity and size to avoid confusion with artifacts, and should be evaluated under appropriate image evaluation conditions. A systematic approach should be followed in the analysis of the diagnostic image. For this, all anatomical formations must be defined before evaluating the radiograph. Bone structures, bone density, height, amount, anatomical formations according to each region, structures associated with teeth, periodontal space, lamina dura should be carefully evaluated (Fig. 1.1).

As there are many different modalities that can be used a thorough understanding on the imaging is important. The chapters in this book elaborate in detail how best to visualize the dentomaxillofacial anatomy and its pathologies, thus instructing the clinicians which examinations to ask for.

1.4 Conclusions

The combination of both clinical and X-ray images provides vital information to the dentist for preparing comprehensive dental treatment plans. The end result is a continual improvement in oral healthcare today. A close collaboration between professions should be made to ensure the correct diagnosis, moreover a standardized terminology and evidence-based guidelines must be taken into consideration for correlation of clinical symptoms and imaging findings.

Further Reading

American Academy of Craniofacial Pain. Craniofacial pain: a handbook for assessment, diagnosis and management. Chattanooga: Chroma; 2009.

Eren H, Kolsuz ME, Orhan K. An overall look for temporomandibular joint pathologies and imaging. Int J Orthop. 2015;2(6):452–61.

Farman AG. Panoramic radiology. New York: Springer; 2007.

Mozzo P, Procacci C, Tacconi A, Martini PT, Bergamo IA. A new volumetric CT machine for dental imaging based on the cone-beam technique: preliminary results. Eur Radiol. 1998;8:1558–64.

Oz U, Orhan K, Abe N. Comparison of linear and angular measurements using two-dimensional conven-

tional methods and three-dimensional cone beam CT images reconstructed from a volumetric rendering program in vivo. Dentomaxillofac Radiol. 2011;40(8):492–500.
Rozylo-Kalinowska I, Orhan K. Imaging of the temporomandibular joint. Cham: Springer; 2019.
Whaites E. Essentials of dental radiography and radiology. 3rd ed. China: Elsevier Science; 2002.
White SC, Pharoah MJ. Oral radiology: principles and interpretation. St. Louis: Mosby/Elsevier; 2009.

2 Basic Principles of Intraoral Radiography

Antigoni Delantoni and Kaan Orhan

2.1 Basic Principles of Intraoral Radiography

X-ray production is made through an **X-rays** tube, which is a vacuum tube that uses a high voltage to accelerate the electrons released by a hot cathode at a high velocity. The high velocity electrons collide with a metal target, the anode, creating the **X-rays**. Basically, the Xrays production occurs in the anode from the energy produced in the anode, only a fraction has enough energy for the production of diagnostic X-rays. Dental X-ray tubes use a static anode unlike medical machines that have a rotating anode. The major difference is that the energy production from a static anode is much lower than that of the rotating anode. As with all machines the amount of milliamperes and Kilovolts has significant effect on image production.

The control of mA regulates the amount of current that passes from the cathode, and this circuit is known as low voltage circuit of the tube. A higher value of mA results to a rise in filament temperature which results to more electrons being released leading in turn to higher quantity of X-rays. As the mA affects the quantity of produced X-rays an increase in the mA leads to more electrons produced which in turn leads to more photons falling on the image plate.

The difference in kilovoltage refers to the levels of thousands of Volts between the cathode and the anode. When more electrons are released and accelerated through the cathode and are attracted to the anode target, a current is formed. The quality of X-rays produced is determined from the KV. The maximum difference is known as the peak of KV through the cathode and anode, thus the KVp. Differences under the KVp accelerate electrons to a smaller degree. Thus X-rays of higher KVp penetrate the tissues easier, leading to a slight increase of the radiographic density. Smaller KVp rays are more likely to get absorbed from the tissues and not give the image we need on the film after they reach it.

Besides the KVp and the mA the time of exposure is of high significance and basically alters the basic features of the image. The exposure time and mA affect the quantity of X-rays produced and we use the time of exposure to regulate the quantity of produced radiation, and in conclusion the density of the image produced.

The authors state that the chapter does not contain any information or images or other third party material that is not copyrighted by the authors.

A. Delantoni (✉)
Department of Dentoalveolar Surgery, Implant Surgery and Radiology, Faculty of Dentistry, Aristotle University of Thessaloniki, Thessaloniki, Greece
e-mail: andelant@dent.auth.gr

K. Orhan
Department of DentoMaxillofacial Radiology, Faculty of Dentistry, Ankara University, Ankara, Turkey
e-mail: knorhan@dentistry.ankara.edu.tr

A. Delantoni, K. Orhan (eds.), *Atlas of Dentomaxillofacial Anatomical Imaging*,
https://doi.org/10.1007/978-3-030-96840-3_2

Besides the production of X-rays and the basic principles the film is the second element that serves to the production of the final image.

Radiographic films are a special design containing chemical radiosensitive materials which are used as the recording media of the image, those chemicals after the effect of radiation undergo a latent chemical alteration, which to become identified, need the additional effect of other chemical agents (developers and fixers) during their manipulation on the dark room.

The major characteristic of intraoral radiographs is that the receptor or film which is the means to produce the image is placed within the oral cavity. Regarding plain film or digital images, the basics of both methods is the same. The only significant difference that may present upon the radiographs themselves is that in direct digital radiography the use of the sensor, in many cases has a smaller size of active area than the corresponding films or PSP plates.

In 1989 Trophy made a major change in the digitization of intraoral radiographs, with the use of CCD sensors. The first research presented on the new sensors was made by Wenzel and Moystadand Van der Stelt at the same time.

The question that arises in relation to digital intraoral radiography is what the disadvantages of conventional radiographic systems are, and whether they should be replaced by a digital system and for which reason.

The disadvantages of conventional film are as follows:

- Cost (films and processing materials).
- Investment cost from the existence of a darkroom.
- Time for the appearance and maintenance of the machine.
- Time for storing and archiving the material.
- Environmental costs from the use of chemicals.
- Reproducing the image where needed requires time and multiple processes while the copy of the tile is of lower quality than the original.
- Quality materials are rarely of a high standard in everyday practice.
- The main disadvantage remains the significantly higher radiation dose to which the patient receives when taking a conventional X-ray compared to the corresponding digital X-ray.

Digital images are made up of digits and are essentially distinct in terms of the resolution of the image elements (pixels) and in terms of the different shades of gray of each element (pixels) of the image. Essentially a digital image consists of horizontal and vertical pixel arrays. Each pixel has a column and row mapping in the image that marks its position in the image and represents a shade of gray.

2.2 How the Digital Image Is Produced

The production of the digital image requires certain steps that start with the conversion of the image from analog to digital (analog to digital conversion) according to the amount of radiation received. This value is stored on the computer and represents the image. This defines the parameters and monitors the images during their production. The difference in this absorption is detected and recorded by special detectors, which are located directly opposite to the X-ray tube.

2.3 How the Doctor Sees the Picture

The detectors convert the absorption into an electrical signal, which with the appropriate amplification is transferred to the computer. The computer organizes and assigns the pixels to their correct position. There the absorption data is converted into a digital signal, which, after being processed by the computer, gives the image of the predetermined section of the body that has been selected. To store the image, the computer uses eight memory locations (8 bits = 1 byte). Each byte can represent 256 [1] shades of gray, from value 0 to value 255 [2, 3]. After processing with a computer, each number corresponding to a different shades of gray is converted into an image. The final image consists of a set of small squares called pixels (picture element). Each of these elements has, as mentioned, values that express the absorption of radiation that passes through the specific tissues and thus the diagnostic information which is included in the original image. This defines a value of gray from 0 to 256 which corresponds to the number initially determined based on the amount of radiation absorbed. But the ability to see the data depends not only on the image but also on the lighting in the space [4–6].

2.4 Digital Screen

The screen on which it is projected plays an important role in the presentation of a digital image. Although the gold standard for the assessment of image quality remains the conventional radiological film, mainly in terms of resolution, (spatial resolution) when it is projected in a proper transparency and in an area with dim lighting [7].

This is interpreted simply by saying that the screen displays the data it receives from the receiver accurately. But what is this data?

This data is detailed data that to be displayed correctly on the screen, the pixels of the receiver must be matched with the pixels of the screen. Ideally, there should be a 1:1 correlation and ratio at diagnosis [8, 9].

These data, therefore, based on the value they have in their mapping when displayed on the screen, correspond to differences in optical density, contrast, and resolution. This is in levels and shades of gray and is a function of the "screen depth" like the number of bits used to represent the shade of a pixel (bit depth or bits per pixel) [4, 10].

The screen is good to have a depth of 12 bits, i.e., to be able to display 4096 (212) instead of 256 shades of gray in the images produced and to have increased contrast resolution as well as allows the dentist to use if he wants special programs advanced diagnostics such as for caries etc [7].

Ideally the screen dentists use to view radiographs, should correspond to the diagnostic screens used by radiologists when they view radiographic images. This is because the dentist must have the same criteria as doctors, since it is thim, who sets the radiographic diagnosis (plays the role of the patient's radiologist). The differences between medical screens and conventional screens are that special medical screens give a maximum brightness of 600–900 cd/m^2 as opposed to the good conventional screens on the market which give only about 235 cd/m^2 [11–14].

Finally, in relation to the screens it should be noted that the special medical screens are available in the market while there are also dual performance screens where it can be adjusted with a scale for the diagnostic display and a second scale for the patient data and other data.

Also, the elements of the existing lighting of the room where the image is projected are particularly important.

The basic combinations that the dentist should know are the following three: [15–17].

- Bright screen and low room lighting give us a high-quality diagnostic result.
- Bright screen and medium power room lighting gives us a lower quality diagnostic result.
- Bright screen and high-power room lighting gives us a low quality diagnostic result.

2.5 Types of Dental Digital X-Ray

Direct digital detectors are CCD (Charge Coupled Device) and CMOS (Complementary Metal-oxide Semiconductors) where the receptor is connected to the computer directly, and and there is an image produced simultaneously [18, 19].

Indirect digital systems are PSP (Photostimulable Phosphor) also known as SPS (Storage Phosphor Systems) where the image must be "scanned digitally to be dispayed" and there is a small time difference from receiving the image and presenting it on the screen (closer as a technique to conventional intraoral X-ray) [1, 20–24].

As for direct digital systems, CMOS technology is newer technology than CCD and both have been in the market since 1967, although CMOS were introduced into dental X-rays only in recent years by Trophy and Schick [12, 20, 25, 26].

CCD receptors are generally considered better for dental radiology while CMOS are still under research [27].

In general, CCD receptors have a better light response with the X-ray photons used for this, they are more efficient than CMOS, but CMOS receptors have a better "optical" package (microfiches and scintillators) with similar efficiencies, although this makes them more expensive [28, 29].

CMOS sockets are the basis of video operation and are the same as silicon-based CCD semiconductors but differ in the way the pixel is read since in CMOS each pixel is isolated from the neighbors and directly connected to the transducer [30].

The key features of digital receivers are:

- Contrast resolution,
- Spatial resolution,
- Detector latitude,
- Detector sensitivity.

Contrast analysis is the ability to distinguish different optical frequencies in the radiographic image.

It is a function of the following factors:

- The effect of tissue weakening characteristics depicted.
- The ability of the receptor to distinguish differences in the number of X-ray protons coming from different parts of the object being irradiated.
- The ability of the computer screen to show differences in density.
- The ability of the observer to recognize the differences presented on the screen by the system.

The receptors receive the data at 8- or 16-bit depth, and thus theoretically receive 256 [1] or 65,536 (216) different shades of gray, respectively, although the exact number of shades they cover is limited by inaccuracies in image capture (noise) [4, 31–34]. Respectively, the conventional screens where the images are projected can only display 256 tones of gray and are usually 8 bit images [3].

Spatial resolution is the ability to discern detail (resolution). A theoretical limitation in digital imaging is the function of the pixel size of the image measured in line pairs per millimeter [4, 5]. Theoretically the image analysis is based on the size of the pixels only, not taking into account the data loss due to diffusion from the scintillator, and the electronic systems of the receptor. At the highest CCD resolution, 20 μm per pixel have been measured corresponding to a ratio of 8 μm Ag grain. At these receptors, 20 μm per pixel gives a theoretical resolution of 25 pairs of lines per millimeter [5]. So because the human eye can distinguish 6 pairs of lines per millimeter most digital systems perform very well (more than 7 pairs of lines per millimeter).

The limitations of digital image resolution become visible and apparent when an image is magnified (often in cases over ten) where at very large magnifications a square image corresponding to the "pixel" image of the image is observed.

In such cases of very large magnification of the image it has been observed that we do not have a diagnostic improvement but often the observer dentist may have more difficulty in diagnosis [9].

Receptor amplitude is the ability of a receptor to receive a range of radon photon energy, which clinically varies from the gums to the enamel and allows slight variations in radius permeability to be apparent in the image.

Receptor sensitivity is the ability to respond to small amounts of radiation. In conventional tiles this has been categorized based on the velocity system of the tile (A to F) according to criteria of the International Organization of Standardization (International Organization of Standardization) while the extra film has a corresponding classification based on the Kodak system while there is no corresponding classification for digital receptors [35].

2.6 Image Manipulation

Digital image processing is called whichever function improves, analyzes or modifies the original image in any way.

Some of those image modifications and enhancements are included in the image acquisition by the manufacturers, but are not all known to the user since as in many programs, they are often fixed functions of the machine operating programs. Still others are controlled by the program user in order to improve the image and analyze its content.

2.7 Image Restoration

The image is restored because in many cases the original data is not ready for storage or presentation. This often requires a series of pre-processing steps to be displayed on the computer screen. These steps are programmed by the manufacturers and are NOT changed or modified. However, it is necessary to correct the image from known defects (defective pixels) as well as to improve the image for optimal presentation [36].

2.8 Saving the Image

The image is stored in sizes from 200 KB for intraoral X-rays to about 6 MB for high-resolution panoramic X-rays. Although storage is becoming more and more economical nowadays, in many cases it needs to be compressed.

The image is compressed without the loss of image elements in the format (TIFF/JPEG) for compression up to 3:1 and in CBCT files (conical beam computed tomography) which are automatically saved by compression without loss of data [2]. The image is compressed with data loss in cases where the files are in JPEG format and are not in the original desired format [37].

However, the evidence for image compression in dentistry is insufficient as there are currently only few literature with the first from Eraso that showed that compression of the original image at a final rate of 2% had to be made to have significant loss of diagnostic data and the detection of peripheral lesions [38]. For this reason and until there are sufficient studies regarding the images compression, it is best to keep all the image files in their original form or in a form that does not have compression or possible loss of the elements of the original image.

2.9 Advantages of Digital Radiography

Digital X-ray has several advantages which are mentioned by Farman and Farman [39, 40] in the files of the American Society of Maxillofacial Diagnosis and are as follows:

- Immediacy in image production, resulting in better ergonomics (for CCD and CMOS sensors) [41].
- The presentation of the image on the computer helps the patient to understand the disease.
- Ease of storing images and archiving them.
- Ease of making copies where necessary.
- The simplification of the measurements required mainly for endodontics.
- There are no chemicals or other materials in the doctor's office.
- Ability to communicate with colleagues and discuss the diagnosis.
- The low radiation dose.

2.10 Disadvantages of Digital Radiography

The main disadvantages of intraoral digital radiography are as follows:

- The lack of knowledge of the programs by the staff and lack of familiarity with the sensors which may result to multiple repetitions in the production of the images.
- The technique of digital radiography has low sensitivity in cases where the patient is irradiated more than he should be (although it is not easy

since many radiological machines now have a choice of digital or non-digital image) [42].

- When the image is printed on plain paper diagnostically there may be loss of original image info.
- It is possible to modify and edit the image so that digital images are not accepted as evidence.
- This in the future can be solved as a problem with techniques such as in medical radiological files where after the image is entered in the program it is not possible to process the image.

2.11 Conclusions

In conclusion, we can say that technology is evolving rapidly, and the dentist must monitor it.

Sensors must be capable of producing high-resolution X-rays with radiation doses lower than conventional films, the time required to produce the image should be less than that required with conventional films, and the images stored in safe and accurate formats. Files that have no data loss. Dentists must emphasize not only the purely radiological part of the machine but also the image taken and the screen on which it is projected.

References

1. Huda W, Rill LN, Benn DK, et al. Comparison of a photo stimulable phosphor system with film for dental radiology. Oral Surg Oral Med Oral Pathol Oral Radiol Endod. 1997;83(6):725–31.
2. Frederiksen NL. Specialized radiographic techniques. In: Pharoah MJ, White SC, editors. Oral radiology principles and interpretation. 4th ed. St. Louis: Mosby; 2000. p. 223–4.
3. Fifadara DH, Averbukh A, Channin DS, Badano A. Effect of viewing angle on luminance and contrast for a five-million-pixel monochrome display and a nine-million-pixel color liquid crystal display. J Digit Imaging. 2004;17(4):264–70.
4. Fetterly KA, Blume HR, Flynn MJ, Samei E. Introduction to grayscale calibration and related aspects of medical imaging grade liquid crystal displays. J Digit Imaging. 2008;21(2):193–207.
5. Bushong SC. Radiologic science for thecnologists: physics, biology, and protection. 7th ed. St. Louis: CV Mosby; 2001. p. 374.
6. van der Stelt PF. Principles of digital imaging. Miles DA. Applications of digital imaging modalities for dentistry. 2000;44(2):237–248.
7. Sim L, Manthey K, Stuckey S. Comparison of performance of computer display monitors for radiological diagnosis; "diagnostic" high brightness monochrome LCD, 3MP vs "clinical review" colour LCD, 2MP. Australas Phys Eng Sci Med. 2007;30(2):101–4.
8. Abreu M Jr, Tyndall DA, Ludlow JB. Detection of caries with conventional digital imaging and tuned aperture computed tomography using CRT monitor and laptop displays. Oral Surg Oral Med Oral Pathol Oral Radiol Endod. 1999;88(2):234–8.
9. Krupinski EA, Roehrig H, Dallas W, Fan J. Differential use of image enhancement techniques by experienced and inexperienced observers. J Digit Imaging. 2005;18(4):311–5.
10. Heo MS, Choi DH, Benavides E, Huh KH, Yi WJ, Lee SS, Choi SC. Effect of bit depth and kVp of digital radiography for detection of subtle differences. Oral Surg Oral Med Oral Pathol Oral Radiol Endod. 2009;108(2):278–83.
11. Ludlow JB, Abreu M Jr. Performance of film, desktop monitor and laptop displays in caries detection. Dentomaxillofac Radiol. 1999;28(1):26–30.
12. Lacević A, Vranić E, Bosn J. Different digital imaging techniques in dental practice. Basic Med Sci. 2004;4(2):37–40.
13. Park CM, Lee HJ, Goo JM, Han DH, Kim JH, Lim KY, Kim SH, Kang JJ, Kim KG, Lee CH, Chun EJ, Im JG. Comparison of observer performance on soft-copy reading of digital chest radiographs: high resolution liquid-crystal display monitors versus cathode-ray tube monitors. Eur J Radiol. 2008;66(1):13–8.
14. Liang H, Park S, Gallas BD, Myers KJ, Badano A. Image browsing in slow medical liquid crystal displays. Acad Radiol. 2008;15(3):370–82.
15. Langer S, Fetterly K, Mandrekar J, Harmsen S, Bartholmai B, Patton C, Bishop A, McCannel C. ROC study of four LCD displays under typical medical center lighting conditions. J Digit Imaging. 2006;19(1):30–40.
16. Geijer H, Geijer M, Forsberg L, Kheddache S, Sund P. Comparison of color LCD and medical-grade monochrome LCD displays in diagnostic radiology. J Digit Imaging. 2007;20(2):114–21.
17. Krupinski E, Roehrig H, Furukawa T. Influence of film and monitor display luminance on observer performance and visual search. Acad Radiol. 1999;6(7):411–8.
18. Sanderink GC, Miles DA. Intraoral detectors CCD, CMOS, TFT, and other devices. Dent Clin N Am. 2000;44(2):249–55.
19. Paurazas SB, Geist JR, Pink FE, Hoen MM, Steiman HR. Comparison of diagnostic accuracy of digital imaging by using CCD and CMOS-APS sensors with E-speed film in the detection of periapical bony lesions. Oral Surg Oral Med Oral Pathol Oral Radiol Endod. 2000;89(3):356–62.

20. Gröndahl HG. New radiographic imaging technologies: a challenge for the dental profession. Oral Surg Oral Med Oral Pathol. 1994;77(5):437.
21. Borg E. Some characteristics of solid-state and photostimulable phosphor detectors for intra-oral radiography. Swed Dent J Suppl. 2000;139:i–viii:1–67.
22. Svanaes DB, Møystad A, Sisnes S, et al. Intraoral storage phosphor radiography for approximal caries detection and effect of image magnification: comparison with conventional radiography. Oral Surg Oral Med Oral Pathol Oral Radiol Endod. 1996 Jul;82(1):94–100.
23. Cederberg RA, Tidwell E, Frederiksen NL, et al. Endodontic working length assessment: comparison of storage phosphor digital imaging and radiographic film. Oral Surg Oral Med Oral Pathol Oral Radiol Endod. 1998;85(3):325–8.
24. Benediktsdottir IS, Hintze H, Petersen JK, Wenzel A. Image quality of two solid-state and three photostimulable phosphor plate digital panoramic systems, and treatment planning of mandibular third molar removal. Dentomaxillofac Radiol. 2003;32:39–44.
25. Mouyen M, Benz C, Sonnabend E, et al. Presentations and physical evaluation of RadioVisioGraphy. Oral Surg Oral Med Oral Pathol. 1989;68(2):238–42.
26. Williams CP. Digital radiography sensors: CCD, CMOS, and PSP. Pract Proced Aesthet Dent. 2001;13(5):395–6.
27. Wallace JA, Nair MK, Colaco MF, et al. A comparative evaluation of the diagnostic efficacy of film and digital sensors for detection of simulated periapical lesions. Oral Surg Oral Med Oral Pathol Oral Radiol Endod. 2001;92(1):93–7.
28. Kitagawa H, Scheetz JP, Farman AG. Comparison of complementary metal oxide semiconductor and charge-coupled device intraoral X-ray detectors using subjective image quality. Dentomaxillofac Radiol. 2003;32:408–11.
29. Tsau JN, Mupparapu M. Reliability of CCD and CMOS (APS) digital sensors compared with D and E-plus-speed films in the detection of dental pathology: an in vitro study. Penn Dent J (Phila). 2001;101:10–1.
30. Hellén-Halme K, Rohlin M, Petersson A. Dental digital radiography: a survey of quality aspects. Swed Dent J. 2005;29(2):81–7.
31. Samei E, Ranger NT, Delong DM. A comparative contrast-detail study of five medical displays. Med Phys. 2008;35(4):1358–64.
32. Samei E, Wright SL. Viewing angle performance of medical liquid crystal displays. Med Phys. 2006;33(3):645–54.
33. Saunders RS Jr, Samei E. Resolution and noise measurements of five CRT and LCD medical displays. Med Phys. 2006;33(2):308–19.
34. Schulze D, Rother UJ, Fuhrmann AW, Tietke M. A comparison of two intraoral CCD sensor systems in terms of image quality and interobserver agreement. Int J Comput Dent. 2003;6:141–50.
35. Nair MK, Nair UP. An in-vitro evaluation of Kodak Insight and Ektaspeed Plus film with a CMOS detector for natural proximal caries: ROC analysis. Caries Res. 2001;35(5):354–9.
36. Kimpe T. Defective pixels in medical LCD displays: problem analysis and fundamental solution. J Digit Imaging. 2006;19(1):76–84.
37. Schulze RKW, Richter A, d'Hoedt B. The effect of wavelet and discrete cosine transform compression of digital radiographs on the detection of subtle proximal caries. ROC analysis. Caries Res. 2008;42:334–9. https://doi.org/10.1159/000151328.
38. Eraso FE, Analoui M, Watson AB, Rebeschini R. Impact of lossy compression on diagnostic accuracy of radiographs for periapical lesions. Oral Surg Oral Med Oral Pathol Oral Radiol Endod. 2002;93:621–5.
39. Farman AG, Farman TT. A comparison of 18 different x-ray detectors currently used in dentistry. Oral Surg Oral Med Oral Pathol Oral Radiol Endod. 2005;99(4):485–9.
40. Farman AG, Farman TT. Extraoral and panoramic systems. In: Miles D, editor. Applications of dental imaging modalities in dentistry. Dent Clin N Am. 2000;44(2):257–72, v-vi.
41. Miles DA. Imaging using solid-state detectors. In: Miles DA, Van Dis ML, (Eds). Advances in dental imaging. Dent Clin N Am. 1993;37:531–40.
42. Webber RL, Messura JK. An in vivo comparison of diagnostic information obtained from tuned-aperture computed tomography and conventional dental radiographic imaging modalities. Oral Surg Oral Med Oral Pathol Oral Radiol Endod. 1999;88(2):239–47.

Intraoral Radiographic Anatomy

3

Antigoni Delantoni and Kaan Orhan

3.1 Intraoral Radiographic Anatomy

In this chapter the authors will deal with the normal radiographic anatomy of teeth and periapical tissues seen in intraoral radiographs, which include periapical bitewing and occlusal radiographs which are basically radiographs taken with the image receptor placed in the oral cavity. Intraoral radiographs have been used for dental diagnosis since the 1920s [1].

It is of high significance to select the technique appropriate for the correct diagnosis thus the application of selection criteria for intraoral radiography [2, 3]. Which are used where needed intraoral radiographs are the initial diagnostic tool for dentists prior to more advanced imaging which are used where needed [2, 3].

Intraoral radiographs are the same for digital sensors and analogue films when it comes to anatomical features but the positioning may be slightly compromised in direct digital radiography due to a smaller size of active area of receptor in comparison with a PSP plate and conventional film packet.

The following intraoral radiographs are available:

- Periapical (taken by means of paralleling technique or bisected angle technique).
- Bitewing (taken by means of paralleling technique or bisected angle technique).
- Occlusal—maxillary and mandibular, standard, lateral, and axial.

3.2 Periapical Radiographic Anatomy

In normal periapical radiography there are a few initial features seen in all radiographs that should be described and are seen in Fig. 3.1 [4, 5].

- Enamel, which is the hardest structure of the human body, is depicted with high radiopacity and is seen to cover the crown of the tooth. Its thickness is greater in the posterior teeth and smaller in the anterior teeth, and this is the reason its radiopacity varies among teeth groups.

A. Delantoni (✉)
Department of Dentoalveolar Surgery, Implant Surgery and Radiology, Faculty of Dentistry, Aristotle University of Thessaloniki, Thessaloniki, Greece
e-mail: andelant@dent.auth.gr

K. Orhan
Department of DentoMaxillofacial Radiology, Faculty of Dentistry, Ankara University, Ankara, Turkey
e-mail: knorhan@dentistry.ankara.edu.tr

A. Delantoni, K. Orhan (eds.), *Atlas of Dentomaxillofacial Anatomical Imaging*,
https://doi.org/10.1007/978-3-030-96840-3_3

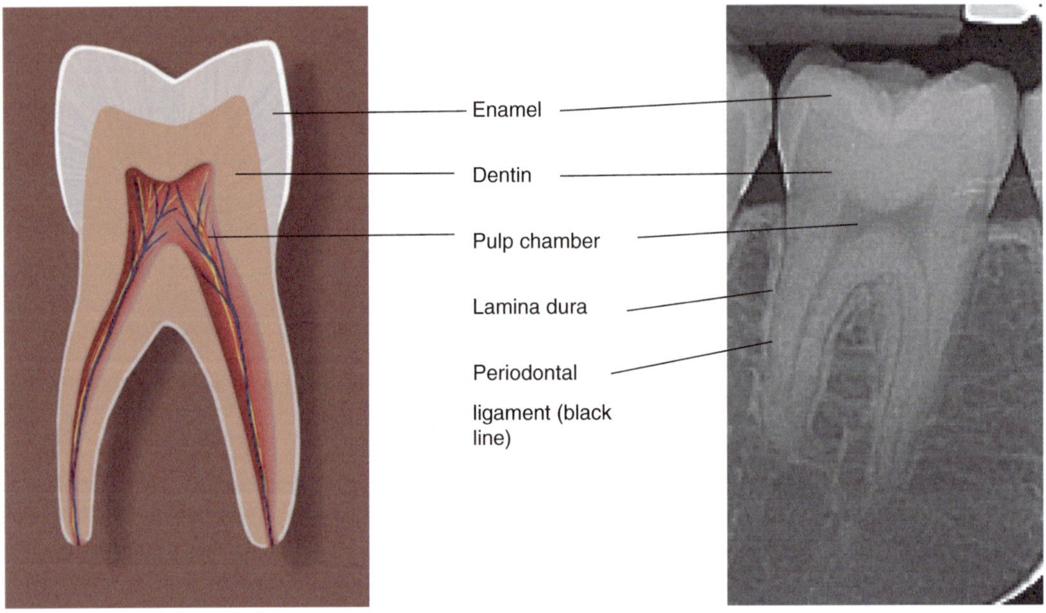

Fig. 3.1 A sketch of the tooth with the basic anatomical features and a radiograph providing the same anatomy

- Dentin, constitutes the largest part of tooth structure (hard dental tissues), is less calcified than enamel, and is depicted less radiopaque than enamel. Root cementum is the structure of similar radiopacity covering the root of the teeth. Root cementum and dentin are basically same in structure and radiopacity.
- The pulp chamber and the tooth's roots which are seen as radiolucent structures in the central section of the tooth and consist of soft tissues.
- The periodontal ligament consists of periodontal fibers and is seen as a thin radiolucent line surrounding teeth. It consists of unique specialized connective tissue between the cementum covering the tooth root and the lamina dura of the alveolar bone.
- Lamina dura is the part of the compact bone laying adjacent to the periodontal ligament in the root pocket. Basically, it surrounds the tooth socket and provides the attachment surface of the tooth in the bone. In images it is seen as a radiopaque line surround the tooth root.

One should note that the study of intraoral images, and particularly the periapical section and periodontal imaging, can provide valuable information on the height of the existing alveolar bone, the periodontal condition of the teeth and the periapical condition too.

3.3 Normal Radiographic Anatomy of the Maxilla

The most frequently visualized anatomical structures of the maxilla than can be seen in periapical radiographs are from anterior to posterior teeth [4–6]:

3.3.1 Anterior Teeth

The *median palatine suture* or intermaxillary suture (Fig. 3.2) which is the cranial suture between the right and left palatine bones or maxilla in the oral cavity. It courses it the midline from the alveolar crest to the posterior part of the hard palate. Radiographically, it appears as a thin vertical radioluscent line in the midline and it is seen inperiapical and between the two central maxillary incisors.

The *anterior nasal spine* (Fig. 3.2), is a bony projection of the skull in the maxillary midline,

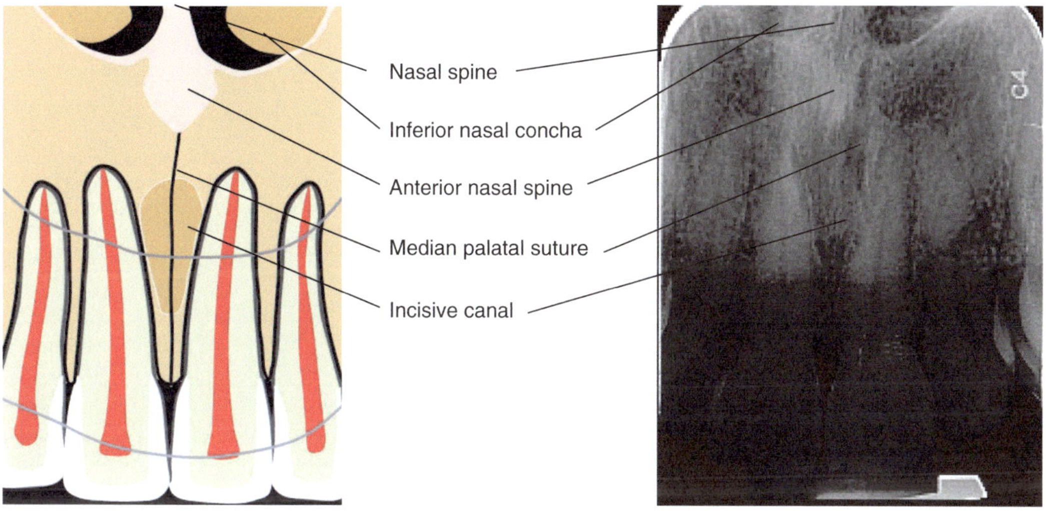

Fig. 3.2 A sketch and a corresponding radiograph of the maxillary incisors teeth

and it is formed from the fusion of the two maxillary bones. It is the most anterior part of the floor of the nose and the beginning of the median palatine suture. In radiographs it appears as a V shaped or triangular bony radiopacity. It is also seen on maxillary central incisors periapical radiographs.

The *nasal fossae* or nasal cavities (Fig. 3.2) are the nasal openings located above the maxillary anterior teeth. They are divided by the midline onto right and left chambers. In radiographs, they are seen as radiolucent structures bounded by bone. They are clearly seen in central incisor periapical radiographs and partially or sectional in lateral incisor or canine periapical radiographs.

Nasal septum, or nasal diaphragm (Fig. 3.2), is seen as a thin bony structure vertical in position, dividing the nasal cavity into right and left chambers. Radiographically in intraoral radiographs it is a radiopaque line above the anterior nasal spine visible in anterior incisor radiographs in the midline.

The *inferior nasal concha* or inferior turbinate bone (Fig. 3.2) is a scroll shaped paired bone (right and left) that rests in the lateral wall of the nasal cavity. It is one of the three paired nasal conchae in the nose, it is radiographically seen slightly radiopaque and in the floor of the nasal cavity.

Incisive foramen or nasopalatine foramen (Fig. 3.2) is a funnel shaped opening in the hard palate, in the midline behind the incisor teeth. It is basically the termination of the nasopalatine canals from the floor of the nasal cavity. In radiographs, it is the most common radiolucency between the two central incisors, of oval or round shape at the periapical part of the teeth.

Inverted Y (Figs. 3.3 and 3.4): The inverted Y is a radiographic landmark that depicts where the nasal fossa meets the maxillary sinus. The border between them is shaped like an upside-down letter Y, hence its name. The periapicals often demonstrate the inverted Y, a classic radiographic landmark of the right and left anterior maxilla. The fossa is positioned toward the midline while the sinus extends toward the posterior aspect of the maxilla. Typically, the inverted Y sits at the area of the maxillary lateral incisor and canine teeth.

3.3.2 Posterior Teeth

Sinus: The maxillary sinus (or *antrum of Highmore)* is seen in the intraoral radiographs of posterior upper teeth, it is a paired pyramid shaped sinus (part of the paranasal sinuses) within the maxillary bone, which drains via the maxillary ostium in the infundibulum, then

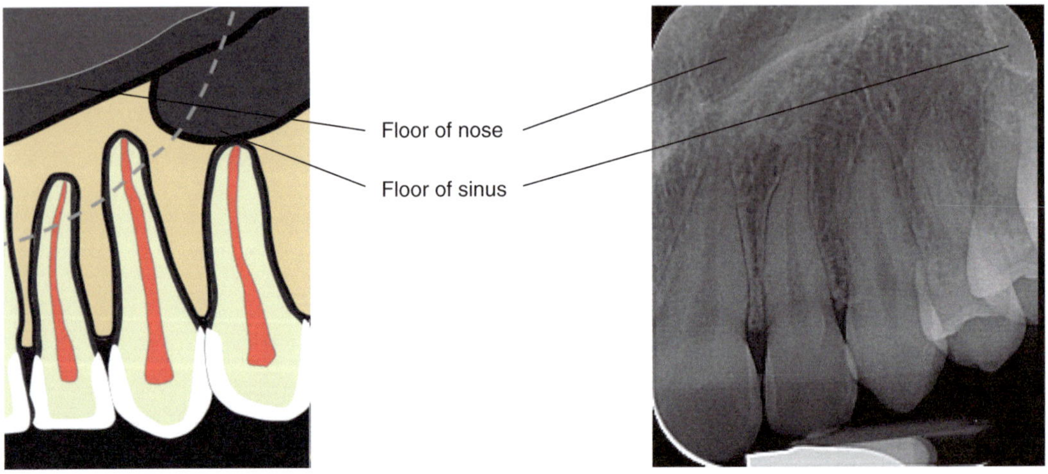

Fig. 3.3 A sketch and a corresponding radiograph of the maxillary canine

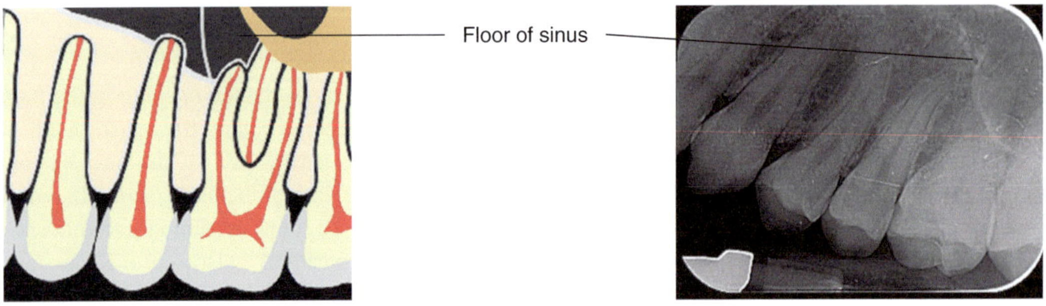

Fig. 3.4 A sketch and a corresponding radiograph of the maxillary premolar region

through the semilunar hiatus into the middle meatus (Fig. 3.4).

Described as a pyramid, the maxillary sinuses have a base on the lateral border of the nose, with the apex pointing toward the zygomatic process of the maxilla. The floor is formed by the alveolar process of the maxilla. The roof is the orbital floor. The posterior wall forms the anterior border of the pterygopalatine fossa.

There are several recesses of the maxillary sinus,

- infraorbital recess (superiorly),
- zygomatic recess (laterally),
- alveolar recess (inferiorly),
- palatine recess (variable extension of alveolar recess).

Like the other paranasal air sinuses, these can vary in size.

Large maxillary sinuses can extend to the alveolar process of the maxilla to the point where the roots of the molar teeth can project into the space. Unlike the other paranasal air sinuses, the opening of the sinus is found on its superior end.

Zygomatic bone: It is the bone that is attached to the right and left sides of the posterior maxilla. The zygomatic bone is quadrangular and widens posteriorly. It is superimposing the apices of maxillary premolars and molar teeth (Fig. 3.5).

Zygomatic process: The zygomatic process is the radiopaque U-shaped structure indicating the area where the zygomatic bone attaches to the maxilla. The zygomatic process of the maxilla is the most anterior aspect of the zygomatic bone. It

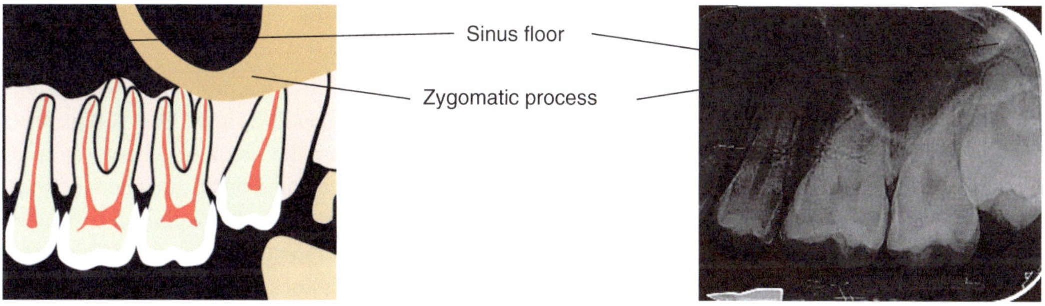

Fig. 3.5 A sketch and a corresponding radiograph of the maxillary molar area

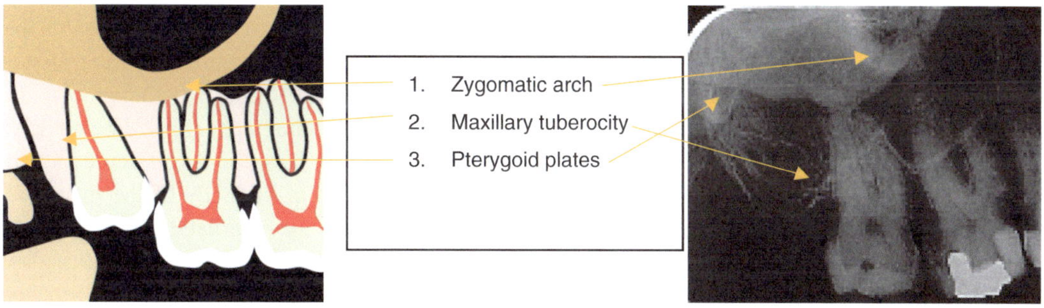

Fig. 3.6 A sketch and a corresponding radiograph of the maxillary wisdom tooth

is positioned toward the midline while the bone extends posteriorly away from the midline. It can also be seen on maxillary premolar and molar periapicals, often superimposing other areas and making the pathological diagnoses more difficult to set (Fig. 3.5).

Maxillary tuberosity: The maxillary tuberosity is the rounded end of the alveolar process of the maxilla. It is the most posterior part of the maxilla posterior to the last tooth This radiopaque structure appears bilaterally on maxillary molar periapicals and often on maxillary premolar periapicals, it can also be seen on molar bitewing radiographs. The tuberosity gives a smile appearance to the maxilla by curving upwards (Fig. 3.6).

Pterygoid plates: The lateral and medial pterygoid plates are located behind the maxillary tuberosity. They project an image configured like a thin wing of bone extending posteriorly from the tuberosity. This bilateral radiopacity is occasionally recorded on maxillary molar periapicals (Fig. 3.6).

Pterygoid hamulus: The hamular process or pterygoid hamulus is a tiny finger or hook-like projection of bone that extends inferiorly from the medial pterygoid plate. This bilateral radiopacity occasionally appears on maxillary molar periapicals (Fig. 3.6).

3.4 Normal Radiographic Anatomy of the Mandible

The most frequently visualized anatomical structures of the mandible than can be seen in periapical radiographs are the following from anterior to posterior teeth [4–6]:

3.4.1 Anterior

Genial tubercle or genial tuberosity (also known as mental spine or genial apophysis) are one or sometimes two small eminences of bone on the lingual section of the mandible at the midline below the level of apices of the anterior mandibular teeth. They form important points and anatomical landmarks for maxillofacial surgeons prosthodontists, radiologists and general dentists. The genial tubercle serves as an attachment point of the genioglossus and geniohyoid muscles (Fig. 3.7).

Radiographically it often produces a circular ring like radiopaque structure at the level or mandibular incisors apices. Laterally it may radiographically superimpose the mental spine which is located in the buccal side of the mandible (Fig. 3.7).

Lingual foramen: A small opening in the mandible lingually. It is in the midline and it is the point where the lingual arteriew and nerve pass through, It is seen in the midline between the apices of the anterior central incisors, and is radioluscent in appearance. Often one can see around it a small radiopacity corresponding to the genial tubercle (Fig. 3.7).

Mental fossa: It is a bone depression in the labial aspect of the mandible. It is not always present since its appearance is diffused (Fig. 3.7).

Mental ridge: An inverted V shaped radiopacity of the prominence of the bone in the labial surface of the anterior mandible (Fig. 3.7).

3.4.2 Posterior

Mental foramen: It is the primary landmark anatomically in the mandible, it is a radiolucent structure located below the premolars' roots. It is the anterior end of the mandibular canal and the mental nerve and vessels pass through it, it is bilateral and should be differentially diagnosed from periapical premolar lesions (Figs. 3.8 and 3.9).

Mandibular canal: it is the pathway of the inferior alveolar nerve in the mandible. It rises from the ramus of the mandible as the mandibular canal and proceeds from interiorly and lingually to palatally and exteriorly to the mental foramen. It is readily visible in both premolar and molar periapical radiographs (Figs. 3.8 and 3.9).

Submandibular fossa: it is the depression in the lingual aspect of the body of the mandible, bilaterally below the internal oblique ridge or mylohyoid line where the submandibular glard rests. The submandibular fossa is recorded on premolar and molar periapicals. This structure is also referred to as the submandibular gland fossa or mandibular fossa.

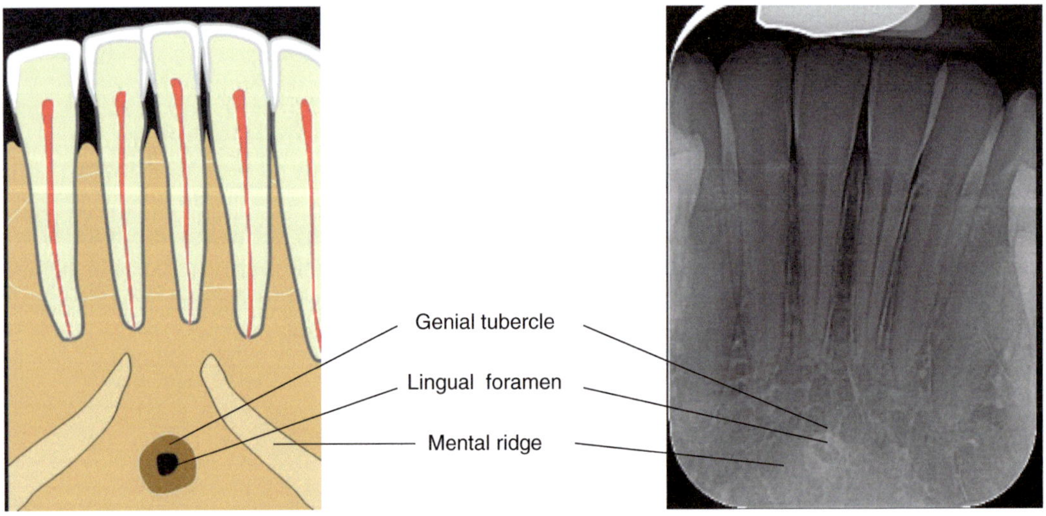

Fig. 3.7 A sketch and a corresponding radiograph of the mandibular incisors

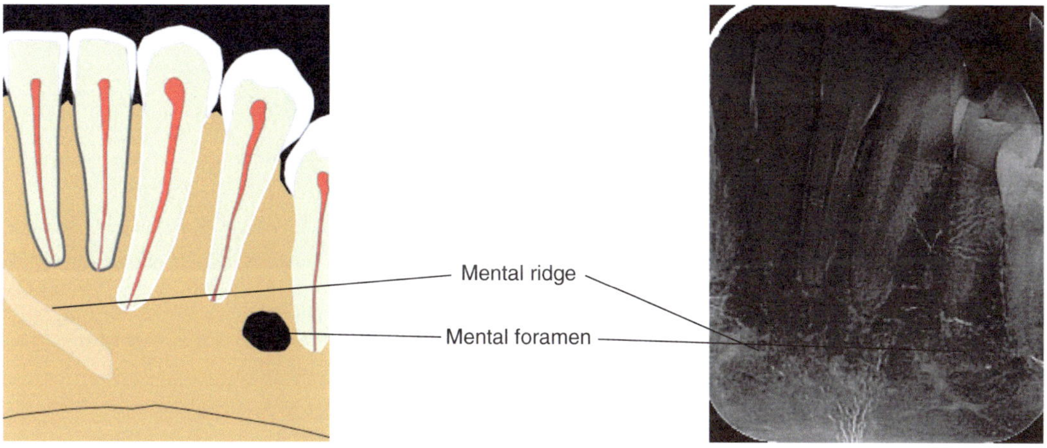

Fig. 3.8 A sketch and a corresponding radiograph of the mandibular canine

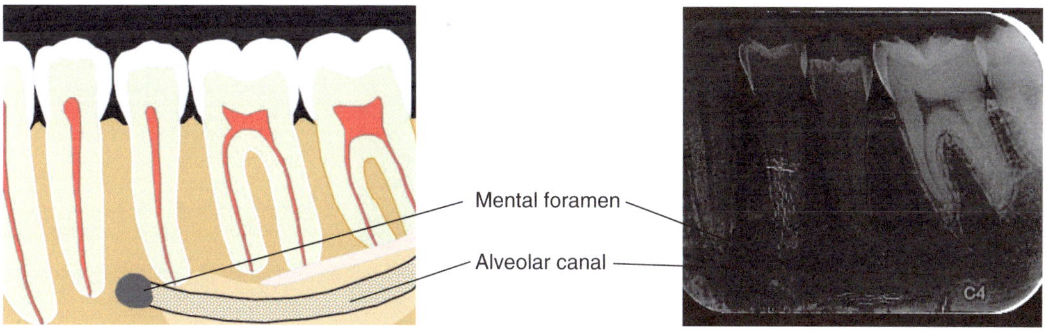

Fig. 3.9 A sketch and a corresponding radiograph of the mandibular premolar region

3.5 External and Internal Oblique Ridges

The external oblique ridge or line is the bony anterior border of the ramus located on the outer aspect of the mandible. It is in the retromolar area and it is seen in radiographs more frequently than the internal oblique line. The internal oblique ridge is found on the lingual aspect of the retromolar area of the mandible. It is radiopaque and ranges from well defined to barely visible. It is below or parallel to the external oblique line and serves as a mylohyoid attachment of the mandible (Fig. 3.10).

Lower border of the mandible: it is a radiopaque band of dense bone delineating the inferior aspect of the mandible.

To complete this section there are a few more images added that demonstrate the anatomical features not always or frequently seen in intraoral radiographs (Figs. 3.11, 3.12, 3.13, 3.14, 3.15, 3.16, and 3.17).

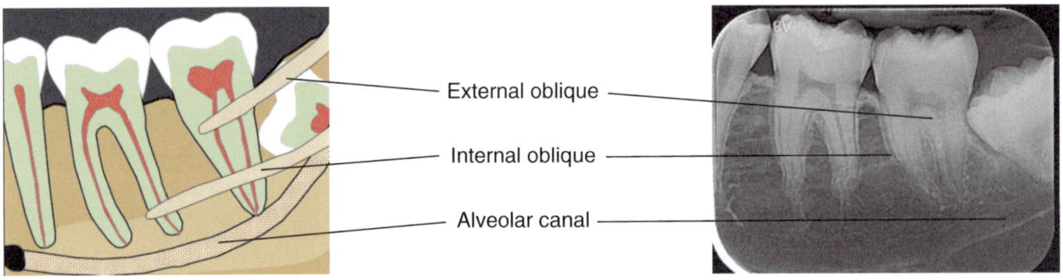

Fig. 3.10 A sketch and a corresponding radiograph of the mandibular wisdom tooth

Fig. 3.11 A radiograph of the anterior maxillary teeth taken with the bisecting angle technique, demonstrating a large number of features not readily seen with the use of the paralleling technique

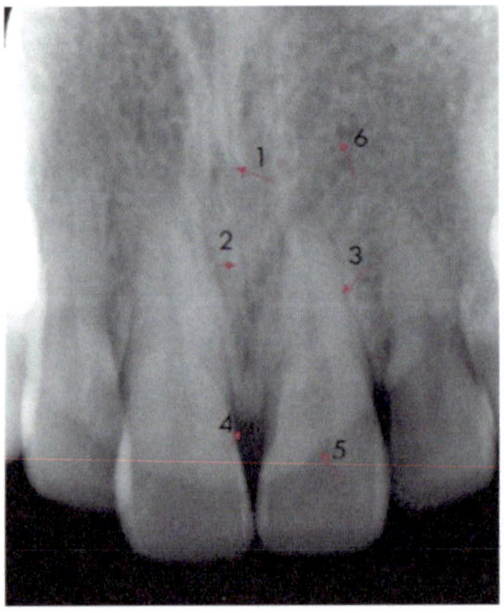

1. ANTERIOR NASAL SPINE
2. INTERMAXILLARY SUTURE
3. RADICULAR LAMINA DURA
4. CRESTAL LAMINA DURA
5. SOFT TISSUE OUTLINE (NOSE)
6. BONE TRABECULATION

Fig. 3.12 A radiograph of the anterior maxillary teeth taken with the bisecting angle technique, demonstrating features not readily seen with the use of the paralleling technique but frequent in the bisecting angle technique

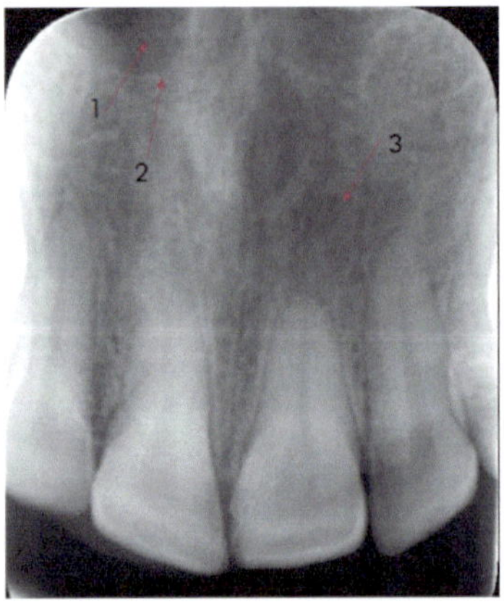

1. NASAL CAVITY
2. NASAL CAVITY INFERIOR BORDER
3. NASOPALATINE CANAL

Fig. 3.13 A radiograph of the maxillary posterior taken with the paralleling technique clearly and very well demonstrating the differences between sinus and zxygomatic arch imaging

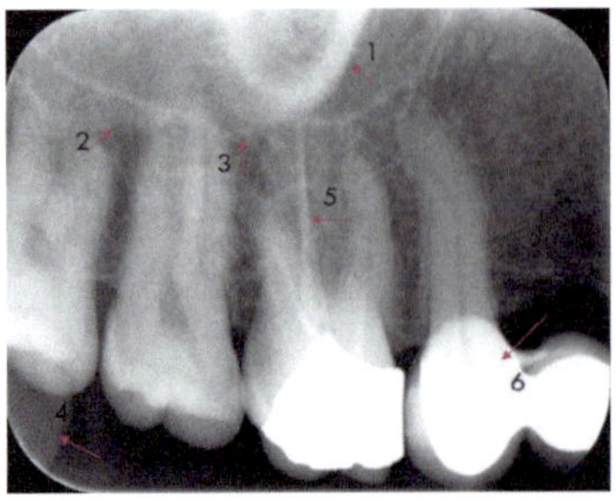

1. ZYGOMATIC PROCESS
2. ZYGOMATIC ARCH
3. MAXILLARY SINUS INFERIOR BORDER
4. CORONOID PROCESS
5. ROOT CANAL FILLING MATERIAL
6. PORCELAIN RESTORATION

Fig. 3.14 Anterior mandibular radiograph clearly showing the anatomical landmarks of the region

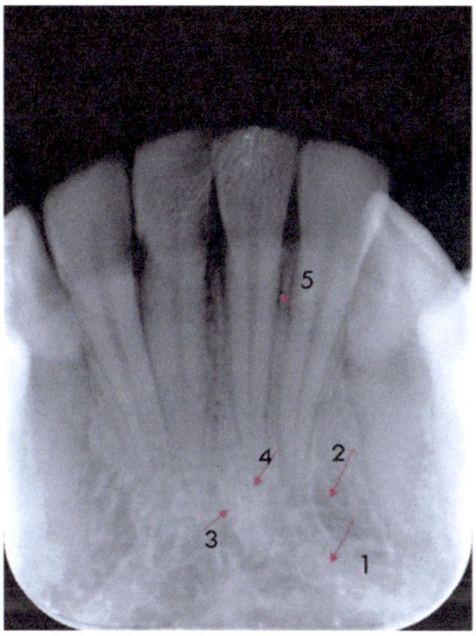

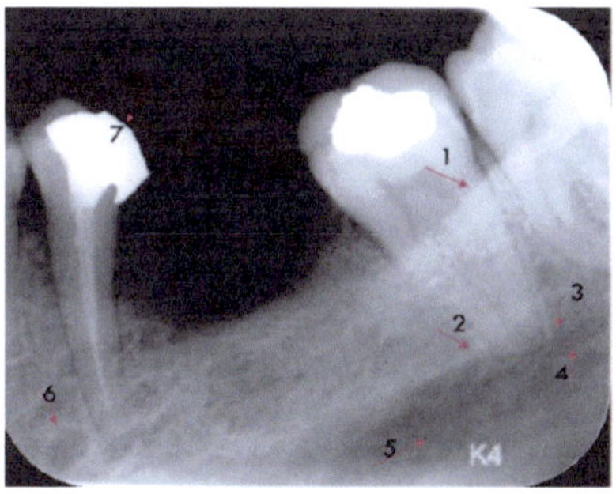

Fig. 3.15 Radiograph of the posterior mandibular teeth very well depicting the internal and external oblique lines of the mandible

Fig. 3.16 A radiograph of mandibular premolar region well demarcating the inferior border of the mandible which is seen upon placement of the film deep into the floor of the mouth all the way to the osseous border

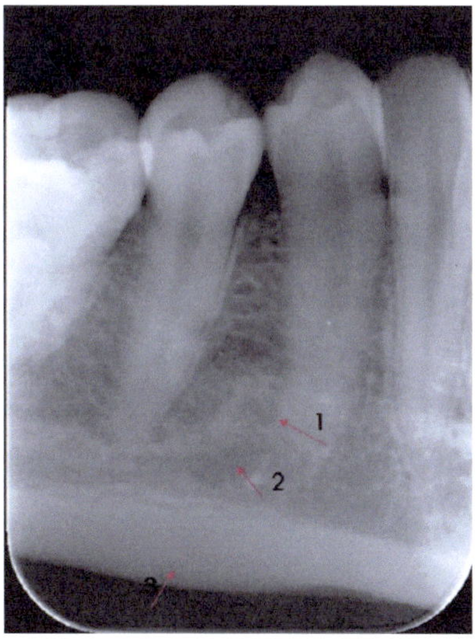

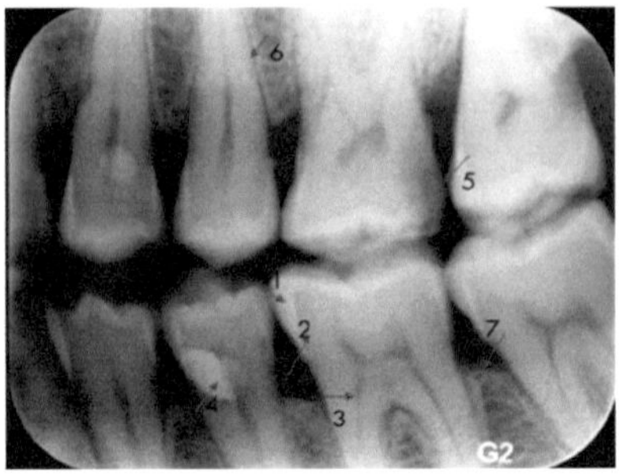

1. ENAMEL
2. DENTINE
3. PULP
4. DENTAL RESTORATIVE MATERIAL
5. DENTAL CARIES
6. RADICULER LAMINA DURA
7. CRESTAL LAMINA DURA

Fig. 3.17 A typical bitewing radiograph with all the anatomical seen features

References

1. McCormack FW. A plea for a standardized technique for oral radiography, with an illustrated classification of findings and their verified interpretations. J Dent Res. 1920;2:467.
2. Brooks SL. A study of selection criteria for intraoral dental radiography. Oral Surg Oral Med Oral Pathol. 1986;62(2):234–9.
3. Brooks SL, Cho SY. Validation of a specific selection criterion for dental periapical radiography. Oral Surg Oral Med Oral Pathol. 1993;75(3):383–6.
4. Berry HM. VIII. Mandibular intraoral radiographic anatomy. In: Radiologic anatomy of the jaws. Philadelphia: University of Pennsylvania Press; 2018. p. 77–90.
5. Sadrameli M, Mupparapu M. Oral and maxillofacial anatomy. Radiol Clin North Am. 2018;56(1):13–29.
6. Atchison KA, White SC, Flack VF, Hewlett ER, Kinder SA. Efficacy of the FDA selection criteria for radiographic assessment of the periodontium. J Dent Res. 1995;74(7):1424–32.

4 Basic Principles of Panoramic Radiography

Kaan Orhan and Antigoni Delantoni

4.1 Panoramic Radiography

The idea of showing all dental arcs on a single film was introduced by Bouchacourt in 1904. Bouchacourt considered recording the image of the arcs on a film outside the mouth, giving the X-ray source through inside the mouth. Then, in 1949, panoramic radiography technique has been developed with the efforts of Prof. Dr. Yrjo V. Paatero [1].

Panoramic radiography is a technique that enables imaging of a single tomographic image of both dental arches and adjacent anatomic structures with minimal geometric distortion and superposition ([2], s. 7). Panoramic radiography is a technique that shows all teeth and jaws, the maxillary region up to the 1/3 upper part of the eye socket, maxillary sinuses, mandible and temporomandibular joint together [1] (Fig. 4.1).

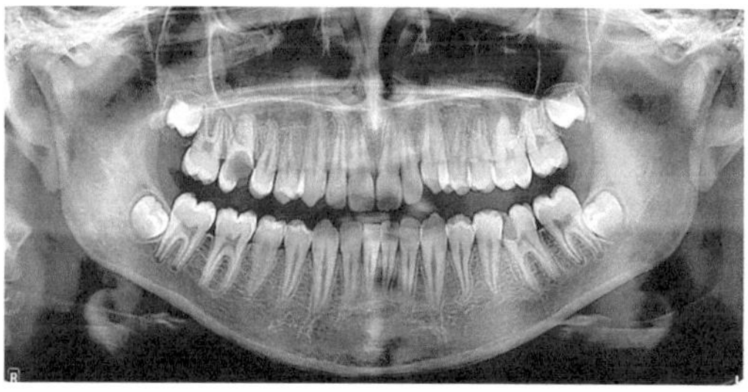

Fig. 4.1 Representative Panoramic Image showing the entire maxilla, mandible and dentomaxillofacial region

4.2 Panoramic Devices Used in Dentistry

Panoramic devices used in dentistry are divided into four basic groups as **single rotation centers (rotograph)**, **two rotation centers (panorex)**, **three rotation centers (ortopantomograph)**, and **continuous rotation centers (GE-Panel IPS)** according to the rotation center, number, and localization of the X-ray [3] (Fig. 4.2).

4.2.1 Single Rotation Centered (Rotograph)

In this technique, the cassette is prepared in a curved shape in accordance with the shape of the jaw. The beam source is constant and emits a very fine beam. The patient and the film rotate in front of the beam at the same speed but in the opposite

K. Orhan (✉)
Department of DentoMaxillofacial Radiology, Faculty of Dentistry, Ankara University, Ankara, Turkey
e-mail: knorhan@dentistry.ankara.edu.tr

A. Delantoni
Department of Dentoalveolar Surgery, Implant Surgery and Radiology, Faculty of Dentistry, Aristotle University of Thessaloniki, Thessaloniki, Greece
e-mail: andelant@dent.auth.gr

A. Delantoni, K. Orhan (eds.), *Atlas of Dentomaxillofacial Anatomical Imaging*,
https://doi.org/10.1007/978-3-030-96840-3_4

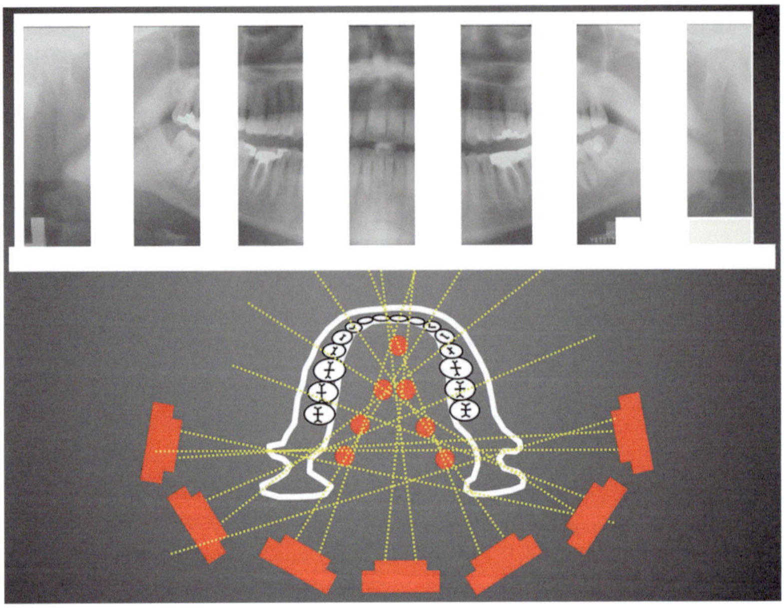

Fig. 4.2 The development of panoramic radiography devices. (Courtesy of Prof. Dr. Dobó-Nagy Csaba)

direction. The image of the lower and upper jaws is obtained on an X-ray film that is displaced by a narrow beam [1].

In this technique, since the dental arch is accepted as a circle and a single rotation center is created and the jaws cannot be represented with such a single circle, a great amount of distortion occurs [3].

4.2.2 Two Rotation Centered (Panorex)

This technique is based on the tomography of curved surfaces. These are also used in flat cassettes. The head of the patient is fixed and the X-ray tube and film cassette rotate around the patient's head [1]. In this device, the right and left sides of the tooth curve are considered as separate parts of a circle and two separate rotation centers are created accordingly [3]. The first center of rotation is in the right molar area. The X-ray tube and cassette rotate around the patient's head, creating an image of the left side up to the midline on the film. In the meantime, the X-ray is automatically cut and the patient is shifted 7.5–10 cm to the right with the seat on which he sits, thus creating a second center of rotation. Meanwhile, the exit point of the central beam is shifted to the left side of the patient's spine. The tube and cassette start moving again.

The image of the right side of the chin is obtained from the back. In radiographs obtained with this technique, the image formed in the lateral parts of the dental arch is satisfactory. However, cutting the beam for a while as the tube moves behind the cervical vertebra leaves an empty space in the middle of the radiograph. These radiographs are either left as they are, or the two sides are combined with each other by cutting the empty part in the middle [1].

4.2.3 Three Rotation Centered (Ortopantomography)

The diameters of the jaw arcs are more in the posterior region and less in the anterior region. For this reason, there are three separate rotation centers corresponding to two posterior regions and one anterior region. A segment between the condyle and the premolar region is considered as an anterior segment, and a rotation center is available for each segment. While the jaws are examined with these three separate segments, a continuous, view is obtained from condyle to condyle [3]. There is a special cephalostat on this appliance. The head of the patient is fixed here.

The X-ray tube and the film cassette are rotated in proportion to each other around the patient's head. The cassette also revolves around itself [1].

The slit-shaped lead collimator placed on the X-ray source and the film holder allows the central beam to reach the film as a vertical beam by narrowing the X-ray beam [3]. When the X-ray machine starts up, the X-ray tube and rotation center are on the right side of the patient, and the cassette is on the left. Image recording starts from the patient's left side and continues towards the midline. When the central beam reaches the left canine, the center of rotation changes. This second center is a point in the middle of the two canines. The region between canine and canine is recorded on the film while rotating around the center. When the central beam reaches the right side canine, the center of rotation changes again. This third center of rotation is around the left third molar. The image of the part from the right canine to the upper part of the right temporomandibular joint is obtained [1].

4.2.4 Continuous Rotation (GE-Panel IPS)

Normally, the fact that the teeth are lined up in the jaw arches in a semielliptical manner has led to the selection of an elliptical rotation center and this system is called elipsopantomography. With this system, superpositions between neighboring teeth are tried to be minimized [3]. Today, panoramic devices with a continuous rotation center are preferred instead of multi-rotational panoramic devices. This feature optimizes the shape of the image layer and reveals the teeth and the structures that support it. The center of rotation starts from the right side of the body near the lingual surface of the mandible, continues from the back of the patient, the midline is visualized when it comes to the neck, then the arc continues in the sagittal plane and the image is complete ([4], p. 166) (Fig. 4.3).

4.3 Indications of Panoramic Radiographs

- For initial diagnostic purposes.
- Comprehensive evaluation of maxilla and mandible.
- Trauma.
- Wisdom teeth localizations.
- Known or suspected large lesions.
- Dental development examinations in the mixed dentition period.
- TMJ pains.
- In people who cannot tolerate intra-oral radiographs.

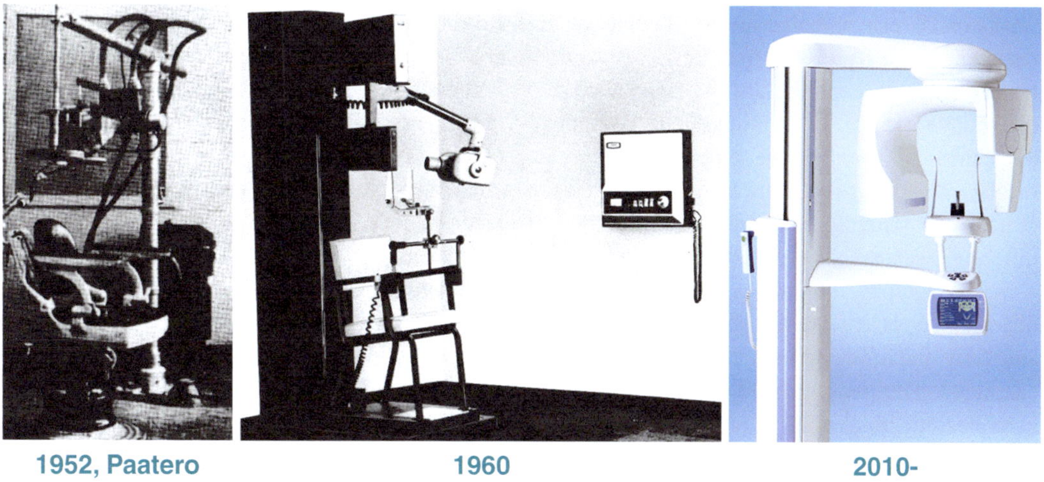

Fig. 4.3 Image showing panoramic device with a continuous rotation center

Panoramic radiography has many advantages including short time for the procedure, greater patient acceptance and cooperation, overall coverage of the dental arches and associated structures (more anatomic structures can be viewed on a panoramic film than on a complete intra-oral radiograph series), simplicity, low patient radiation dose.

The dose to the patient is approximately ten times less than full-mouth survey using the long cone and E+ film and it is four times less than four bitewings using the long round cone and E+ film.

The panoramic radiograph is less confusing to the patient than a series of small separate intra-oral radiographs, making it easier for the dentist to explain the diagnosis and treatment plan to the patient.

The panoramic radiograph is an excellent imaging modality in patients with trismus or trauma, because such patients cannot open their mouths and this is not required to take a panoramic film. It is an excellent projection of diverse structures on a single film, which no other imaging system can achieve.

In such cases, the high resolution and detail available in intra-oral radiographs is not required. Panoramic imaging is also an imaging technique that can often be used in the initial evaluation of situations that require further projections ([5], p. 175).

Although panoramic radiography is a curvilinear variant of conventional tomography, it works on the principle that there is also an image receiver with a reciprocal moving X-ray source located around a central point or plane called the image layer ([5], p. 175). In classic radiography, the entire thickness of the object between the focal spot and the film is seen on the film in two dimensions. Therefore, images of structures at different levels are superposed on each other.

In tomography, the images of the structures at different levels are prevented from overlapping and only the layer whose image is desired is examined. The parts in front of and behind this layer become blurred.

The image layer is an invisible layer in space between the radiation source and the image receptor. The image layer is a 3-dimensional "focal trough" and the dentition and related structures must be positioned within this layer in order to be clearly seen in the panoramic radiography [1]. The structures outside of this layer are seen as blurry, magnified or smaller than normal and distorted ([5], p. 177).

4.4 Technical Considerations of Panoramic Radiography

4.4.1 Image Layer (Focal Through)

The image layer is an invisible layer in space between the radiation source and the image receptor. The image layer is a three-dimensional "focal trough" and the dentition and related structures must be positioned within this invisible layer.

The structures outside of this layer are seen in the image that is blurry, magnified, or smaller than normal and distorted [6] (Fig. 4.4).

4.4.2 Projection Geometry

Projection geometry explains the effect of the size and position of the focal spot point on image clarity, distortion, and magnification ([5], p. 46).

4.4.2.1 Image Resolution

Resolution describes the sharpness of the boundary between two different radiodensity fields. Although the sharpness and resolution of the image have different properties, they are affected by the same geometric variables. For a correct clinical diagnosis, the radiography should be taken under high resolution and optimized conditions.

In order not to lose resolution and improve image quality;

1. *Focal spot point*: The focal spot point used in dental X-ray devices should be ≤1 mm. The larger the focal spot point, the less clear the image.

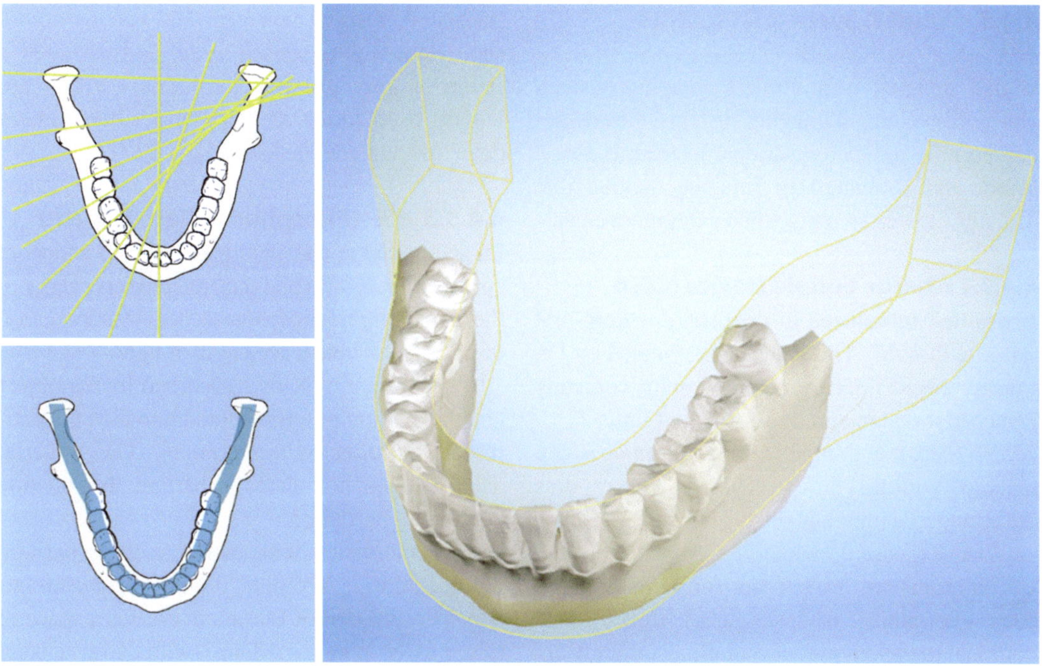

Fig. 4.4 Representative İmage of focal through

2. *Distance between object-focal spot point*: The greater the distance between the object-focal spot point, the more image blur is reduced.
3. *Distance between object and film*: The shorter the distance between the object and the film, the better the image clarity [1].

4.4.2.2 Distortion

Distortion is formed as a result of magnification at different points of the same object. This is because all parts of the object are not equal to the same focal spot point-to-object distance.

If it is not equal, distortion occurs in two ways;

1. *Shortening*: It develops due to unequal distances between different parts of the object and the film.
2. *Elongation*: Elongation occurs when the X-ray focus is passed through the right corner of the object, not directly onto the film.

Things to do to minimize distortion;

- The film should be positioned parallel to the long axis of the object. When the long axis of the film and tooth are parallel, the deformation in the image is minimized.
- It should be ensured that the central X-ray is perpendicular to the film and object. The film and the object are parallel to each other, but if the X-ray is not perpendicular to them, distortion occurs in the image. In cases where X-rays are sent vertically but at an angle, the palatinal roots of the teeth are seen to be longer than the buccal roots ([5], p. 46).

4.4.2.3 Magnification

Magnification means obtaining an image larger than the actual size of the object in radiography. The passing of photons in different ways causes the image on the radiography to grow. Magnification is related with the focal spot point-film distance and object-film distance. When the distance between the focal spot point and the film is increased and the distance between the object and film is decreased, the image undergoes magnification.

4.4.3 Digital System Detectors

Digital imaging is a filmless imaging system. Unlike conventional imaging systems, they do not require film and bath solutions. Instead, it uses a sensor and computerized imaging method that instantly creates an image on a computer screen.

4.4.3.1 Charge Couple Device (CCD)

It was first introduced to dentistry for intra-oral imaging in 1987. The system was created by Dr. Frances MOUYENS and the Trophy company launched it commercially for the first time.

CCD uses a thin silicon layer. Images are recorded with this silicon layer. Silicon crystals are arranged within a pixel.

When exposed to radiation, the bonds between silicon atoms are broken and form electron-gap pairs. The number of these gaps is directly proportional to the amount of radiation coming from the X-ray source.

The resulting electrodes are then drawn towards the most positive part of the device. Here they form electron packets called charge or charge packets. Each packet corresponds to one pixel. Here, these charge packets made up of each pixel (one pixel in the matrix) form the latent image. The image is created by transferring each pixel one after another in sequence. When the charge (load) reaches the end of the row, a reader is supplied to the amplifier and transmitted as a voltage to the ADC.

For panoramic imaging, CCDs (charge couple devises) of several pixels wide in either linear rows or one dense pixel length (one row) were produced.

4.4.3.2 CMOS (Complementary Metal Oxide Semiconductor)

CMOS forms the basis of typical consumer video cameras. These detectors are silicon-based semiconductors, but technically the way pixel charges are processed is different from CCD. Each pixel in the sensor is directly connected to the neighboring pixel via the transistor.

As in CCD, electron gaps due to X-ray are created depending on the amount of incident beam. These charge packs are transferred to the transistor as small voltages. The voltage across each transistor is sensed, read, and assigned a shade of gray just like the CCD. CMOSs are widely used today as chips and video camera detectors and are cheaper ([5], p. 213).

4.4.3.3 PSP (Phosphorus Plate System)

Photostimulable phosphor plates absorb and store energy from X-rays and then release this energy in the form of light (phosphorescence) by stimulation of another suitable wavelength of light.

The amount of X-rays absorbed by the object and the amount of light emitted into the phosphorescent is directly proportional. The material used in phosphor plates is barium fluorohalide containing europium.

In combination with metals such as barium, iodine, chlorine, bromide, it creates a crystal lattice. The addition of Europium creates a space in this weave. When irradiated with X-rays, electrons in the europium absorb energy and are displaced. These electrons migrate into nearby halogen spaces (called f centers), into the fluorohalide lattice and remain there in a metastable state. The number of electrons remaining here increases in proportion to the X-ray value and forms a latent image. Excitation with red light at the rate of 600 nm releases barium fluorohalide electrons. Electrons return to europium. During this turn an energy is released from the 300–500 nm green spectrum. This energy is captured by photomultiplier tube and converts light into electrical energy. The resulting voltage occurs according to the changes in the light coming from the latent image. The voltage signal is digitized with an analog–digital converter and displayed as a digital image ([5], p. 224).

PSP systems can be used for panoramic viewing. The PSP systems named below are used most frequently.

- *Fixed scanning system*: These systems have preferred to reflect red laser light with a versatile separate system. There is a mirror inside the system. When the mirror rotates, laser light passes through the plate, and as the plate advances, scanning occurs on the adjacent phosphor plate.

- *Rotating plate system.*
- *Photon collection system*: In this system, the scanner laser beam rotates instead of plates. It has a resolution of up to 20 lp/mm and 16 bits and about 65,000 gray tones were targeted at 40 lp/mm as an achievable technology ([5], p. 225).

4.4.3.4 Flat Panel Detectors

It is mostly used in the field of medicine and is now being used as routine in extra-oral imaging devices. These detectors create larger matrix areas with a pixel size of less than 100 μm. They can be used for these larger areas, especially head and neck examinations.

In these detectors, there are two approaches to X-ray sensitive material selection. Indirect detectors: They are sensitive to visible light and are used to convert an amplifying X-ray energy into light. The detector thickness of these devices is limited. The display size of thick screens is small, but as they absorb more photons, the image sharpness decreases.

This material is similar to selenium silicon, and its atomic number is higher than similar materials. The higher the atomic number, the more effective X-ray absorption.

The electrons released by the electric field effect (during selenium irradiation) are directly sent to the thin-film detector located at the bottom. Selenium is generally used in direct detectors, they provide very high resolution, their efficiency is less than the indirect. Electrical energy is directly proportional to X-ray power. Energy is processed and turned into an image by applying appropriate rows and columns. It is an expensive system, but it is used in specialized imaging procedures or devices such as digital panoramic and CBCT ([5], p. 240).

4.4.4 Digital Detector Features

4.4.4.1 Contrast Resolution

Contrast resolution is the difference in density in the radiographic image. This depends on the X-ray absorption characteristic of the imaged tissue, the capacity of the image receptor, the capacity of the computer to display them, and the ability of the examiner to notice them.

Current digital detectors can capture 8-10-12 or 16 bit deep data. Since the bit depth is a multiple of 2, theoretically detectors can capture 65,536 different density. However, in practice, the real number is limited by the errors in image formation, which is called noise. Regardless of how much gray difference a detector will catch, conventional computer monitors can only display an 8-bit gray scale. Therefore, the density that can be monitored on a monitor is 256.

Another limitation is that the human eye can detect only 60 shades of gray under favorable conditions. If this radiography examination is not suitable, it falls below 30.

4.4.4.2 Spatial Resolution

Spatial resolution is the capacity to separate fine details. Theoretically, pixel size in digital imaging systems limits resolution.

Currently, the highest CCD resolution is 20 μm. Approximately 25 lp/mm can be achieved at 20 μm/pixel. Observers can easily distinguish 6 lp/mm without any magnification. 20 lp/mm is usually what can be observed in a conventional intra-oral film. Current digital systems, on the other hand, can show a resolution of 8–12 lp/mm.

4.4.4.3 Detector Sensitivity

Detector sensitivity is the ability to respond to lower radiation. The sensitivity of digital receptors is not fully standardized. It is affected by a number of factors. Detector efficiency varies with pixel size and system image ([5], p. 231).

4.4.4.4 Image Processing

Image processing is the name given to the enhancement, analysis, processing, and modification processes made on a digital image. There are many processing methods available in dental digital imaging. Some of these processes come automatically in image processing software. Others are under the control of the operator.

4.4.4.5 Image Storage

The use of digital images in dentistry requires image archiving and examination systems. The storage of images can most simply be done on magnetic or disk media. However, the problem arises in what format and how the images will be stored in these processes. Generally, digital imaging can have a data size of 200 kB to 6 MB (extra-oral images). The storage of these data is not a trivial matter at all. However, the important issue should be in a way that prevents deletion or modification of the original image data of the software, since digital images are stored in digital format. Not all software is suitable for this. Therefore, it is attempted to be made a standard. However, image storage should generally be done on hard-disks, CD and DVD's.

4.4.4.6 Image Compression

The purpose of image compression is to reduce the size of the image (for archive and transmission). This becomes a big problem, especially in busy clinics that store extra-oral images, because storing data can take up a lot of space. Compression refers to the meaningful compression of data without loss of image information. Compression methods are expressed as lossy and lossless. There is no loss in image data in the lossless method. Many compression techniques take advantage of removing the excess in the image. It creates the same but simpler regions. The maximum compression ratio is typically 1/1 for lossless compression. However, in lossy compression, image data is compressed more.

Studies have shown that these compressions generally do not affect image quality. A noticeable effect on 12/1 and 14/1 compression has not been found, especially for the diagnosis of caries. In endodontic treatment, for canal length calculations, 25/1 is the same rate of diagnostic as uncompressed images. Generally, the simplest compression technique is the JPEG compression method. Apart from that, the JPEG 2000 format is one such image compression technique. Its main difference is that it prevents blurring that occurs at high compression value in JPEG ([5], p. 240).

4.5 Major Concerns in Panoramic Imaging

Advantages of Panoramic Imaging

- Comprehensive display of facial bones and teeth.
- Minimal radiation dose application.
- Patient positioning.
- Providing convenience for the patient in examination.
- It enables us to easily take radiography in patients with mouth-restriction.
- Short duration.
- Useful in informing patients.

Disadvantages of Panoramic Imaging

- Low image quality compared to intra-oral radiographs.
- Shadows created by soft tissues and the airway.
- Ghost images and artifacts.
- Distortion and magnification.
- Long exposure time.

In addition, the main disadvantage of panoramic imaging is that it is not suitable for children under 5 years of age and disabled people due to the long exposure time ([4], s. 172). The development of superpositions on the approximal surfaces of premolar teeth is another disadvantage of panoramic. Sometimes the superposition of cervical vertebrae hides odontogenic lesions, especially in the anterior region.

4.6 Patient Positioning

Position of the patient is very important in panoramic radiographs. To obtain diagnostically useful panoramic radiographs, it is necessary to prepare patients properly and to position their heads carefully in the focal through. Teeth and dental arches must be in the image layer. In this way, the image is obtained with the least distor-

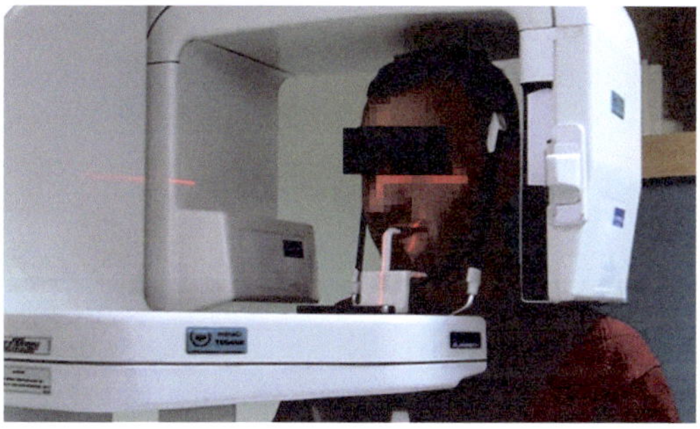

Fig. 4.5 Figure showing the correct positioning of the patient in panoramic imaging

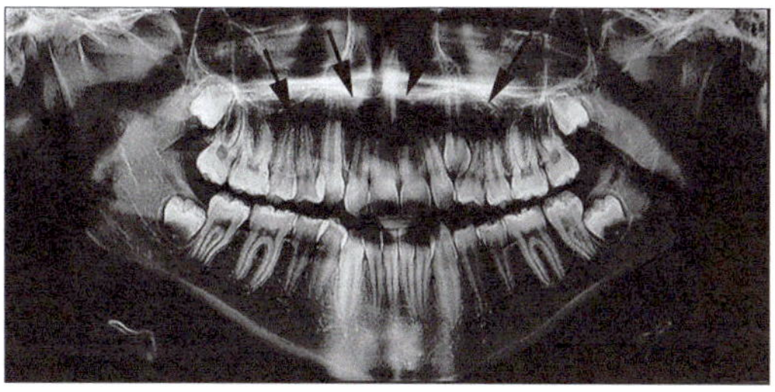

Fig. 4.6 Figure showing the patient's tongue does not touch the palate, resulting in the formation of a radiolucent band that shadows the apices of the maxillary teeth (arrows)

tion [1]. If the patient is wearing glasses, they should be asked to remove their glasses, as well as all jewelry and other metallic items ([4], p. 166). After the machine settings are made in orthopantomography, the patient puts his chin on the support so that the patient's Frankfurt plane is parallel to the ground and the sagittal line is in the middle of the chin support [1]. The patient should be informed about how to bite the bite block, then he should be told to close his lips and swallow and stick his tongue to the palate [6]. After the patient is placed on the cephalostat in this way, he is asked to take a step forward and hold the holders on the machine with his hands. This position is called skiing position [1]. During the irradiation period, he should be told to keep his tongue on his hard palate and not to move at all ([4], p. 166) (Fig. 4.5).

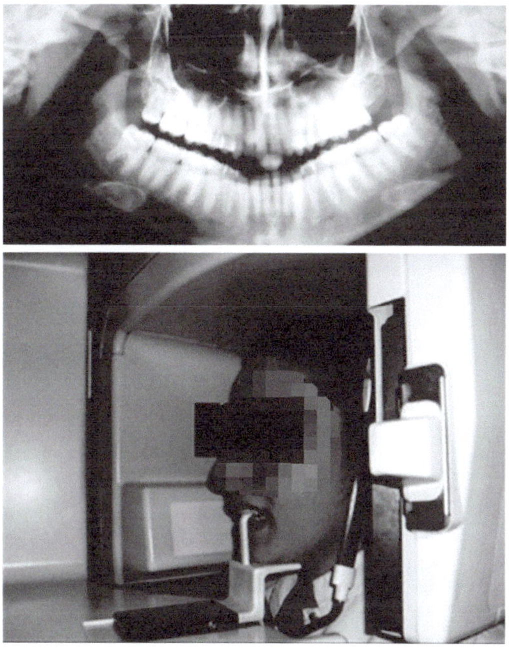

Fig. 4.7 The patient bites the bite block forward so that the notch is inside the mouth, both dental arches and teeth remain outside of the image layer. In the radiographs taken in this position, all of the front teeth are blurred, but the premolars are superposed on each other

4.6.1 Common Errors in Panoramic Radiography

Positioning errors do not depend solely on the patient or the person taking radiography, there is a need for devices designed to facilitate patient positioning.

During irradiation, the patient's tongue does not touch the palate, resulting in the formation of a radiolucent band that shadows the apices of the maxillary teeth and overlook periapical pathological lesions, root resorption, and non-odontogenic lesions close to the apex of the maxillary teeth [7] (Fig. 4.6).

If the patient bites the bite block too far forward so that the notch is inside the mouth, both dental arches and teeth remain outside of the image layer. In the radiographs taken in this position, all of the front teeth are blurred, while the premolars are superposed on each other (Fig. 4.7). If the patient has bitten the bite block from behind, the anterior teeth are also blurred but wider (Fig. 4.8) [1].

When the patient's head is tilted too low (Fig. 4.9), excessive inclination in the occlusal

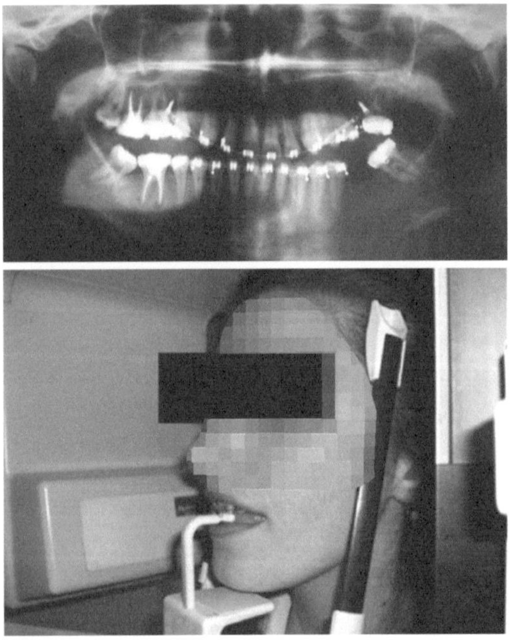

Fig. 4.8 The patient has bitten the bite block from behind, the anterior teeth are also blurred

plane, blurring of the apex of the mandibular anterior teeth, narrowing of the intercondylar distance, sometimes inability to trace the condyle heads, and superposition in the posterior contacts of the teeth can occur [7].

When the patient's head is tilted backwards (Fig. 4.10), too much, the upper incisors will stay out of the image layer, so these teeth appear blurry. As a result of the superposition of the hard palate on the roots of the teeth, a radiopaque line forms on the apex of these teeth. In addition, condyles protrude towards the edges of the film.

If the sagittal line deviates from the midline to the right or left, that is, if the head turns to the right or left, the teeth and dental arches on one side give a wider image than the other side (Fig. 4.11). During the radiography, the neck of the patient should be stretched well, in which the patient should be given a ski position. If this position is not given, the ghost image of the vertebrae cannot be prevented and as a result, a radiopaque

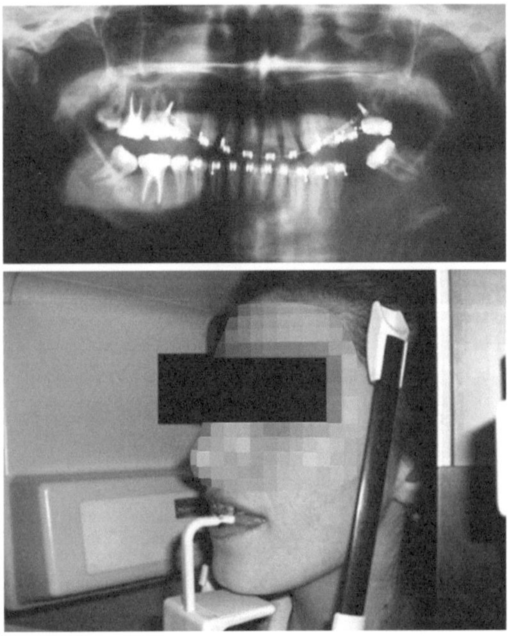

Fig. 4.9 When the patient's head is tilted too low. excessive inclination in the occlusal plane, blurring of the apex of the mandibular anterior teeth

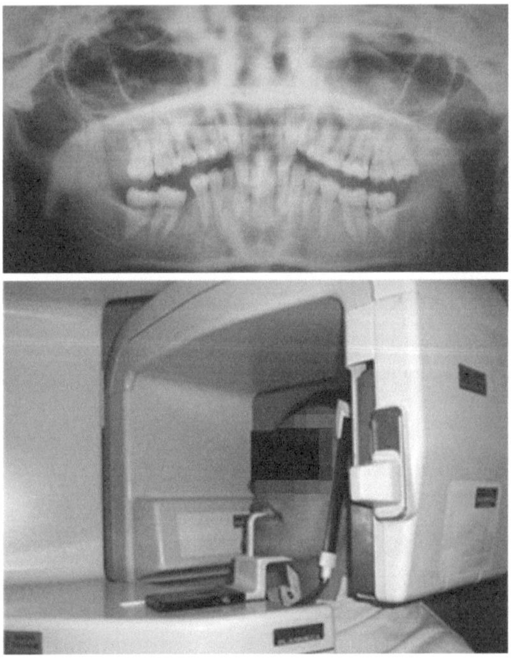

Fig. 4.10 When the patient's head is tilted backwards too much, the upper incisors will stay out of the image layer, so these teeth appear blurry

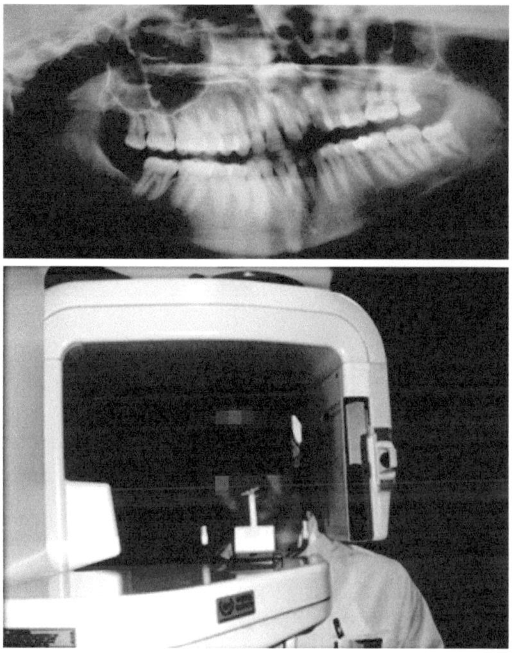

Fig. 4.11 If the sagittal line deviates from the midline to the right or left, that is, if the head turns to the right or left, the teeth and dental arches on one side give a wider image than the other side

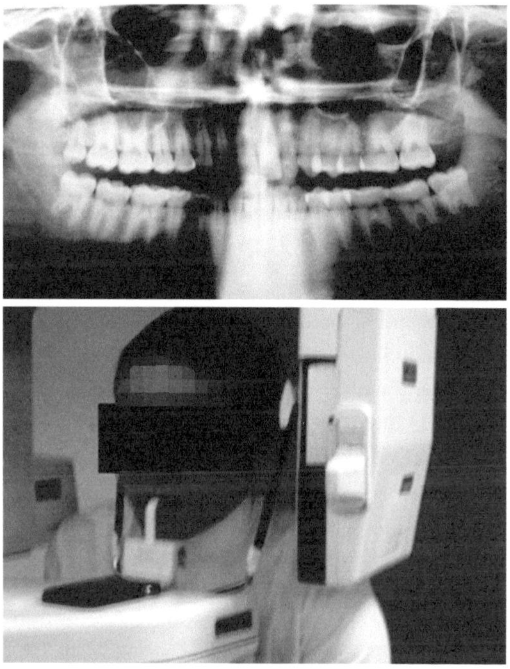

Fig. 4.12 During the radiography, the neck of the patient should be stretched well, in which the patient should be given a ski position. If this position is not given, the ghost image of the vertebrae cannot be prevented

area is seen in the middle of the radiographs (Fig. 4.12). During the radiography, after the patient is positioned, it is requested not to move during the exposure. If patient moves, irregular parts occur on the radiography [1].

4.6.1.1 Ghost Images

- Cervical vertebra (CV),
- Corpus of the mandible, ramus, and contralateral shadow of its angulus (Md),
- Hard palate (PI) ([4], p. 161).

In fact, many ghost images originate from normal anatomical tissues. Although ghost images caused by some anatomical formations cannot be prevented, most ghost images can be eliminated or reduced. The most common ghost image, which we do not want to occur, is the image formed by the vertebrae in the mandibular incisor region. In order to prevent this, the patient should stabilize his neck straight and stretched during the irradiation. If the patient stands hunched over, the X-rays will cross the cervical vertebrae transversely, so it is seen as a radiopaque shadow in the mandibular incisor area ([4], p. 174).

Since all jewellery, especially earrings have high atomic density and are generally outside the image layer, they cause ghost images. The ghost image of the earrings usually occurs on the maxillary sinus and on the opposite side of the mandible corpus.

If the earring is unilateral, the ghost image of it can be mistaken for an odontoma or another radiopaque lesion. The earrings on the tongue are seen in the form of a radiopaque shadow on the nasal passage. Its actual shadow changes according to the position of the tongue during the irradiation (Fig. 4.13).

In cases where the X-ray device is well calibrated, the use of lead apron, which we use to protect the patient from radiation, has been abolished in many countries. Lead aprons and thyroid protectors are used to protect patients from incoming radiation.

Objects outside of this focal trough that are dense enough to attenuate X-rays will occasionally present twice as the X-ray tube rotates around the patient, this is known as a ghost image. The density will appear at the true location and secondly on the contralateral aspect of the image as a distorted "ghost" image. Motion artifact is a patient-based artifact that occurs with voluntary or involuntary patient movement during image acquisition (Figs. 4.14 and 4.15). Metallic objects esp. Thyroid collars, except aluminum, are opaque, and most animal bones and all glass foreign bodies are opaque on radiographs. Most plastic and wooden foreign bodies (cactus thorns, splinters) and most fish bones are not opaque on radiographs (Figs. 4.16 and 4.17).

Hoogeveen et al. compared newly developed cephalographic thyroid protectors (CTP) and anatomical cranial collimators (ACC) with traditional thyroid collars. In the study, four separate patient groups were formed, in which nothing was used, CTP was used, CTP + ACC was used together, and a thyroid protective collar was used. As a result, while the radiation dose affecting the thyroid was reduced by 85% when groups 2 and 3 were used, an 81% reduction occurred by using only group 4 [8].

Prostheses of the patient must also be removed during panoramic radiography. Apart from this, if our patient is wearing glasses, he/she should definitely remove it as it may hide important details on the image ([4], p. 170).

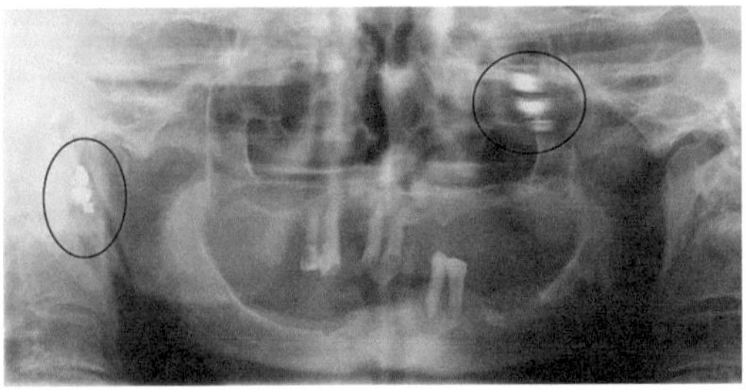

Fig. 4.13 The image of a duplicate 'ghost' image at the contralateral aspect of the image

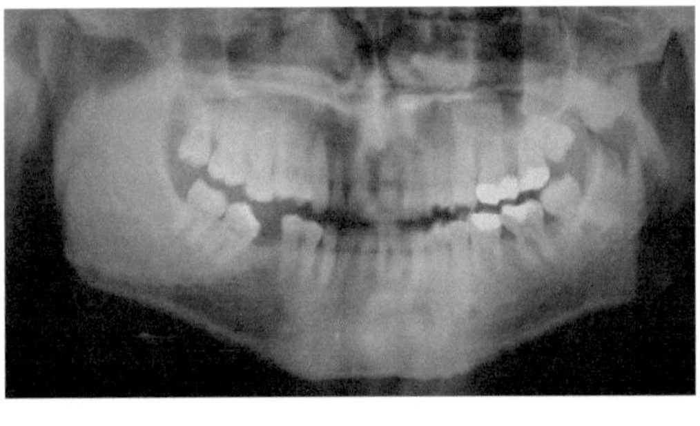

Fig. 4.14 The image of a motion artifact of the patient

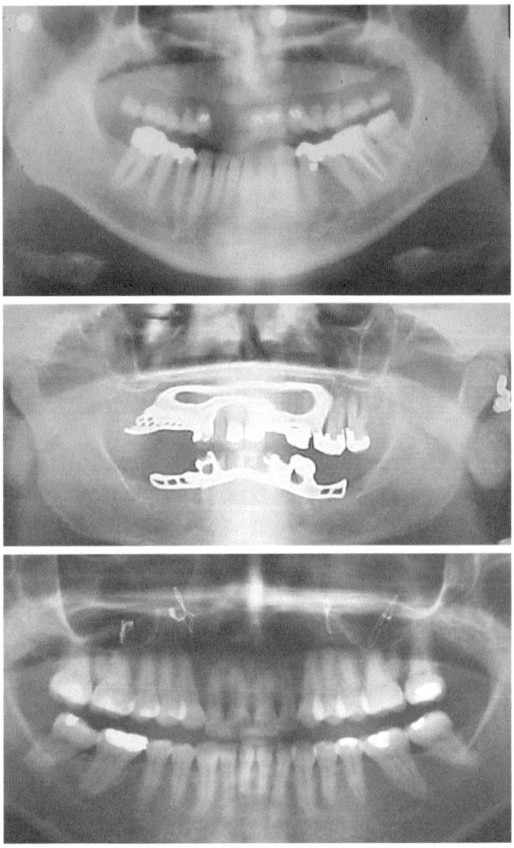

Fig. 4.15 The image of a motion artifact of the pediatric patient

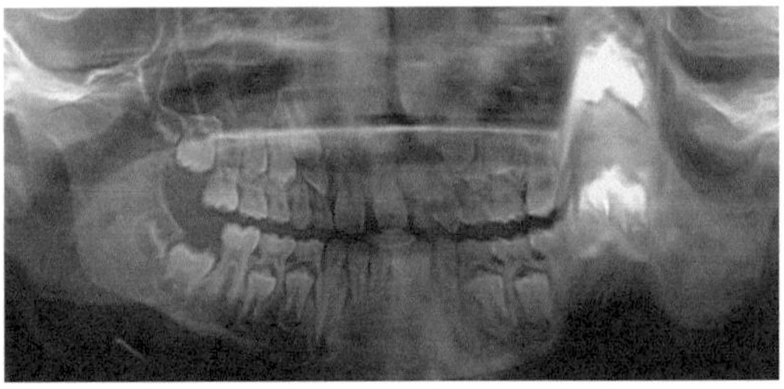

Fig. 4.16 The panoramic images of foreign bodies and motion artifact that appear on the radiographs

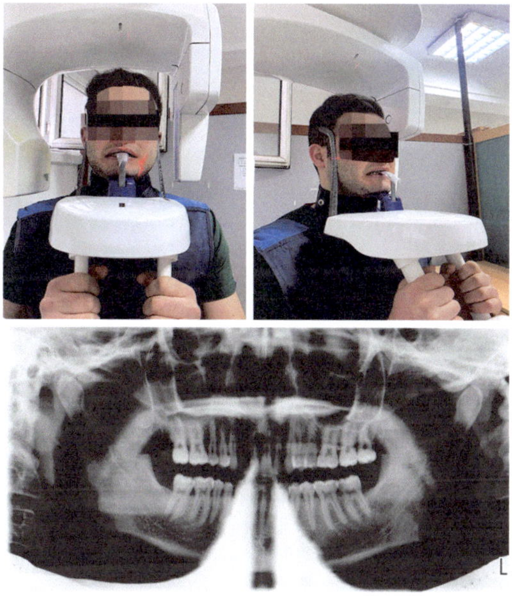

Fig. 4.17 The artifact image of a due to thyroid collar

4.7 Advances in Panoramic Imaging

4.7.1 Volumetric Panoramic Reconstruction

Volumetric panoramic radiography provides the opportunity to create an advanced panoramic image in each section within the focal through area and in its combination. Although volumetric panoramic radiography varies according to the device, 5–8 different sections can be created from a single scan. It provides the opportunity to obtain higher quality images with the same radiation dose and in the same time as conventional panoramic radiography.

With this technique, the superposition section is eliminated with the help of a computer, it is based on the principle of creating images (using the best sections) from multiple sections, not a single section (Fig. 4.18).

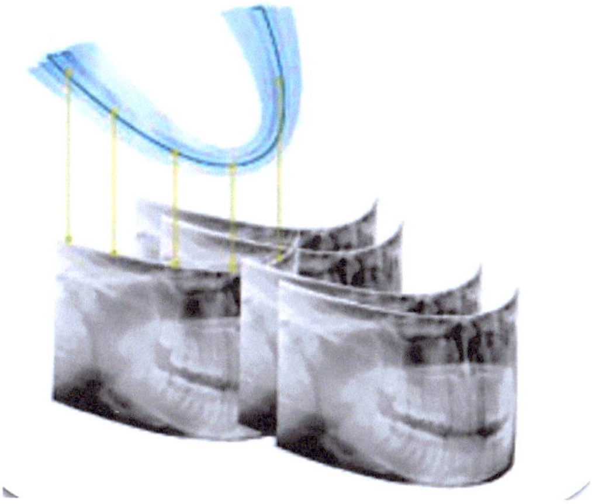

Fig. 4.18 The principle of creating images (using the best sections) from multiple sections of volumetric panoramic image reconstruction

4.8 Panoramic Radiography: Radiation Dose

Depending on the dental radiography, we also observe that the stochastic effects depending on the age. It has less effect in the elderly, mostly in children and young people. When calculating the likelihood of cytocratic effects, it should not be forgotten that individuals under 10 years of age are affected three times more, individuals between 10 and 20 years 2 times and individuals 20–30 years 1.5 times more [9].

Table 4.1 shows the effective radiation dose obtained from dental radiographs used in dental practice, calculated according to the ICRP 1990 norms. Studies conducted in recent years are carried out especially according to the ICRP 2007 criteria. According to ICRP 2007 criteria, it has shown that the amount of radiation dose revealed as a result of dental radiography is higher than ICRP 1990.

Although dental radiography applications give less radiation dose than other medical applications, a verification process should be passed to

Table 4.1 Effective radiation doses obtained from dental radiographsm (ICRP 2007)

X-ray techniques	Effective dose (mSv)	Fatal cancer rate
Intraoral Radiographies (Periapical-Bitewing)	1–8.3	0.02–0.06
Maxillary Anterior Occlusal	8	0.4
Panoramic	3.85–30	0.21–1.9
Lateral Cephalometric Radiography	2.0–3.0	0.34
Sectional Tomography (each section)	1–189	1.0–14.0
CT scan (Maxilla)	364–1202	18.2–88
CT scan (Mandible)	100–3324	8–242

determine whether the specific requirement is really needed or not.

The most important step of this is the selection criteria for patients to be radiographed. Selection criteria are based on multiple factors.

Radiographic examination decision should always be made as a result of anamnesis and clinical examination. The indication and technique appropriate for the patient should be determined. Whether the patient has had a film before and the film has not lost its validity for diagnosis, the use of previous radiographs can also be considered among the selection criteria [9].

Currently, many companies around the world produce high quality films and digital panoramic machines. Nowadays, panoramic devices are multi-rotation centric devices. Panoramic devices can create images of the patient in different positions and localizations, instead of providing only standard panoramic images.

These devices can provide tomographic images of TMJ, maxillary sinuses, and cross-sectional views of maxilla and mandible. Cephalometric radiographs can be easily taken with the same device. Today's devices also have computer controlled automatic dose control, motion speed control, and versatile tomography capabilities. In purchasing these devices with different features, the need of the physician or imaging center and also the effective dose given to the patient should be considered.

References

1. Çağıl H. Serbest Çalışan Diş Hekimlerinin Kullandıkları Radyografik Teknik ve Ekipmanları bitirme tezi. İzmir: Ege Üniversitesi Diş Hekimliği Fakültesi Oral Diagnoz ve Radyoloji Anabilim Dalı; 2009.
2. Farman AG. Panoramic radiology. New York: Springer; 2007.
3. Açıkgöz A. Ortopantomografilerın Klinik Kullanımları. Atatürk Üniv Diş Hek Fak Derg. 1996;6(2):80–5.
4. Whaites E. Essentials of dental radiography and radiology. 3rd ed. China: Elsevier Science; 2002.
5. White SC, Pharoah MJ. Oral radiology: principles and interpretation. St. Louis, MO: Mosby/Elsevier; 2009.
6. Glass BJ. Successful panoramic radiography. 6th ed. Rochester, NY: Eastman Kodak; 1999.
7. Aydın Ü, Aybar Y. Panoramik radyografilerde ortaya çıkan hataların tipleri ve sıklığı. SDÜ Tıp Fak Derg. 2004;11(2):1–5.
8. Hoogeveen RC, Rottke D, van der Stelt PF, Berkhout VER. Dose reduction in orthodontic lateral cephalography: dosimetric evaluation of a novel cephalographic thyroid protector (CTP) and anatomical cranial collimation (ACC). Dentomaxillofac Radiol. 2015;44:20140260.
9. Granlund C, Thilander-Klang A, Ylhan B, Lofthag-Hansen S, Ekestubbe A. Absorbed organ and effective doses from digital intra-oral and panoramic radiography applying the ICRP 103 recommendations for effective dose estimations. Br J Radiol. 2016;89(1066):20151052.

5 Panoramic Radiographic Anatomy

Kaan Orhan and Antigoni Delantoni

5.1 Anatomical Landmarks

A panoramic radiography taken from the patient should be evaluated by the physician as described below;

When evaluating the radiography, first the right-left half segment of the maxilla, midline, nasal cavity, and sinuses are evaluated, then the shadows of the tongue and soft palate are evaluated at this stage. Following this, cervical vertebra and related structures are evaluated. Then start from the midline of the mandible and continue towards the back. The last teeth should be examined. First, it starts from the right or left half of the maxilla or mandible, then passes to the other half, and then the other jaw teeth are examined ([1], p. 168).

5.1.1 Normal Anatomy

Normal anatomical shadows may vary from one radiograph taken with a panoramic device to another. However, it is generally divided into subgroups:

5.1.1.1 **Hard Tissue** (Figs. 5.1, 5.2, 5.3, 5.4, 5.5, 5.6, 5.7, 5.8, 5.9, 5.10, 5.11, 5.12, 5.13, 5.14 and 5.15)

- Teeth.
- Mandible.
- Base of maxilla and antrum, medial and posterior wall (A).
- Hard palate (HP).
- Zygomatic arch (Z).
- Styloid process (SP).
- Hyoid bone (H).
- Nasal septum (NS).
- Orbita (O).
- Skull base.
- Meatus acusticus externus (EAM).

5.1.1.2 Airway Shadows

- Nasal fossa.
- Oral cavity.
- Oropharynx.
- Nasopharynx.

5.1.1.3 Soft Tissue Shades

- Ear lobes (EL).
- Nasal cartilages (NC).

K. Orhan (✉)
Dentomaxillofacial Radiology, Faculty of Dentistry, Department of DentoMaxillofacial Radiology, Ankara, Turkey
e-mail: knorhan@dentistry.ankara.edu.tr

A. Delantoni
Department of Dentoalveolar Surgery, Implant Surgery and Radiology, Faculty of Dentistry, Aristotle University of Thessaloniki, Thessaloniki, Greece
e-mail: andelant@dent.auth.gr

A. Delantoni, K. Orhan (eds.), *Atlas of Dentomaxillofacial Anatomical Imaging*,
https://doi.org/10.1007/978-3-030-96840-3_5

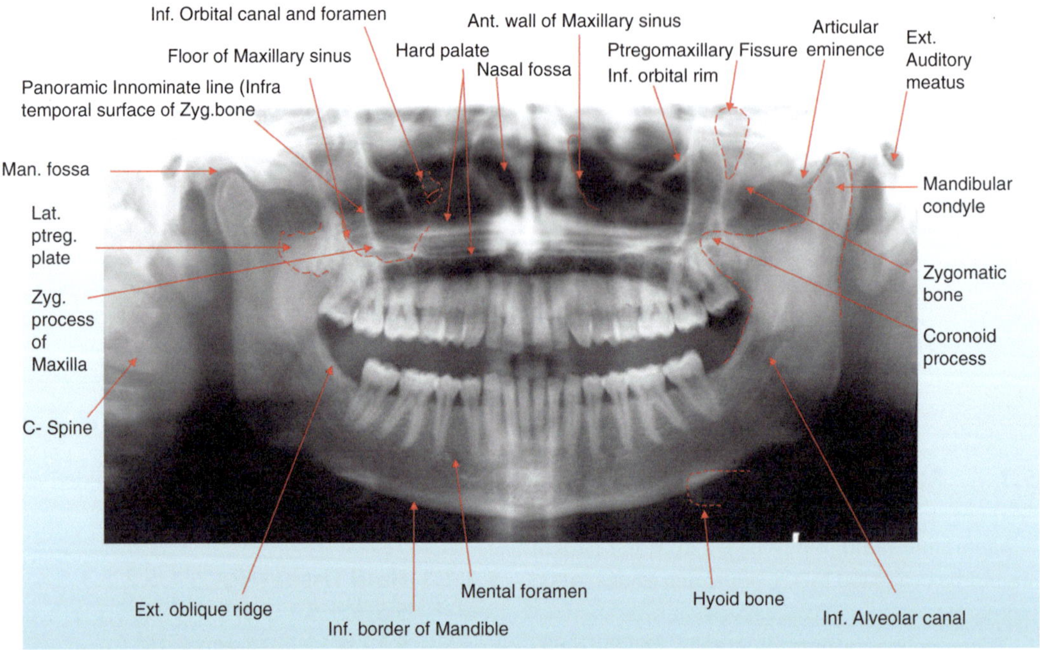

Fig. 5.1 Representative panoramic Images showing the entire maxilla, mandible, and Dentomaxillofacial region, which are indicating hard tissues in the region

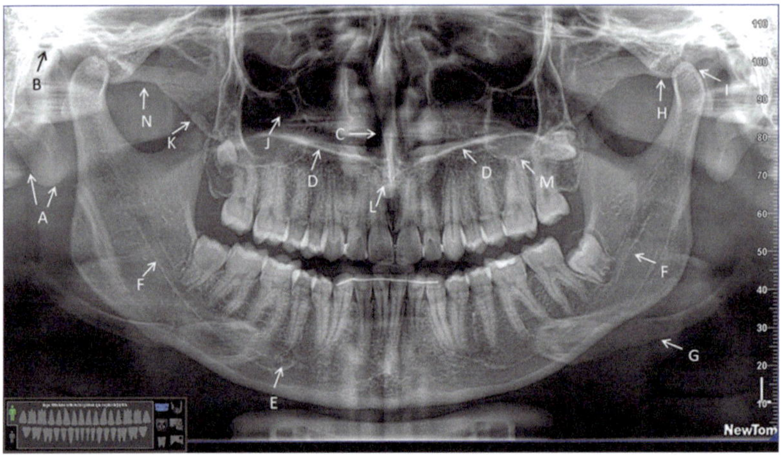

Fig. 5.2 Representative panoramic Images showing anatomical landmarks. A—Ear Lobe, B—External Auditory Meatus, C—Nasal Septum, D—Palate, E—Mental Foramen, F—Mandibular Canal, G—Hyoid Bone, H—Articular Eminence, I—Mandibular Condyle, J—Maxillary Sinus, K—Coronoid Process, L—Spina Nasalis Anterior, M—Inferior Border of Maxillary Sinus, N—Zygomatic Arch

- Soft palate (SP).
- The dorsum of the tongue (DT).
- Cheek and lip mucosa.
- Nasolabial Folt (NF).
- Epiglottis.
- Thyroid cartilage.
- Turbinates (middle and inferior) (Figs. 5.16 and 5.17).

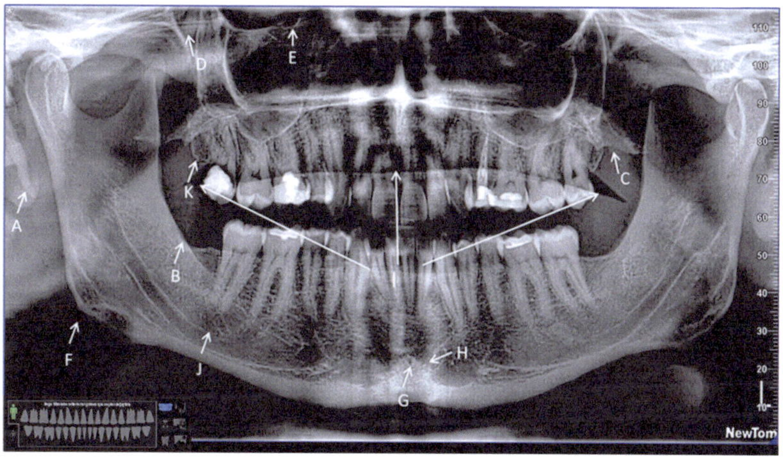

Fig. 5.3 Representative panoramic Images showing anatomical landmarks. A—Styloid Process, B—External Oblique Ridge, C—Pterygoid Plates, D—Pterygomaxillary Fissure, E—Infraorbital Foramen, F—Angulus Mandibula, G—Lingaul Foramen, H—Genial Tubercle, I—Palatoglossal Air Space, J—Submandibular Gland Fossa, K—Tuber Maxilla

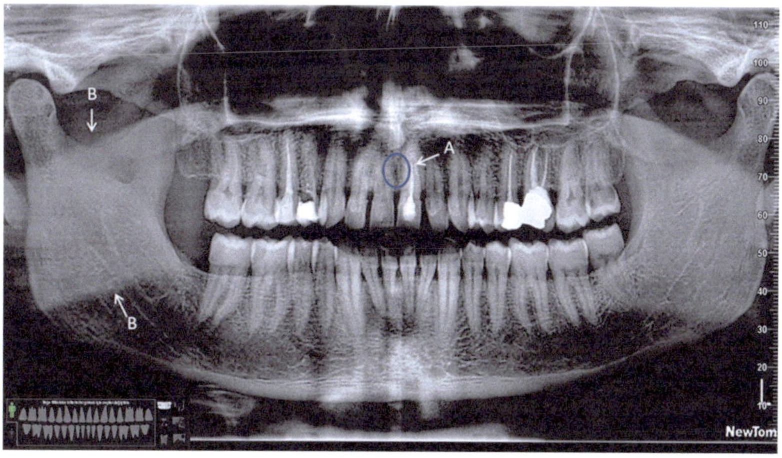

Fig. 5.4 Representative panoramic Images showing anatomical landmarks. A—Incisıve Foramen, B—Ghost of Mandible

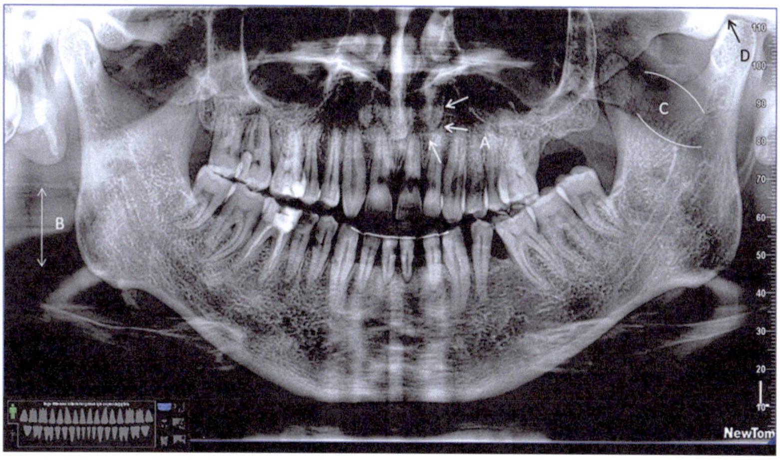

Fig. 5.5 Representative panoramic Images showing anatomical landmarks. A—Soft Tissue of Nose, B—Glossopharyngeal Airway Space, C—Nasopharyngeal Airway Space, D—Glenoid Fossa

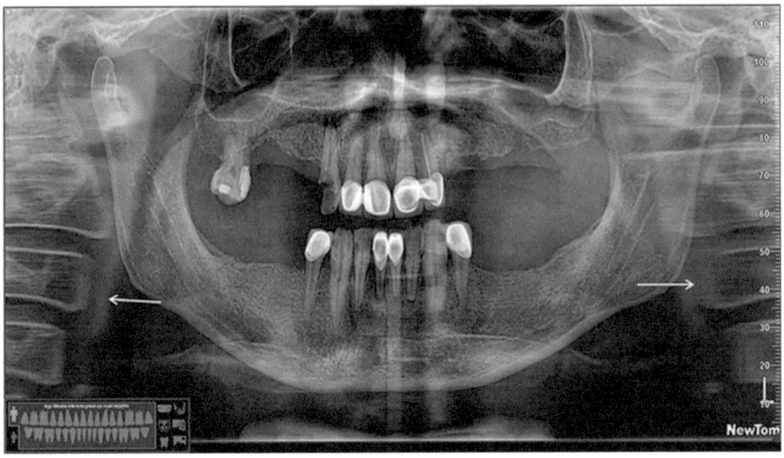

Fig. 5.6 Representative panoramic Images showing anatomical landmarks. Vertebra

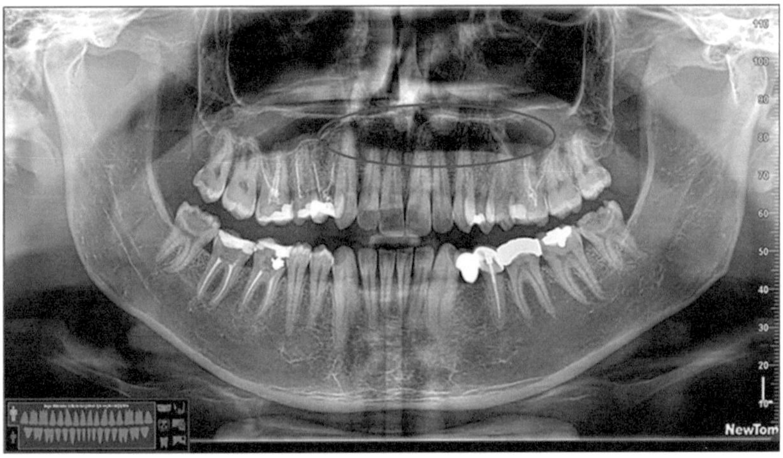

Fig. 5.7 Radiolucent artifact superimposed over the maxillary apices. Patient's tongue not placed against the hard palate

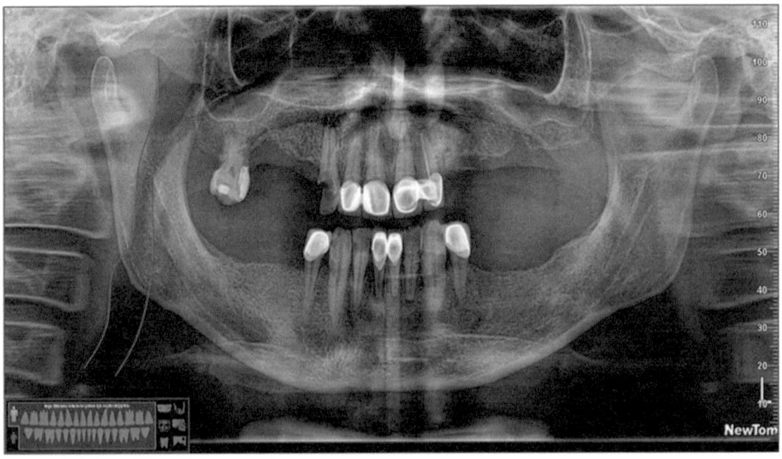

Fig. 5.8 Representative panoramic Images showing anatomical landmarks. POSTERIOR WALL OF PHARYNX

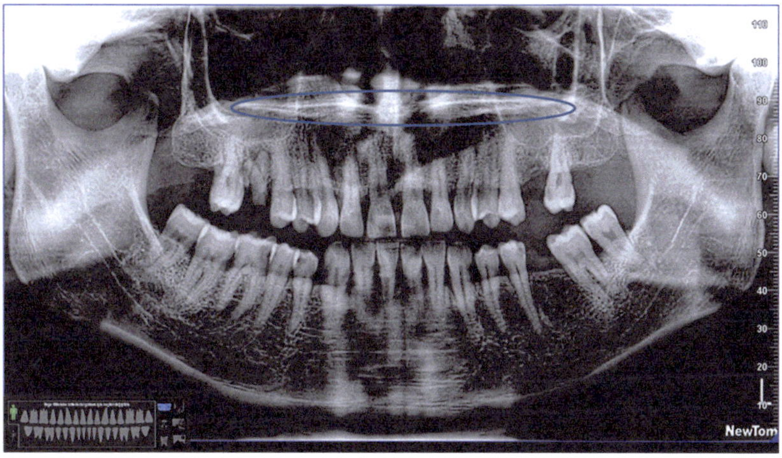

Fig. 5.9 Representative panoramic Images showing anatomical landmarks. HARD PALATE

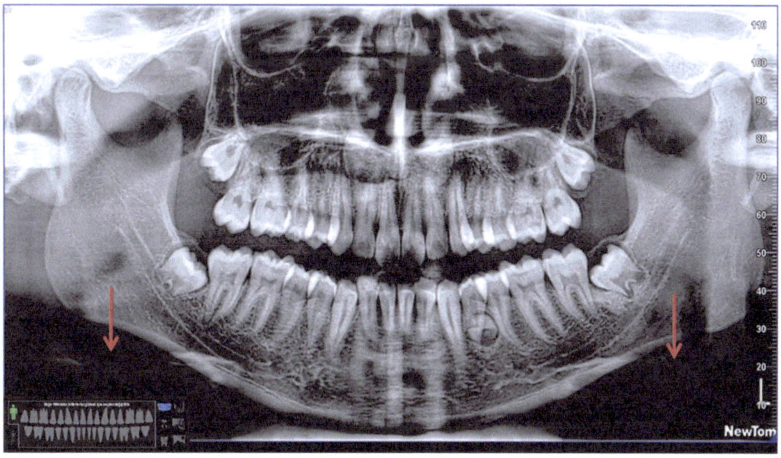

Fig. 5.10 Representative panoramic Images showing anatomical landmarks. HYOID

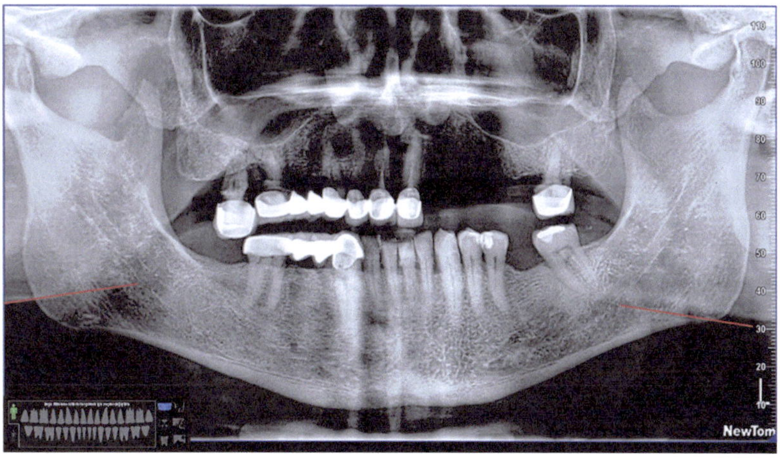

Fig. 5.11 Representative panoramic Images showing GHOST OF MANDIBLE

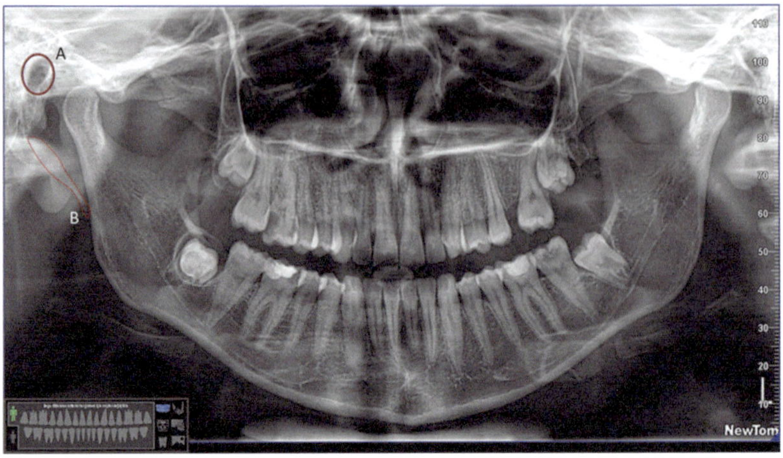

Fig. 5.12 Representative panoramic Images showing anatomical landmarks. A—Meatus Acusticus Externus, B—Styloid Process

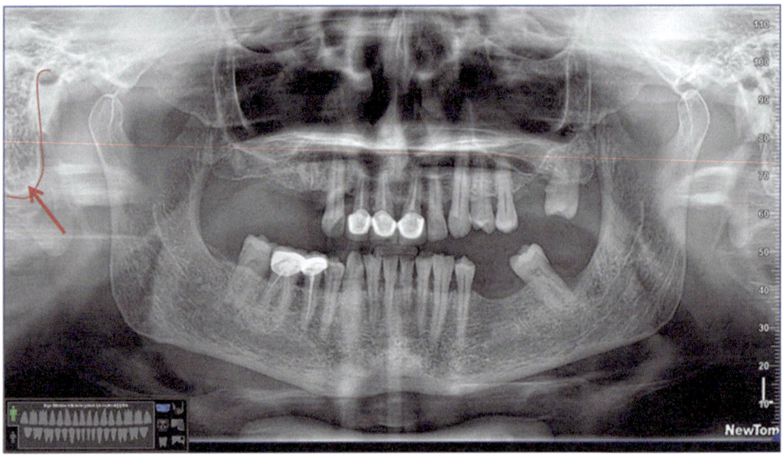

Fig. 5.13 Representative panoramic Images showing mastoid process

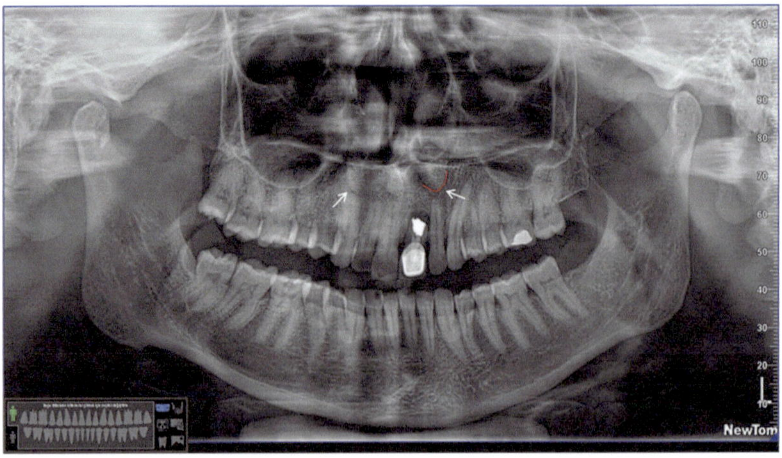

Fig. 5.14 Representative panoramic Images showing soft tissue of nose

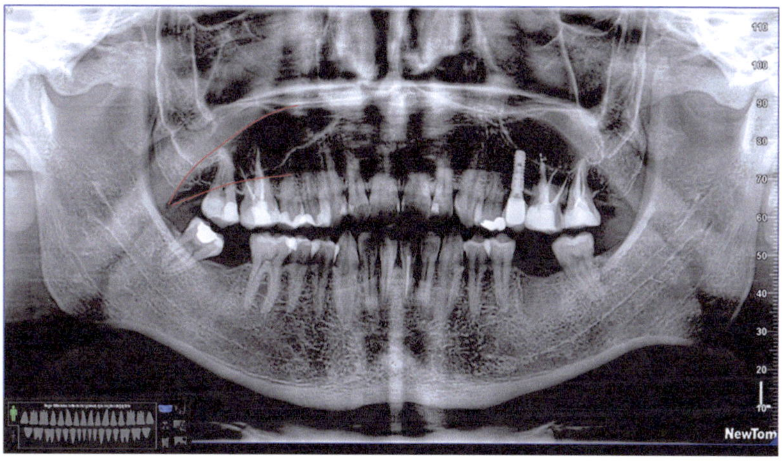

Fig. 5.15 Representative panoramic Images showing palatoglossal airway space

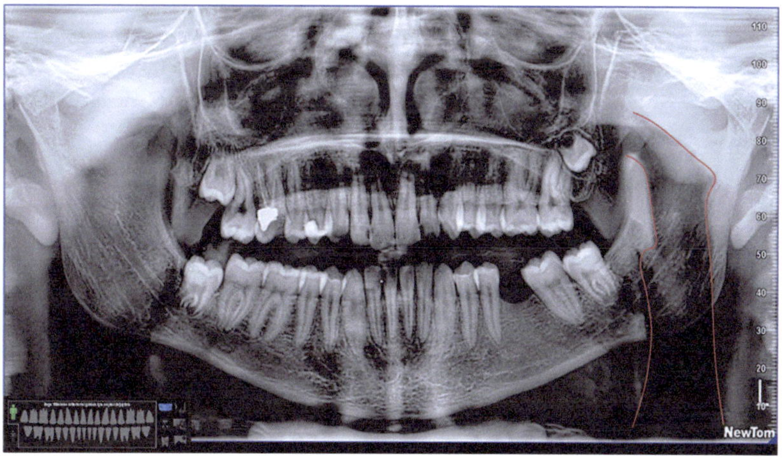

Fig. 5.16 Representative panoramic Images showing air space of pharynx

5.2 Panoramic Radiography: Diagnosing Dentition Anomalies

Dental anomalies are generally anomalies that affect the shape, structure, number, and size of teeth during tooth development. These dental anomalies that occur during tooth development can affect the organization of the dental arches and cause malocclusion.

Accordingly, it affects surgical treatment, orthodontic treatment, endodontic treatment, and restorative dental treatment procedures. Dental anomalies affect both primary dentition and permanent dentition [2].

Panoramic radiography can be used to diagnose these dentition anomalies. In cases where there is hypodontia, hyperdontia, gemination or fusion in primary dentition, anomaly development in permanent dentition is under the high risk group. Due to this close relationship between primary dentition and permanent dentition, early diagnosis of anomalies helps the physician to examine for the future and determine the best treatment plan at the earliest stage.

Panoramic radiography has a very important place in the identification, localization, and surgical removal of supernumerary teeth. In addition, anomalies in the permanent dentition, supernumerary teeth and morphological anomalies of

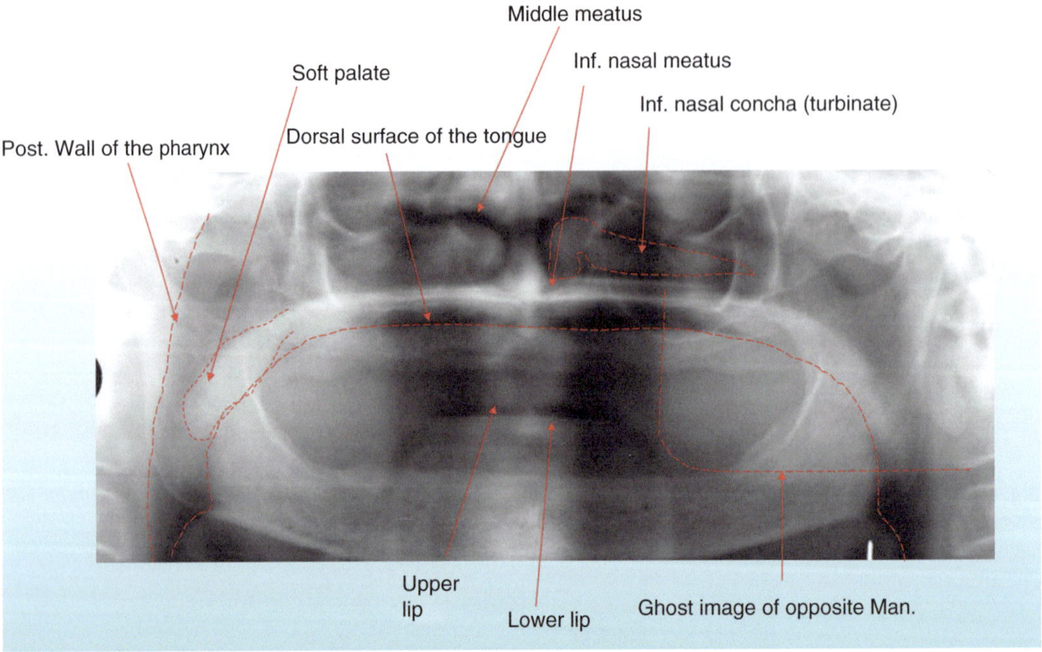

Fig. 5.17 Representative panoramic Images showing the entire maxilla, mandible, and Dentomaxillofacial region which are indicating soft tissue shades and airways tissues in the region

maxilla and mandible seen in cleiocranial dysplasia can diagnosed by panoramic radiography.

Gardner syndrome, which is seen with multiple embedded supernumerary teeth, osteomas in the skull and jaws in long bones, multiple polyps in the intestines, and epidermoid or dermoid cysts, can be diagnosed by panoramic radiography. Fatal malignancy can be prevented by early diagnosis of Gardner syndrome when osteomas and multiple supernumerary teeth are seen in the jaws in panoramic radiography ([3], p. 48).

Early diagnosis of macrodontia is an important place in orthodontic treatment planning. If there is macrodontia and tooth development is not possible due to this reason, if it is impacted or maloccluded, panoramic radiography helps early diagnosis ([3], p. 41). Taurodontism is hereditary morphology anomalies seen in multiroot teeth due to invagination error of the Hertwig epithelial sheath. Taurodontism is the enlargement of the pulp chamber as a result of the displacement of the pulp base and bifurcation towards the apical [4]. Taurodontism is usually seen symmetrically and bilaterally. It is rarely seen when a single tooth is affected. No anomaly is encountered in the relevant teeth during clinical examination. Taurodontism is diagnosed by radiography. Panoramic radiography has been found to be reliable for the diagnosis of taurodontism ([3], p. 53).

Whittington and Durward examined the anomalies of primary dentition and permanent dentition using panoramic radiography in 1680 people aged 5 years. They found hypnodontics in 6 children, supernumerary teeth in 3 children, and fusion and gemination in 14 children. In 14 of these children with primary dentition anomalies, anomalies were also found in permanent dentition. Due to this close relationship between primary dentition and permanent dentition, early diagnosis of anomalies helps the physician to examine for the future and determine the best treatment plan at the earliest stage ([3], p. 41).

Patil et al. conducted a research to determine the diagnosis and prevalence of dental anomalies on panoramic films taken from 4133 patients. As a result of the research, 36.7% of them have dental anomalies. Of these, 16.3% are congenital tooth

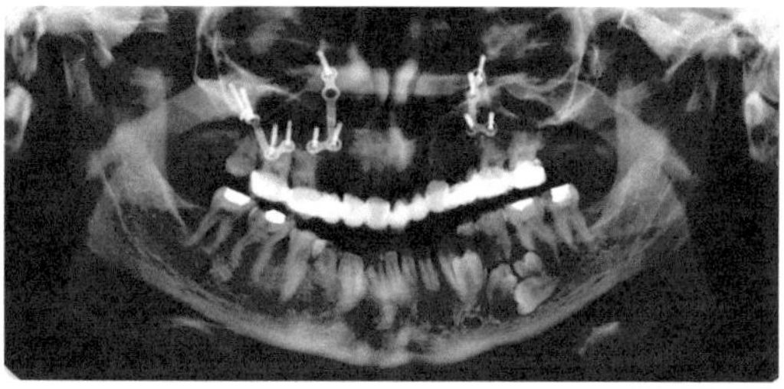

Fig. 5.18 Panoramic image showing supernumerary premolars with a non-syndromic patient

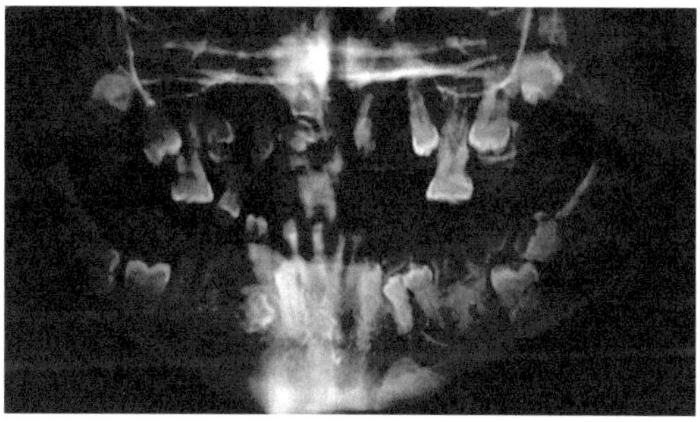

Fig. 5.19 Panoramic image showing a syndromic patient with eruption problems together with cystic lesion

deficiency, 15.5% are impacted teeth, 1.2% are supernumerary teeth, and 1% are microdontia [5].

Panoramic radiography is very effective and useful in diagnosing dental anomalies in addition to clinical examinations. Since dental development anomalies can affect patients' esthetics and self-worth perception, early diagnosis of anomalies enables us to make the necessary treatment planning. Although the treatment of anomalies that are not diagnosed early is more difficult, the prognosis is not good ([3], p. 66) (Fig. 5.18).

5.3 Panoramic Radiography: Evaluation of Tooth Eruption and Impaction

Radiography is of great importance in evaluating whether the tooth eruption process is normal in terms of both position and timing. This is especially important in the evaluation of clinically undetectable teeth with eruption delay or impacted teeth. The impacting of a tooth may develop due to either the surrounding tissues or a pathology.

Eruption delays, affecting both primary dentition and permanent dentition, may be associated with a systemic disease such as rickets, cretinism or cleidocranial dysplasia ([3], p. 73).

Neonatal diseases or postnatal nutrition are closely related to the eruption timing of primary teeth. Delays in tooth eruption are observed in fibromatosis gingiva due to enlarged gingiva. If eruption delays are due to a local cause (fibromatous gingiva, supernumerary teeth, odontome, etc.), eruption can be controlled with early treatment (Fig. 5.19).

In cases where eruption delays are prolonged, they should be examined with panoramic radiography or intraoral radiography. Since panoramic radiology can cooperate during patient exposure, it provides the most appropriate view. Periodic panoramic radiology is useful in the diagnosis of conditions such as tooth eruption anomalies caused by dentigerous cysts around 20-years-old teeth.

The impaction of the third molar teeth is classified according to the Winter Method, depending on the position. Panoramic X-rays show the mesiodistal and vertical position of the impacted tooth, but do not provide information about the buccolingual position or buccolingual angulation. Therefore, when deciding on the treatment plan, we may need to support panoramic radiography with occlusal films or three-dimensional images created using an intraoral detector ([3], p. 74). As a result, although there are some discussions about the monitoring or removal of the third molar tooth with panoramic radiography, panoramic radiography is an important prediagnosis device used in the evaluation of these teeth. In order to evaluate the relationship of the mandibular posterior tooth roots with the mandibular canal, it should be supported by other additional radiographs that provide information bucco-lingually [6] (Fig. 5.20).

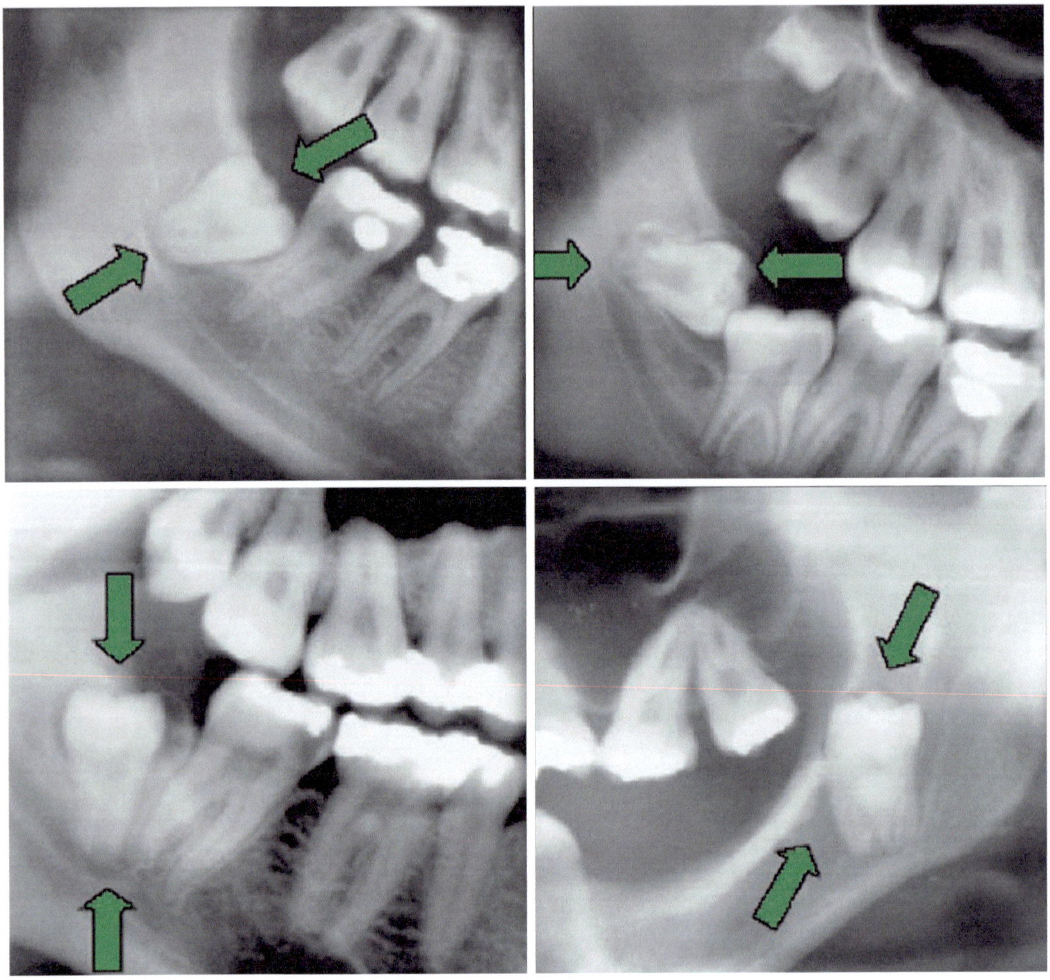

Fig. 5.20 Cropped panoramic image showing third molars positioning in relation to anatomical landmarks

5.4 Panoramic Radiography: Evaluations in Orthodontics

Today, panoramic radiography has become an indispensable diagnostic method in evaluating the success and failure of orthodontic treatment. Panoramic radiography provides information about the presence and absence of the tooth, its morphological and structural variations, and the eruption pattern. In addition, panoramic radiography has become the standard in the evaluation of tooth parallels, especially for orthodontics.

Panoramic radiography is one of the first preferred 2-dimensional imaging methods for patients who will undergo orthodontic treatment. The lack of teeth or the presence of supernumerary teeth in some patients can be understood as a result of clinical examination. However, panoramic radiography provides a wide examination opportunity including all maxillary and mandibular arches of the patient together with the temporomandibular joint. Panoramic radiographs are useful in showing root morphology deviations, eruption times or changes in development, impactedness, loss or supernumerary teeth, as well as any pathological lesions or mandibular asymmetry, while they also provide limited information about sinuses, root parallelism, and periodontal health ([7], p. 35; [8]). It also helps to assess the quality and quantity of alveolar bone for the placement of temporary anchoring devices or implants and to determine their distance to vital structures ([7], p. 35).

5.5 Panoramic Radiography: Mandibular Canal Variations

The mandibular canal, which neurovascular structures pass through, feeding the lower teeth and adjacent anatomical structures, is a bone-surrounded space that starts from the foramen mandible at the back and extends to the foramen mentale in front (Fig. 5.21). It is important to determine the position and course of the canal correctly in terms of evaluating whether there is an anatomical variation and whether there is a bifid mandibular canal. In addition, it provides protection against complications that may occur during surgical operations such as tooth extraction or implant placement [9]. Bifid mandibular canal, rather than being a projection artifact, are real variations affecting approximately 0.5–1% of the population (Fig. 5.22). Although they are usually asymptomatic, they sometimes cause pain and TMJ dysfunction [10].

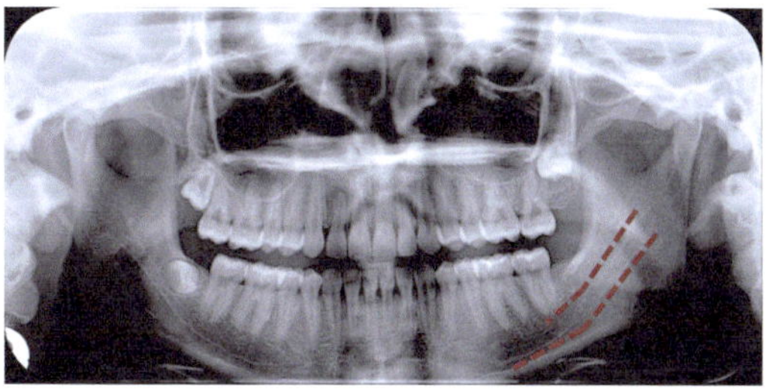

Fig. 5.21 Panoramic image showing mandibular canal

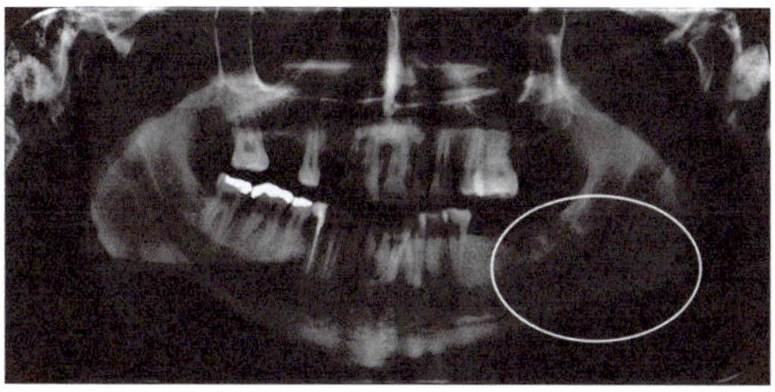

Fig. 5.22 Panoramic image showing bifid mandibular canal

As a result of the study performed on 75 CBCTs from data obtained from private clinics near São Paulo, bifid mandibular canals were classified into four different groups.

1. **Type 1**; It is divided into two subgroups.
   (a) Unilateral bifurcation extends to the third molar and its surrounding tissues,
   (b) The double-sided bifurcation extends to the third molar and its surrounding tissues.
2. **Type 2**; It is divided into four subgroups.
   (a) Unilateral bifurcation extends to the main canal and converges in the ramus of the mandible,
   (b) Unilateral bifurcation extends to the main canal and converges at the mandible corpus,
   (c) The bilateral bifurcation extends to the main canal and converges in the ramus of the mandible,
   (d) Bilateral bifurcation extends to the main canal and converges at the mandible corpus.
3. **Type 3**; It is seen as a combination of type 1 and type 2 bifurcation types.
4. **Type 4**; The two channels start from two completely different foramen mandible and then merge to form a single and wide mandibular canal [11].

The presence of a bifid mandibular canal is large enough to be diagnosed using panoramic radiography. However, since the observation that can be made in panoramic radiography is limited, there is a doubt about the actual existence of the bifid mandibular canal [9].

Orhan et al. examined a total of 484 mandibular canals (right and left) on CBCT scans taken from 242 patients for various reasons and 225 bifid mandibular canals were found. In the studies performed on conventional panoramic radiographs, they stated that, since the bifid mandibular canal can be seen much less, it is necessary to examine with 3D imaging methods before implant placement, 20-year-old tooth extraction and similar surgical interventions [12].

A study was conducted at Chonnam National University on 1000 panoramic radiography and on 40 dry mandibles whether there was a bifid mandible canal. Bifid mandibular canal was found in 1 of them on panoramics taken from 40 dry mandible. According to the results of this study, it was argued that the bifid mandibular canal diagnosed in panoramic radiography should be supported with CBCT before a surgical treatment and should be evaluated in terms of whether it contains neurovascular tissue in both channels [9].

Orhan et al. stated that the course and localization of the incisive canal should be evaluated with 3D imaging methods before surgical interventions such as implant placement in the anterior region in order to prevent complications that may develop due to the incisive canal variations they detected as a result of their study on CBCT images of 356 patients [13].

5.6 Panoramic Radiography: Common Pathological Conditions

It has been observed that the disease process can affect the panoramic radiographic view of the mandibular canal in various ways. While localized losses of the mandibular canal cortex may be associated with chronic apical periodontitis, chronic periodontitis and, rarely, large Stafne bone cavity, generalized losses are usually associated with severe infections and aggressive neoplasms, osteomyelitis, invasive squamous cell carcinoma, multiple myeloma, osteogenic sarcoma, and rarely it may be related with ameloblastoma.

In cases of large radicular cysts, residual cysts, dentigerous cysts, Cemento-ossifying fibroma, benign cystic or neoplastic cases, the displacement of the mandibular canal may occur.

While benign lesions such as neurilemmomas that develop inside the mandibular canal cause the expansion of the mandibular canal, although they are generally of neurovascular origin, they cause the canal to be displaced towards the top or the bottom, while malignant lesions such as leiomyosarcoma cause destruction in the canal cortex ([3], p. 110).

As a result, it is very important for the dentist to be aware of normal anatomy and the changes that various diseases will make to normal anatomy. While some diseases cause the formation of permanent and distinctive radiological changes, others cause variable nonspecific formations. Considering the distinct panoramic radiological features of the lesions, the changes that may occur in the channel are accurately predicted and a diagnosis list can be created based on this information ([3], p. 115).

5.7 Panoramic Radiography: Maxillary Sinus

Panoramic radiography and waters radiography show the upper, lower, lateral walls, soft tissue, and fluid contents, but not the anterior and posterior wall of the maxillary sinus. Therefore, magnetic resonance imaging or computerized tomography is used as an alternative in the examination of the maxillary sinus. Although computerized tomography and magnetic resonance imaging are considered appropriate for examining the maxillary sinuses, these options should be preferred only in cases where there are signs and symptoms. Since most maxillary sinus lesions are asymptomatic, panoramic radiographs taken for dental observations are usually the first cases where maxillary sinus lesions are diagnosed. Although panoramic radiography helps to detect maxillary sinus lesions, it should never be used alone to exclude sinus pathology, because the lesion will only be seen when it remains within the image layer ([3], p. 111) (Fig. 5.23).

5.7.1 Inflammations Involving the Maxillary Sinus

The most common inflammatory condition involving the maxillary sinus is mucus retention cyst. Mucus retention cyst usually affects 5.8% of the population and is usually two times more common in men. Mucus retention cyst is seen on panoramic radiography as a smooth dome-shaped swelling with homogeneous radiodensity. Sinus polyps can only be seen on panoramic radiography if they are located in the image layer. The mucus retention cyst is usually located at the sinus floor and does not cause the sinus floor to displace. It is rarely symptomatic. Usually does not require treatment [14] (Fig. 5.24).

Aspergilloma, which was formed by the aspergillus organism, which was first described at the end of the eleventh century, are the most opportunistic fungal infections in the body after candida infections. The most frequently affected area in the head and neck region is the paranasal sinuses. Although aspergilloma is rarely seen in healthy individuals, it can be seen more in immunosuppressive cancer patients. These patients usually present to us with moderate pain in the area where the lesion is localized and subfertile fever. Since aspergilloma may be invasive, CBCT should be preferred over conventional panoramic radiographs to evaluate lesion margins [15].

Chronic dental abscesses involving the tooth roots in the maxillary posterior region cause loss of continuity of the lower wall of the maxillary sinus and sometimes thickening of the mucosa ([3], p. 120). Benign cysts and neoplasms involving the maxillary sinus cause displacement of the sinus floor and cause maxillary expansion. Apical cysts and residual cysts may cause an upward displacement of the maxillary sinus floor, but do not disrupt the continuity of the maxillary sinus wall. Benign neoplasms such as keratocystic odontogenic tumors are in the form of uniocular or multiloocular radiolucency, causing displacement of the sinus floor and jaw expansion. Primary malignancies involving the maxillary sinus are squamous cell carcinoma, adenoid cystic carcinoma, and adenocarcinoma. Early diagnosis of invasion to the maxillary sinus in malignant neoplasms is very important for the prognosis of the patient.

In conclusion, panoramic radiography alone is insufficient in the diagnosis of maxillary sinus lesions, but it is very important for the initial diagnosis. Experimental studies have shown that computerized tomography is more successful in diagnosing osteolytic lesions involving the posterior wall of the maxillary sinus. However, panoramic radiography is more successful than waters radiography in the diagnosis of lesions affecting the floor of the maxillary sinus and determining their localization [14] (Fig. 5.25).

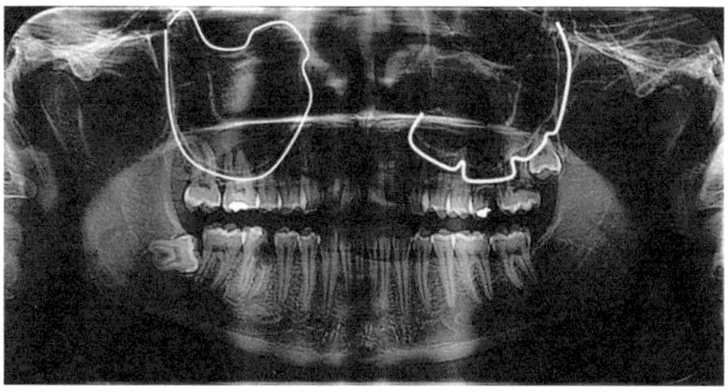

Fig. 5.23 Panoramic image showing maxillary sinus borders

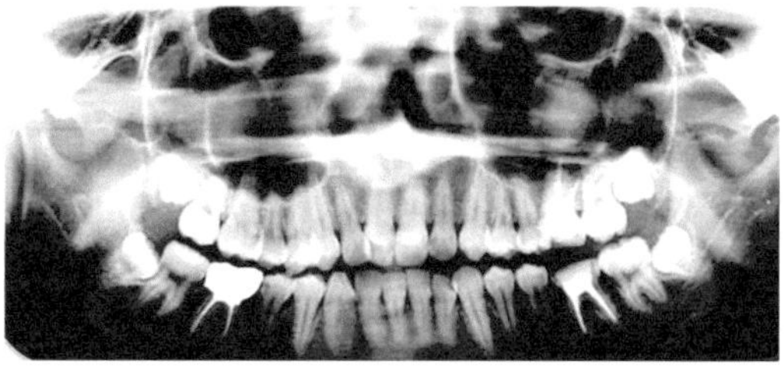

Fig. 5.24 Panoramic image showing a large mucous retention cyst

5.8 Panoramic Radiology: Endodontics

While panoramic imaging can serve as an important endodontic diagnostic tool, it is also used as an important diagnostic tool in evaluating the success of endodontic treatment.

Radiology is particularly important in detecting periapical lesions and evaluating treatment success, including recovery after endodontic therapy. There are no radiological signs in irreversible pulpitis in the early stages. With the spreading of the pulpal inflammation to the periapical tissues, the pain of the patient causes localized and sensitivity in percussion. At this stage, the periodontal interval is seen on the radiograph as enlarged.

In the acute phase of periapical periodontitis, cell activation that will cause bone destruction

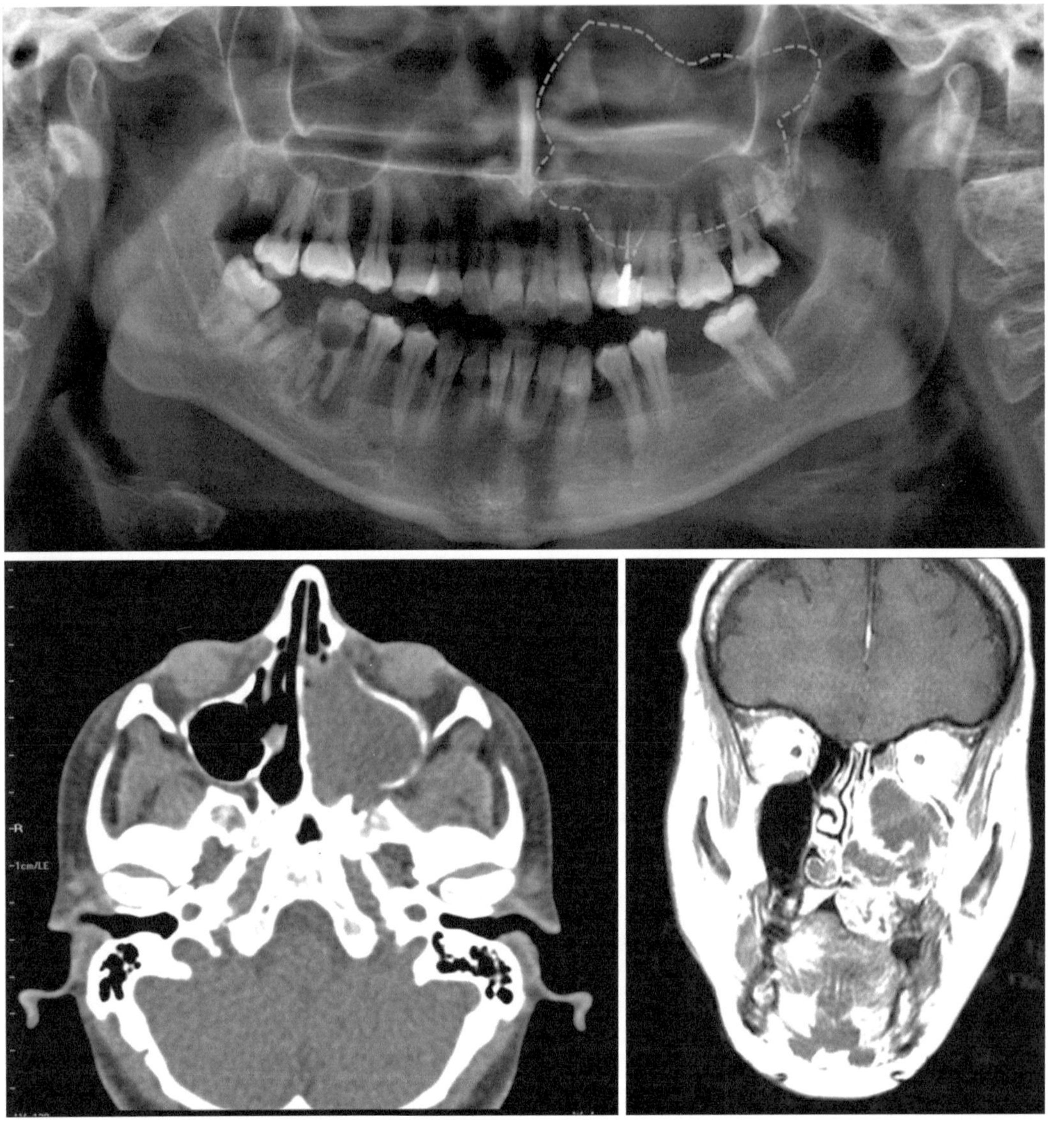

Fig. 5.25 Panoramic image showing a large lesion in the left maxillary sinus. Corresponding CT and MR images of the same patient showing the lesion that was further diagnosed mucoepidermoid carcinoma

has not started yet. If the irritant is strong enough to cause tissue detraction, pus formation and after that, abscess formation will occur. After that, abscess formation will occur. If the lesion remains long enough to form chronic inflammation cells, granulation tissue forms and results in periapical radiolucency. In cases with periapical radiolucencies larger than 1 cm in radiography, the lesion probably contains a cystic component, while smaller lesions may be cystic. Panoramic radiology is more advantageous when the margins of the lesion are too large to be seen on periapical radiography. Therefore, panoramic radiography is more useful when it is necessary to examine the lesion borders. Panoramic radiography is an excellent diagnostic tool that provides information to clinicians about the general appearance of dentoalveolar structures [16].

Ahlqwist et al. conducted an epidemiological study on women to evaluate oral health and compare panoramic and intraoral radiographs. In the study conducted on 75 women, the distribution of teeth, missing teeth, restorations, endodontic treatments with osteolytic lesions in the periapical area, and caries were evaluated. In the comparison between panoramic radiography and intraoral radiographs, 100% correlation was detected for all units, and it was seen that intraoral radiography was more suitable only for determining the caries depth ([3], p. 136). As a result, although periapical radiographs are necessary for the evaluation of root canal morphology, panoramic radiography is useful for the first diagnostic film in the comprehensive evaluation of large periapical lesions, but it is not suitable for the diagnosis of endodontic pathologies ([3], p. 141).

5.9 Panoramic Radiography: Diagnosis of Pericoronal Pathologies

Panoramic radiography has a great role in the diagnosis and evaluation of the pathological conditions present in the jaws. Crowns of unerupted teeth are normally found surrounded by a dental follicle. This dental follicle surrounds the homogeneous radiolucent dental crown in the form of a halo, starting from the enamel-cementum junction. This follicle has a thin radiopaque wall and continues with the lamina dura surrounding the periodontal ligament space. In order to distinguish the normal and abnormal dental follicle area:

Except for the maxillary canine teeth, all teeth have a periodontal space of 2.5 mm in the periapical film and 3 mm in the panoramic. In the absence of clinical symptoms, in cases of large or growing follicles and growth delays, it should be followed up every 6 months. This can be accomplished with the use of panoramic radiography. If the dental follicle undergoes cyst formation, it can turn into a "follicular cyst" If the follicular cyst covers the tooth crown completely and originates from the bone, it is called "dentigerous cyst," and in cases of soft tissue origin, it is called "eruption cyst" [17]. Although dentigerous cyst is the most common development among developmental odontogenic cysts, it is frequently seen in the mandibular third molar teeth, maxillary canine teeth, mandibular premolars followed by the maxillary third molar region in regions where there is a high probability of impacted teeth. While the dentigerous cyst is asymptomatic except for the impacted tooth, it sometimes causes jaw expansion in the locally affected area. While dentigerous cyst usually causes the displacement of the affected tooth, it also causes resorption in the roots of neighboring teeth [18]. Dentigerus cysts are seen on panoramic radiography as uniocular, in different sizes, with well sclerotic margins. While panoramic radiography is sufficient for the diagnosis of dentiginous cysts, more advanced imaging methods should be preferred for treatment planning [19] (Fig. 5.26).

Keratocystic odontogenic tumor is an odontogenic cyst originating from the dental lamina that usually occurs in the second and third decade of life. While it is generally seen as uniocular, well-defined radiolucency on panoramic radiography, it has a thin radiopaque smooth border. Multilocular lesions are seen less frequently and have higher recurrence [20].

Ameloblastomas are benign tumors originating from Malassez epithelial residues that have significant growth potential in bone and cause bone deformity. Ameloblastomas are usually asymptomatic and can sometimes cause jaw expansion, tooth displacement, and root resorption of the affected teeth as they are diagnosed during routine dental radiographs [21]. Ameloblastomas are seen on panoramic radiography as uniocular or multiocular, well-circumscribed. The boundaries of the lesions seen in the mandible are generally well-

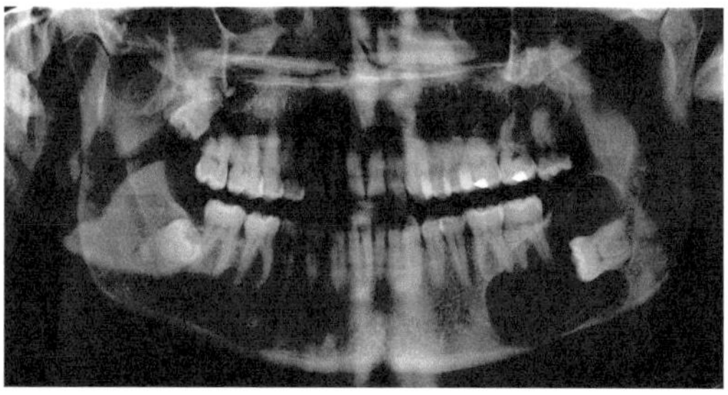

Fig. 5.26 Panoramic image showing large dentigerous cyst due to unerupted third molar

circumscribed, often cortical and sometimes scalloped. On the contrary, lesions in the maxilla are seen with irregular borders. The lesion may give a mixed image radiographically either completely radiolucent or depending on the presence of bone septa.

Calcified epithelial odontogenic tumor (Pindborg tumor) accounts for approximately 1% of odontogenic tumors. Although calcified epithelial odontogenic tumor is less aggressive than ameloblastoma, its only symptom is expansion in the jaws. Similar to ameloblastoma, it is mostly seen in the molar and premolar region in the mandible and is associated with 52% of the impacted teeth. These lesions are seen in uniocular or multiolcular radiolucency with different numbers of radiopaque formations in various shapes and densities. The most characteristic finding is that radiopacities are seen close to the tooth crown. Radiographically, the lesion is called "driven snow" ([22], p. 377).

Adenomatoid odontogenic tumor (AOT) is an epithelial origin, a rare, benign, painless, non-invasive, slow-growing odontogenic tumor. AOT often affects maxillary canine teeth. AOT is a pericoronal well-circumscribed, uniocular, radiopaque-radiolucent, mixed lesion that usually affects an impacted tooth, sometimes involving a few teeth. There are radiopaque foci in 78% of the lesion and they are seen as "conglomerate," while 22% are present in lesions that do not contain radiopaque foci [23].

Odontoma is the most common odontogenic tumor. It is thought that it may be a hamartamatous lesion due to its slow development, its ability to remain in the same size for a long time and not show recurrence. They do not choose gender and generally take shape during dentition. It is divided into two groups as complex and compound odontoma. Odontomas are well-circumscribed, surrounding radiolucent areas containing radiopaque calcified tissue and irregular mass on panoramic radiography. Often they are with the impacted tooth. Since compound-type odontomas have good morphodifferentiation, radiopaque masses can be observed as tooth-like formations, while complex-type odontomas are observed as an accumulation of calcified masses ([22], p. 378).

Although ameloblastic fibromas are benign, mixed odontogenic tumors, they are generally seen as uniocular or multilocular radiolucencies, which are rounded, surrounded by sclerotic margins and associated with the impacted tooth crown ([1], p. 381). Odontogenic mycosoma is a benign odontogenic tumor affecting the jaws.

Plain radiographs and panoramic radiographs are frequently preferred in the diagnosis of hard tissue pathologies in the dentoalveolar region. It is usually seen in a multilocular, spherical form on the panoramic radiography. Its most prominent radiological feature is that it gives an image in the form of "soap bubbles" or "honeycomb" [24].

Sementoblastoma is a benign neoplasm that is frequently seen in the posterior region of the mandible, related to the tooth root. It is seen radiographically that a speckled radiopaque mass surrounds the resorbed tooth root ([22], p. 387).

Cherubism is an autosomal dominant disorder and is a rare fibro-osseous disorder that causes bilateral swelling of the bones in early childhood. Cherubism is usually in the form of bilateral multilocular radiolucencies and is mostly seen in the mandible. It often starts from the angulus mandible and extends into the ramus and corpus [25].

As a result, panoramic radiographs have an important place in the diagnosis and post-operative follow-up of pericoronal lesions, while more advanced imaging methods are preferred for the precise determination of the localization and contour of the lesion, evaluation of invasion into the soft tissue and treatment planning [26].

5.10 Panoramic Radiology: Maxillofacial Trauma

Panoramic radiography has an important role in the diagnosis of suspected jaw fractures, including teeth, and in the evaluation of corpus mandible and angulus mandible fractures. However, panoramic radiographs should not be considered for the diagnosis of temporomandibular joint and condyle head fractures. Diagnosis of maxillary

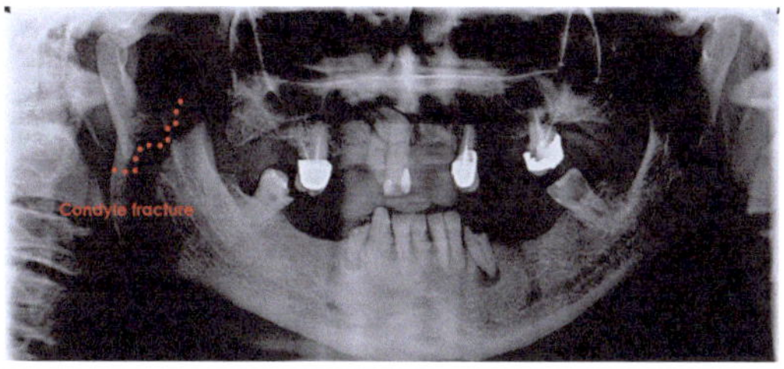

Fig. 5.27 Panoramic image showing condylar fracture

trauma should be supported by computed tomography in addition to panoramic radiography. Although panoramic radiography is useful in demonstrating changes in teeth and alveolar bone, computed tomography is better in evaluating the maxilla (Fig. 5.27).

Panoramic radiography in maxillofacial surgery is helpful in the presence of the following situations;

1. Examination of impacted teeth,
2. Mandible and tooth fractures,
3. In maxillofacial cysts and tumors,
4. In the evaluation of jaw pathologies ([3], p. 155).

Impacted teeth forming a predisposing factor to mandibular fracture;

Many researchers have confirmed that impacted third molar teeth are a risk factor for angulus mandible fractures. Ma'aita and Alwrikat examined 615 panoramic radiographs with mandibular fractures, whether there was a relationship between mandibular fracture and the presence, absence and degree of impaction of the third molar teeth. Angulus mandible fracture was found in 127 of 426 maxillofacial trauma patients with impacted teeth. As a result of the study, the incidence of mandibular fracture was found to be more common in cases where third molar teeth were present than in cases where it was not [27].

In a retrospective study of Meisami et al. Performed on 413 panoramic films, they encountered mandibular fractures in 214 patients. As a result of the study, it was observed that people with embedded third molar were exposed to mandibular fracture 3 times more and it was more common in men than women [28].

Blaeser et al. examined the injury of the n. alveolaris inferior after the extraction of the third molar tooth in a study on panoramic radiography. In the study, eight patients who faced nerve injury after tooth extraction and 17 control patients without nerve injury were compared.

As a result of the study, it was revealed that n.alveolaris inferior injury was more common after impacted third molar tooth extraction in patients with deviations in the canalis alveolaris inferior on the panoramic film and the roots of the third molar teeth appear dark [29].

Sometimes, even in the presence of minor traumas, mandibular fractures can occur due to pathologies such as cysts and tumors that weaken the mandibular bone. Although panoramic radiography helps us about possible diagnoses of pathology, histopathological examination is required for definitive diagnosis. Another factor that causes mandibular fracture may be foreign bodies such as bullets ([3], p. 164).

5.11 Panoramic Radiography: Diagnosis of Systemic Diseases

Atheroma plaques are plaques formed by fat substances, cholesterol, thrombocytes, cell debris, and calcium in the inner layer of carotid and coronary arteries. Plaques within the carotid artery are clinically asymptomatic and subsequently cause late onset of cerebrovascular and cardiovascular disorders.

Atherosclerotic lesions present in the carotid bifurcation area are seen in the lower corners of the panoramic radiography, near the cervical vertebra and hyoid bone. Atheroma plaques are seen on radiography as radiopaque nodular masses or as double radiopaque lines in the neck region. These calcifications are seen in the lower margin of the third or fourth vertebra, approximately 1.5–2.5 cm inferior-posterior part of the angulus mandible. These lesions affect 3–5% of the general dental population. While calcifications in the carotid artery are seen in the lateral parts of the cervical vertebrae, thyroid gland calcifications and epiglottis are seen superposed on the vertebra in the midline.

Freidlander et al. investigated the relationship between the prevalence of atheroma plaques and sleep apnea patients. Atheroma plaque formation occurs as a result of hypoxia in patients with sleep apnea syndrome (Fig. 5.28).

The central nervous system is stimulated and the sympathetic nervous system is activated due to hypoxia. As a result of hypertension, the vessel wall is fragmented and permeability is impaired. During hypoxia, thrombocytes are activated and progress to the fragmented vessel wall and accordingly, growth factors are activated and cause the growth of the muscles in the vessel wall. Due to hypoxia, low-density lipoproteins move towards the damaged vessel wall as oxidized and are swallowed by macrophages.

Macrophages and smooth muscle cells in the damaged vessel wall subsequently cause atheroma plaque formation, as a result, calcium salts are absorbed by the lesion and observed in panoramic radiography [30].

If the dentist suspects calcifications under the mandibular angle, in the panoramic radiography, they should inform the patient, considering that this may be an atheroma plaque, and consultation with the patient's doctor should be made due to the risk of heart attack or ischemia [31].

In hyperparathyroidism where parathyroid hormone levels are above normal values, osteoporosis, weakening or disappearance of the lamina wall surrounding the teeth, as well as unilocular or multilocular cystic radiolucencies, which are called brown tumors, are present in panoramic radiography, which are called brown tumors, are present in panoramic radiography [32, 33].

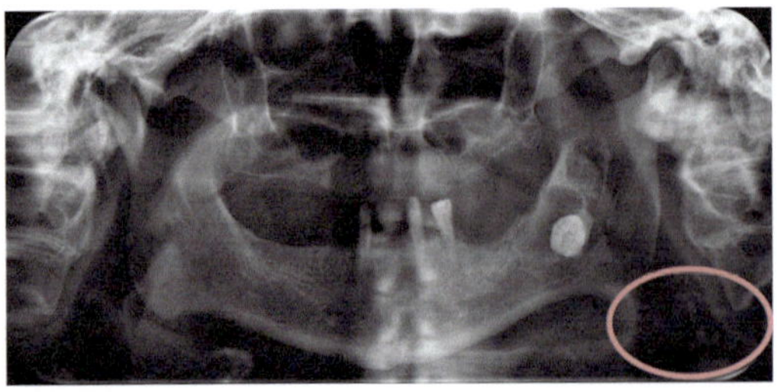

Fig. 5.28 Panoramic image showing carotid artery calcification

Tuberculosis is a specific infection caused by mycobacterium tuberculosis. It is rare for tuberculosis to affect the oral tissues, but it occurs as a result of direct oral inoculation of the bacteria. In cases where this infection affects the jaws, it is seen that patients have persistent toothache-like pain attacks and swelling in the affected area. When it involves the temporomandibular joint, trismus is seen. However, calcifications are seen in the cervical lymph nodes on panoramic radiography.

It is rare for cancers to metastasize to the jaws, and the most metastasis originates from the lung, prostate, breast, and kidneys. Metastasis affects either the soft tissues in the oral area, the jaw bones, or both. The mandibular molar region is the most common metastatic region.

Oral region cancers cause local pain, swelling, numbness, paresthesia in the jaws and lips, and loss of teeth. The radiographic picture of this condition changes depending on the balance between osteoblastic and osteoclastic activity. While osteoblastic lesions usually occur in metastasis caused by prostate cancer, on the other hand, more osteolytic lesions are seen in kidney, lung, and breast metastases. Lesions in the mandible are generally seen as "moth-eaten." Resorption is observed in the cortex in areas adjacent to the lesion, such as the mandibular canal, maxillary sinus, and base of the nose [34].

As a result, although panoramic radiography is useful in the diagnosis of systemic diseases, it is of great importance for the dentist to be able to see the changes caused by systemic diseases in panoramic radiography. Early diagnosis of such conditions is of great importance in terms of providing the necessary treatment and increasing the quality of life of the patient.

5.12 Panoramic Radiology and Oncology

Dental oncology is a focus of dentistry dedicated to meet the unique dental and oral health care needs that arise as a result of cancer therapy. It is an area of oral medicine devoted to improving the well-being and quality of life of people battling cancer.

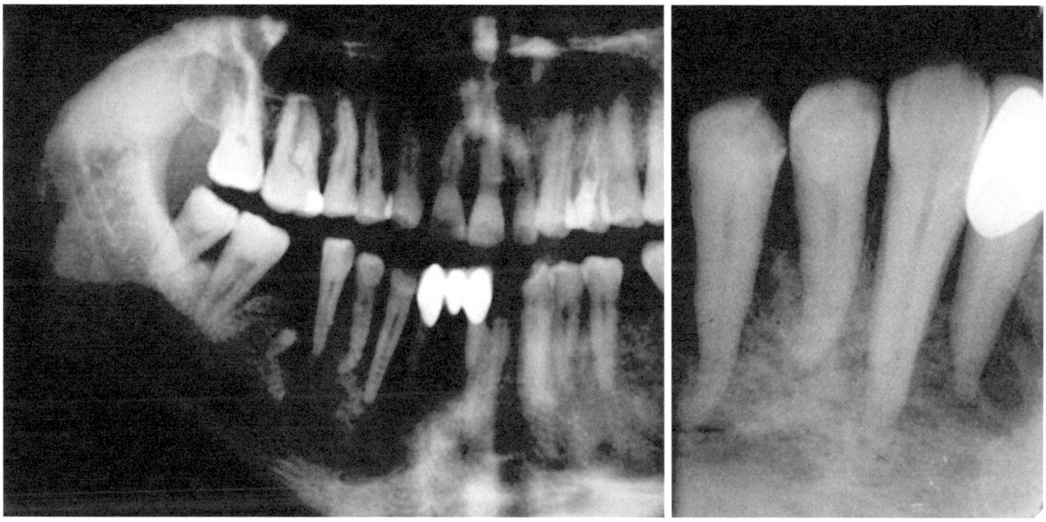

Fig. 5.29 Panoramic and intraoral periapical images showing a prostate cancer metastasis to the mandible

Panoramic radiology plays a role as an important factor in supporting oncological dentistry practice. Panoramic radiography is not only for diagnosing malignancies;

1. Preparing the oral cavity before chemotherapy and radiotherapy to reduce and prevent complications that may occur,
2. Early diagnosis of complications in the maxillofacial region as a result of cancer treatment,
3. It has an important place in the diagnosis of recurrent cancers in the maxillofacial region [35].

Oncological dentistry is a branch of dentistry that deals with the oral and dental health of individuals who have been treated for cancer, especially chemotherapy and radiotherapy.

5.12.1 Oncological Approach

- Before cancer treatment, to ensure that oral health is ready against potential side effects that may occur due to treatment,
- Educating sick individuals against complications that may occur in the face of short- and long-term treatment,
- Providing the necessary oral hygiene training for patients to protect their oral health,
- It has responsibilities such as keeping the patient under follow-up for a long time due to the possibility of cancer recurrence after treatment ([3], p. 183).

Panoramic radiography is a key diagnostic tool for the oncological dentist (Fig. 5.29). It makes an important contribution to the initial diagnosis of maxillofacial cancers. Panoramic radiography is preferred over intraoral radiographs because the oral cavity of individuals undergoing cancer treatment can be extremely sensitive and painful due to chemotherapy and radiotherapy [36].

References

1. Whaites E. Essentials of dental radiography and radiology. 3rd ed. China: Elsevier Science; 2002.
2. Kathariya MD, Nikam AP, Chopra K, Patil NN, Raheja H, Kathariya R. Prevalence of dental anomalies among school going children in India. J Int Oral Health. 2013;5:10–4.
3. Farman AG. Panoramic radiology. New York: Springer; 2007.
4. Köşger H, Konarılı M, Ay S. Taurodontizm (vaka raporu). Atatürk Üniv Diş Hek Fak Derg. 2003;13(2):51–5.

5. Patil S, Doni B, Kaswan S, Rahman F. Prevalence of dental anomalies in Indian population. J Clin Exp Dent. 2013;5(4):e183–6.
6. Neves FS, Souza TC, Almeida SM, Haiter-Neto F, Freitas DQ, Boscolo FN. Correlation of panoramic radiography and cone beam CT findings in the assessment of the relationship between impacted mandibular third molars and the mandibular canal. Dentomaxillofacial Radiol. 2012;41:553–7.
7. English JD, Peltomaki T, Pham-Litscel K. Mosby's orthodontic review. St. Louis, MO: Mosby; 2009.
8. Quintero JC, Trosien A, Hatcher D, Kapila S. Craniofacial imaging in orthodontics: historical perspective, current status, and future developments. Angle Orthod. 1999;69(6):491–506.
9. Kim MS, Yoon SJ, Park HW, Kang JH, Yang SY, Moon YH, diğerleri. A false presence of bifid mandibular canals in panoramic radiographs. Dentomaxillofac Radiol. 2011;40:434–8.
10. Haghnegahdar AA, Bronoosh P, Khojastepour L, Tahmassebi P. Prevalence of bifid mandibular condyle in a selected population in south of Iran. J Dent Shiraz Univ Med Sci. 2014;15(4):156–60.
11. Correr GM, Iwanko D, Leonardi DP, Ulbrich LM, de Araújo MR, Deliberador TM. Classification of bifid mandibular canals using cone beam computed tomography. Braz Oral Res. 2013;27(6):510–6.
12. Orhan K, Aksoy S, Bilecenoglu B, Sakul BU, Paksoy CS. Evaluation of bifid mandibular canals with cone-beam computed tomography in a Turkish adult population: a retrospective study. Surg Radiol Anat. 2011;33:501–7.
13. Orhan K, İçen M, Aksoy S, Ozan O, Berberoğlu A. Cone-beam CT evaluation of morphology, location, and course of mandibular incisive canal: considerations for implant treatment. Oral Radiol. 2014;30(1):64–75. https://doi.org/10.1007/s11282-013-0138-0.
14. Mathew LA, Sholapurkar AA, Pai KM. Maxillary sinus findings in the elderly: a panoramic radiographic study. J Contemp Dent Pract. 2009;10(6):E041–8.
15. Orhan K, Kocyigit D, Turkoglu K, Kartal Y, Arslan A. Aspergillosis of maxillary sinus in immunocompromised patient: case report. N Y State Dent J. 2012;78(1):46–9.
16. Molander B, Ahlqwist M, Grondahl HG, Hollender L. Comparison of panoramic and intraoral radiography for the diagnosis of caries and periapical pathology. Dentomaxillofac Radiol. 1993;22:28–32.
17. Farah CS, Savage NV. Pericoronal radiolucencies and the significance of early detection. Aust Dent J. 2002;47(3):262–5.
18. Gonzalez SM, Spalding PM, Payne JB, Giannini PJ. A dentigerous cyst associated with bilaterally impacted mandibular canines in a girl: a case report. J Med Case Rep. 2011;5:230.
19. Kasat VO, Karjodkar FR, Laddha RS. Dentigerous cyst associated with an ectopic third molar in the maxillary sinus: a case report and review of literature. Contemp Clin Dent. 2012;3(3):373–6.
20. Srivatsan KS, Kumar V, Mahendra A, Singh P. Bilateral keratocystic odontogenic tumor: A report of two cases. Natl J Maxillofac Surg. 2014;5(1):86–9.
21. Paikkatt VJ, Sreedharan S, Kannan VP. Unicystic ameloblastoma of the maxilla: a case report. J Indian Soc Pedod Prev Dent. 2007;25(2):106–10.
22. White SC, Pharoah MJ. Oral radiology: principles and interpretation. St. Louis: Mosby/Elsevier; 2009.
23. More CB, Das S, Gupta S, Bhavsar K. Mandibular adenomatoid odontogenic tumor: radiographic and pathologic correlation. J Nat Sci Biol Med. 2013;4(2):457–62.
24. Friedrich RE, Scheuer HA, Fuhrmann A, Zustın J, Assaf AT. Radiographic findings of odontogenic Myxomas on conventional radiographs. Anticancer Res. 2012;32:2173–8.
25. Wagel J, Łuczak K, Hendrich B, Guziński M, Sąsiadek M. Clinical and radiological features of nonfamilial cherubism: a case report. Pol J Radiol. 2012;77(3):53–7.
26. More C, Tailor M, Patel HJ, Asrani M, Thakkar K, Adalja V. Radiographic analysis of ameloblastoma: a retrospective study. Indian J Dent. 2012;23:698.
27. Maaita J, Alwrikat A. Is the mandibular third molar a risk factor for mandibular angle fracture? Oral Surg Oral Med Oral Pathol Oral Radiol Endod. 2000;89:143–6.
28. Meisami T, Sojat A, Sandor GKB, Lawrence HP, Clokie CML. Impacted third molars and risk of angle fracture. J Oral Maxillofac Surg. 2002;31:140–4.
29. Blaeser BF, August MA, Donoff RB, Kaban LB, Dodson TB. Panoramic radiographic risk factors for inferior alveolar nerve injury after third molar extraction. J Oral Maxillofac Surg. 2003;61(4):417–21.
30. Friedlander AH, Altman L. Carotid artery atheromas in postmenopausal women. Their prevalence on panoramic radiographs and their relationship to atherogenic risk factors. J Am Dent Assoc. 2001;132:1130–6.
31. Barkhuysen R, Berge SJ, van Damme PA. Non ordinary radiopacity on a panoramic radiograph. Ned Tijdschr Tandheelkd. 2006;113:148–9.
32. Morano S, Cipriani R, Gabriele A, Medici F, Pantellini F. Recurrent Brown tumors as initial manifestation of primary hyperparathyroidism. An unusual presentation. Minerva Med. 2000;91:117–22.
33. Ganibegovic M. Dental radiographic changes in chronic renal diseases. Med Arh. 2000;54:115–8.
34. Kumar GS, Manjunatha BS. Metastatic tumors to the jaws and oral cavity. J Oral Maxillofac Pathol. 2013;17(1):71–5.
35. Huber MA, Terezhalmy GT. The head and neck radiation oncology patient. Quintessence Int. 2003;34(9):693–717.
36. Marsiglia H, Haie-Meder C, Sasso G, Mamelle G, Gerbaulet A. Brachytherapy for T1-T2 floor-of-the-mouth cancers: the Gustave-Roussy institute experience. Int J Radiat Oncol Biol Phys. 2002;52(5):1257–63.

Cephalometric Radiography

6

Athina Chatzigianni

6.1 Basic Principles and Interpretation

In the medical and dental science, radiographic examination of patients' bony, dental, and soft tissue structures has been an important diagnostic adjunct tool to clinical examination to reach a final diagnostic assessment of a disease or condition. Many radiographic techniques have been proposed, with divergent outcome, depending on the target structures under investigation and the orientation of the head to the X-ray beam.

The first X-ray images of the whole skull in a standardized lateral view were taken in 1922 by Pacini and Carrera [1]. Pacini's method consisted of a large, fixed distance from the X-ray source to the cassette. Cephalometric radiography gained full acceptance in 1931, when Broadbent [2] in the USA and at the same time Hofrath [3] in Germany introduced radiographic films of the head, taken under standardized conditions. The method consisted of mounting film, positioning the subject and setting the X-ray source in a fixed standardized reproducible position.

A. Chatzigianni (✉)
Department of Orthodontics, Faculty of Dentistry, Aristotle University of Thessaloniki, Thessaloniki, Greece
e-mail: achatzigianni@dent.auth.gr

By means of a standardized cephalometric radiograph, it was possible to study the craniofacial skeleton through time. The craniofacial growth changes in the size and shape of craniofacial skeleton and soft tissue with age could be studied [4]. In 1988, cephalometry was defined by Moyers [5] as a radiographic technique for converting the human skull into a measurable geometric shape.

Moreover, craniofacial variation within a population sample of same or different ethnic origin could be analyzed and anatomical differences between males and females could been examined. For example, the comparison of the craniofacial morphology between the sexes showed that on average, the cranium was significantly smaller in women than in men, except as regard to the nasal bone, the foramen magnum and the inner orbital distance. Regarding the cranial shape a more prominent frontal bone and a less prominent nasal bone were found for females. The average sex determined shape differences revealed that the female skull is significantly smaller than the male [6].

Cephalometric radiographs are also indicated for cephalometric tracing of anatomical structures and have a significant importance in the field of orthodontics and in orthodontic and orthognathic treatment planning. For many decades cephalometry has been one of the main diagnostic tools available to the orthodontist. A variety of cephalometric analysis applied on

A. Delantoni, K. Orhan (eds.), *Atlas of Dentomaxillofacial Anatomical Imaging*,
https://doi.org/10.1007/978-3-030-96840-3_6

cephalometric radiographs have been proposed throughout the years with the aim to describe the dental, skeletal, and facial characteristics of patients. Relationships between teeth, bone, and soft tissue based on cephalometric anatomic landmarks are being analyzed according to many different methods. It has been widely used for the identification and measurement of the craniofacial structures, not only in patients with normal craniofacial development, but also in patients with deviated craniofacial shape. With the use of cephalometric radiographs, the comparison of a patient's dentofacial relationships with a normal reference group of the same racial or ethnic groups was possible, while deviations from norms are revealed. Cephalometric radiographs are used to evaluate the craniofacial complex, dentofacial proportions, malocclusion, soft tissue, and the changes related to growth or treatment, all of which are crucial for orthodontic treatment planning and evaluation.

To obtain cephalometric radiographs, ear rods are used to prevent the rotation of the head about the vertical, sagittal, and transverse axes. Additionally, a nasal stabilizer may be used to prevent the nose from rotating about the transverse axis [2, 7]. Despite all those, a slight rotation of the head may be inevitable and occur, despite the technical configuration. Thus a major limitation of cephalometric radiography is the difficulty in the correct and reproducible position of the head. In the limitations the identification of landmarks due to the superimposition of anatomical structures or poor radiographic quality are included, and also the exposure of patient to radiation [8–12]. Another concern arises in cases where the size of an anatomic structure is calculated, or angular or linear measurements are applied. It is essential to know whether the measurements accurately reflect the true dimensions of the object and, if not, whether the error can be calculated and corrected. The standardized film-object distance eliminates the problem of magnification errors, while the incorporation of a ruler in the radiograph is a common method to control magnification levels.

Moreover, it is worth mentioning that there are inherent limitations in two-dimensional (2D) radiographic projections: magnification, distortion, superimposition, and misrepresentation of anatomic structures [13]. Recently, the validity of 2D cephalometry was examined and it was found that scientific evidence on the usefulness of this radiograph technique in orthodontics is still lacking [14].

The traditional cephalometric radiographs provide a partial description of the overall craniofacial shape, due to the 2D projection of a three-dimensional (3D) object. Unfortunately, despite the wide acceptance and use of 2D cephalometric imaging, it seems that much information of the 3D anatomic elements is missing, while detailed description of anatomic structures is not possible. To solve the above-mentioned problems the transition from 2D to 3D cephalometry has been introduced [15, 16].

Computed tomography (CT) and cone beam computed tomography (CBCT) are available to provide a 3D reconstruction of the craniofacial complex, nevertheless, their application in dentistry and orthodontics has been limited until now in the everyday practice, mainly because of cost and dose considerations compared to traditional radiography [13]. It is however of no doubt that advances in 3D software have led to actual 3D imaging and measurements becoming a reality.

Despite the limitations of cephalometric radiographs, the deep knowledge of the craniofacial anatomical structures that can be identified in different cephalograms is of great importance for the interpretation of the images, as well as for the identification of anatomic landmarks and proper cephalometric analysis by the clinicians. Through knowledge of the anatomy of the skull and the comprehension of the radiographic appearance of each structure, which are described below, errors in the identification of each anatomical cephalometric point will be minimized [17].

6.2 Cephalometric Radiographic Anatomy

6.2.1 Lateral Cephalometric Radiograph

Lateral cephalometric radiographs (Fig. 6.1) are taken with the X-ray beam perpendicular to the midsagittal plane of the patients' skull and the midsagittal plane in turn parallel to the radiographic film. Many different distances between the X-ray source, patients' head, and film cassette have been introduced for enlargement compensation, however, the most widely used distance between the X-ray source and the patient's midsagittal plane is around 150 cm, while the distance between the midsagittal plane and the film is 13–15 cm [18–20].

The lateral cephalometric radiograph is providing information of the craniofacial skeleton in the sagittal and vertical plane. In short, the application of lateral cephalometric analysis and cephalometric tracing can contribute to the following:

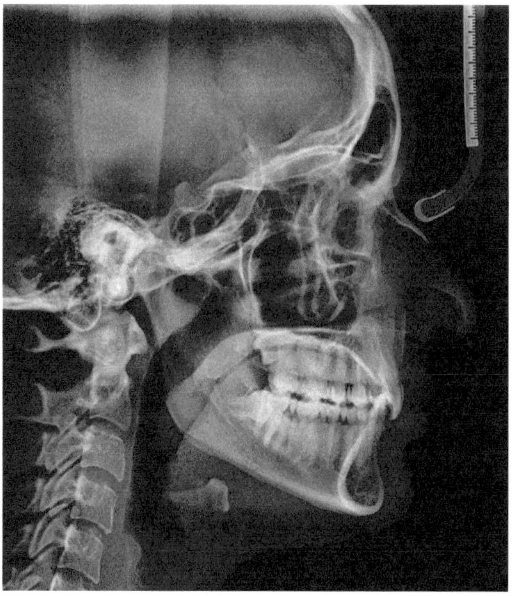

Fig. 6.1 Lateral cephalometric radiograph

1. Study of craniofacial growth in the sagittal and vertical dimension.
2. Study of the soft tissue in the sagittal and vertical dimension.
3. Study of upper airways, sinuses and tongue.
4. Establishment of lateral cephalometric norms specific for a group of people.
5. Study of the craniofacial differences between genders or between people of different racial/ethnic origin.
6. Study on the ageing of the craniofacial skeleton and the soft tissue in the sagittal and vertical dimension.
7. Diagnosis of malocclusions, craniofacial anomalies, and skeletal deformities in the sagittal and vertical dimension.
8. Orthodontic and orthognathic treatment planning of sagittal and vertical problems.
9. Evaluation of orthodontic treatment results on the hard and soft tissue.
10. Skeletal age assessment with the analysis of cervical vertebrae.
11. Detections of abnormalities of the skull or spine.

    By means of lateral radiographs many unilateral, midline or bilateral anatomic structures can be depicted. It is of great importance to understand that bilateral anatomic structures will be seen as one single projection of the two anatomic parts. In many cases, two lines can be seen, which represent the contour of the two bilateral elements, either due to inherent asymmetry between the two parts or due to head rotation in the cephalostat.

The position of the patient in a natural head position, with natural bite, natural lip seal, physiologic rest, and good head orientation can help visualize anatomy of the cranium, joint and soft tissue. Essentially two main components are necessary for description on lateral cephalometric radiographs, i.e., the hard tissue, where the bony elements and the denture are included, and the soft tissue together with the sinuses, airways, and nerve canals.

6.2.1.1 Hard Tissue Anatomic Elements

The most important hard tissue anatomic structures that can be identified on a lateral cephalometric radiograph can be divided in the following categories (Fig. 6.2a):

- Cranial and upper facial anatomic structures.

1. *Frontal bone*: a bone of the skull that forms the forehead and the superior part of the orbits. It has an inner (1a) and an outer (1b) cortical plate.
2. *Nasal bones*: The *nasal bones* are two small, symmetrical bones in the midline, which form the bridge of the nose. On the lateral cephalometric radiograph, only one of the two nasal bones can be depicted.
3. *Ethmoid bone*: The ethmoid bony complex is located between the two orbits and on the lateral cephalometric radiograph it is located superiorly to the nasal cavity, separating it from the brain.
4. *Cribriform plate*: It consists of a lot of small foramina located between the anterior cranial fossa and the nasal cavity.
5. *Anterior cranial base*: it extents anteriorly to the posterior wall of the frontal sinus and posteriorly to the planum sphenoidale and the anterior clinoid process. It forms the floor of anterior cranial fossa, the roof of the nasal cavity, the roof of the frontal sinus, the roof of the ethmoid and sphenoid sinus, and the roof of the orbits.
6. *Middle cranial base:* it extends from the anterior cranial base to the dorsum sellae.
7. *Posterior cranial base*: it extends from the dorsum sellae to the occipital bone.
8. *Planum sphenoidale*: it is the part of the anterior cranial base that forms the roof of the sphenoid sinus and lies anterior to the anterior clinoid process.
9. *Anterior clinoid process*: it is one of the two bony projections of the lesser wings of the

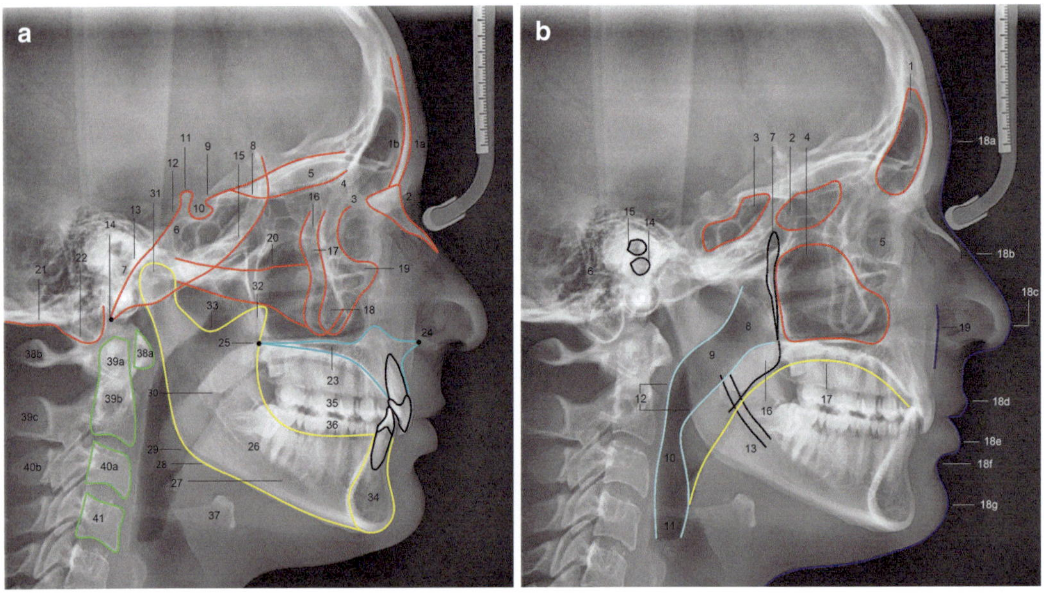

Fig. 6.2 (**a**) Identification of the most important skeletal and dental anatomic parts on the lateral cephalometric radiograph and (**b**) recognition of the main non-hard tissue elements of the craniofacial complex. Numbering corresponds to the text. (Images were created by Dr. Athina Chatzigianni with the use of Viewbox 4 Software (dHAL Software, Kifissia, Greece) [28])

sphenoid bone. It is the border between the anterior and middle cranial base and fossa.

10. *Sella Turcica*: it is the pituitary fossa, where the pituitary gland is located. It has a curved shape and its boarders are the anterior and posterior clinoid process.
11. *Posterior clinoid process*: together with the anterior clinoid process it surrounds the sella turcica. It is one of the two tubercles of the dorsum sellae.
12. *Dorsum sellae*: it is a part of the sphenoid bone and is located posterior to the sella turcica.
13. *Clivus*: it is a bony surface between the dorsum sellae and the foramen magnum and is seen as a straight line sloping downwards and backwards.
14. *Anterior border of foramen magnum*: it is the anterior border of the opening in the occipital bone of the *skull.*
15. *Greater wings of the sphenoid*: these are bony processes of the sphenoid bone.
16. *Zygomatic process of frontal bone:* it articulates inferiorly with the frontal process of the zygomatic bone through the zygomaticofrontal suture.
17. *Frontal process of zygomatic bone*: it articulates superiorly with the zygomatic process of the frontal bone through the zygomaticofrontal suture.
18. *Maxillary process of zygomatic bone*: it articulates inferiorly with the maxilla and forms the orbital surface of the maxilla.
19. *Orbital rim*: it is the cyclic bony margin surrounding the orbit.
20. *Zygomatic arch*: *it is a horizontal* bone at the side of the head around the maxilla and is figured posteriorly to the orbit and zygomatic bone.
21. *Occipital bone*: it is the bone posterior to the foramen magnum and the mastoid process.
22. *Mastoid process*: it is the lower bony projection of the occipital bone.

- Maxillary anatomic structures.

23. *Hard palate (floor of nasal cavity)*: it is the line that separates the oral cavity from the nasal cavities and the maxillary sinuses and extents from the anterior nasal spine to the posterior nasal spine.
24. *Anterior nasal spine*: it is the most anterior point of the hard palate in the midline.
25. *Posterior nasal spine*: it is the most posterior point of the hard palate in the midline.

- Mandibular anatomic structures.

26. *Mandible*: it is also referred as lower jaw and is the only mobile bone of the craniofacial complex, which articulates with the skull through the temporomandibular joint. It consists of a body, two rami, two condyles, two coronoid processes, two gonial angles, and one symphysis. In the lateral cephalometric radiograph only one projection of the bilateral structures is identified, except in cases of mandibular asymmetries or incorrect head position in the cephalostat, where two borders of each bilateral mandibular bone element could be present on the radiograph.
27. *Body of the mandible*: it is also called mandibular body and is the horizontal part of the bone extending to the mandibular angles bilaterally.
28. *Antegonial notch*: it is a concavity of the lower border of the mandible, anteriorly to the gonial angle.
29. *Gonial angle of the mandible*: it is also called mandibular angle and it describes the angle formed by the lower border of the mandibular body with the posterior border of the ramus.
30. *Ramus of the mandible*: the mandibular bone has two rami. Each of them includes the mandibular nerve canal and has two processes, the condylar and coronoid process.

31. *Condyle*: it is the part of the mandible that articulates with the skull in the temporomandibular junction.
32. *Coronoid process*: it is the process of the mandible, which is located mesially to the condyle.
33. *Sigmoid notch of mandible*: it is a deep concavity in the upper border of the mandible, which is surrounded by the condyle and the coronoid process.
34. *Symphysis*: it is the most mesial and lower part of the mandible and includes an external cortical plate and an internal cortical plate.

- Dental elements.

35. *Upper dentition*: it describes the teeth of the upper jaw (maxilla).
36. *Lower dentition*: it describes the teeth of the lower jaw.

- Neck skeleton.

37. *Hyoid bone*: it is located inferiorly and posteriorly to the mandibular bone at the height of the third and fourth cervical vertebra.
38. *first cervical vertebra (atlas)*: it is an atypical cervical vertebra located radiographically below the mastoid process and posteriorly to the mandibular ramus. The anterior arch (38a) and the posterior arch (38b) of atlas are seen on the radiograph.
39. *second cervical vertebra (axis)*: it is an atypical vertebra located below the atlas. Radiographically a vertical process (odontoid process) (39a), a body (39b), and a spinous process (39c) can be identified. The odontoid process of axis (dens) is a large vertical projection of the second cervical vertebra and is seen on the radiograph to intersect with the body of the first cervical vertebra.
40. *third cervical vertebra*: it is a typical vertebra, located between the second and fourth cervical vertebra. Radiographically the body (40a) and the spinous process (40b) can be identified.
41. *fourth cervical vertebra*: it is atypical vertebra like the third cervical vertebra.

6.2.1.2 Soft Tissue and Other Anatomic Elements

The soft tissue together with the sinuses, the air cavities, the tubes, and the nerve canals that can be identified on a lateral cephalometric radiograph are shown in Fig. 6.2b.

- Paranasal sinuses. There are four pairs of air spaces in the craniofacial complex. There are two frontal sinuses, two ethmoid sinuses, two sphenoid sinuses, and two maxillary sinuses:

1. *Frontal sinus*: There are two frontal sinuses in the frontal bone. In the lateral cephalometric radiograph, the projection of the two sinuses is seen as one air chamber located superiorly to the nasal bone.
2. *Ethmoid sinus*: There are two ethmoid sinuses, which can be better seen on the anteroposterior cephalometric radiograph around the nose. On the lateral cephalometric radiograph only one of the two ethmoid sinuses can be seen posteriorly to the orbit, superiorly to the zygomatic arch and inferiorly to the anterior cranial fossa.
3. *Sphenoid sinus*: There are two large sphenoid sinuses in the sphenoid bone. On the lateral cephalometric radiograph, the projection of the two sinuses can be seen as one sphenoid sinus, which lies inferior to the sella turcica and between the dorsum sellae and the greater wings of sphenoid bone.
4. *Maxillary sinus*: There are two maxillary sinuses in the maxillary bone, and these are the largest of the paranasal sinuses. On the lateral cephalometric radiograph, the projection of the two sinuses can be seen as one large air cavity, which is surrounded by the hard palate, the orbit, the floor of the ethmoid sinus, and the pterygomaxillary fissure.

- Cavities.

5. *Orbit:* it is a bony cavity (socket) of elliptical shape, where the eyeball is enclosed.
6. *Mastoid air cells*: these are tiny air cavities within the mastoid process of the cranium.

7. *Pterygomaxillary fissure*: it is a vertical opening on the lateral cephalometric radiograph, just above and posteriorly to the posterior nasal spine and the soft palate. It is a bilateral opening and the midline between the two shadows should be traced.

- Upper airways. They are the air passages, which start from the nasal cavity and end up to the larynx:

8. *Nasopharynx*: it is the nasopharyngeal airway area and is the most superior part of the pharynx, which starts radiographically posterior to the nasal cavity and maxillary sinus and ends to the height of the hard and soft palate.
9. *Velopharynx*: it extends from the posterior part of the hard palate to the posterior pharyngeal wall.
10. *Oropharynx*: it is the part of the airways that is located between the soft palate to the superior border of the epiglottis.
11. *Laryngopharynx:* it is in the inferior part of the pharynx and is extended to the sixth cervical vertebra.
12. *Pharynx wall*: Radiographically the anterior and posterior pharyngeal walls are seen.

- Nerve canals.

13. *Mandibular nerve canal*: there are two nerve canals, which are located within the mandibular bodies and include the inferior alveolar nerve, artery, and vein. Each nerve canal can be perceived on the radiograph as two distinguished lines running through the mandibular body.
14. *External auditory meatus*: it is a bony canal of sigmoid shape, which starts from the outer surface of the head. It has a cyclic shape and is located posteriorly and superiorly to the mandibular condyle on the cephalogram.
15. *Internal auditory meatus*: it is a canal starting from the internal acoustic porous. It has a cyclic shape and is located superiorly to the external auditory meatus on the cephalogram.

- Soft tissue and muscles.

16. *Soft palate*: it is comprised by muscles and connective tissue and lies posteriorly to the hard palate.
17. *Tongue dorsum*: it is the upper surface of the tongue and can be seen as a concave line inferior to the hard palate, starting from the front teeth and ending to the hyoid bone.
18. *Soft tissue profile*: This is the patient's profile marking of the soft tissue that surrounds the craniofacial complex. The soft tissue of the forehead, the nose bridge, the tip of nose, the upper and lower lip, the labiomental fold and the chin are shown (a to g respectively).
19. *Cheek*: it is the patient's fleshy part of the face below the eye.

6.2.2 Posteroanterior Cephalometric Radiography

Posteroanterior cephalometric radiographs (Fig. 6.3a) are taken with the X-ray beam perpendicular to the coronal plane of the patient's skull. The source of the X-ray beam is behind the patient's head, and the film in front of the patient's face, with the forehead and nose against the cassette [21, 22]. The patient's canthomeatal line forms a 10-degree angle with the horizontal plane and the Frankfurt plane is perpendicular to the image receptor [23].

The posteroanterior cephalogram (PAC) analysis and tracing may provide information on bilateral anatomic structures in the transverse and vertical plane and could be used in the following applications:

1. Study of craniofacial growth in the transverse and vertical dimension.
2. Study of skeletal asymmetries.
3. Study of the sinuses bilaterally.
4. Establishment of posteroanterior cephalometric norms specific for a group of people.
5. Study of the craniofacial differences between genders or between people of different racial/ethnic origin.
6. Study on the ageing of the craniofacial skeleton.

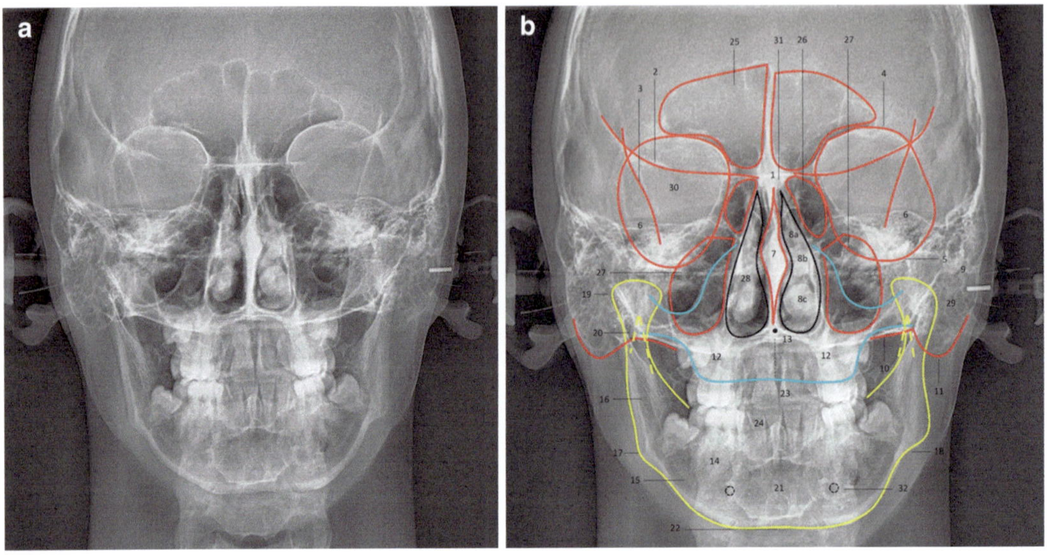

Fig. 6.3 (**a**) Posteroanterior cephalometric radiograph and (**b**) identification of the most important skeletal, dental and non-hard tissue anatomic parts. Numbering corresponds to the text. (Images were created by Dr. Athina Chatzigianni with the use of Viewbox 4 Software (dHAL Software, Kifissia, Greece) [28])

7. Diagnosis of malocclusions, craniofacial anomalies, and skeletal deformities in the transverse and vertical dimension.
8. Orthodontic and orthognathic treatment planning of transverse and vertical problems.
9. Evaluation of orthodontic treatment results on the transverse and vertical plane.

Like in the lateral cephalograms, two main components are necessary for description on posteroanterior cephalometric radiographs, i.e., the hard tissue (bone and teeth) and the non-hard tissue parts, like the sinuses and the cavities.

6.2.2.1 Hard Tissue Anatomic Elements

The hard tissue anatomic structures that can be identified on a posteroanterior cephalometric radiograph (Fig. 6.3b) can be divided in the following categories:

- Cranial and upper facial anatomic structures.

1. *Crista galli*: it is a triangular process in the midline above the ethmoid bone.
2. *Lesser wing of sphenoid:* these are two bony projections of the upper part of the sphenoid bone.
3. *Greater wings of sphenoid*: these are bony processes of the lower part of the sphenoid bone.
4. *Orbital roof*: it is the superior border of the orbit.
5. *Inferior orbital rim*: it is the inferior border of the orbit.
6. *Petrous ridge*: it is a part of the temporal bone separating the anterior from the middle cranial fossa.
7. *Nasal septum*: it is a vertical line dividing the two nasal cavities.
8. *Nasal conchae*: these are three bony projections of the lateral wall of the nasal cavity. They are divided in superior (a), middle (b), and inferior (c) nasal conche.
9. *Zygomatic arch*: *it is the horizontal* bone at the side of the head and is figured bilaterally around the maxilla.
10. *Occipital bone*: it forms the base of skull and can be seen radiographically at the level of the maxillary bone.
11. *Mastoid process*: the same as in lateral cephalogram, it is the lower bony projection of the occipital bone.

- Maxillary anatomic structures.

12. *Maxilla*: it is the upper jaw formed by the two maxillary bones, which are fused together through the intermaxillary suture.
13. *Anterior nasal spine*: it is the most anterior point in the midline where the two maxillary bones are fused.

- Mandibular anatomic structures.

14. *Mandible*: it is the lower jaw and in this radiographic image a mandibular body, two rami, two condyles, two coronoid processes, two gonial angles, and one symphysis can be detected.
15. *Body of the mandible*: it is also called mandibular body and is the horizontal part of the bone extending from the midline to the mandibular angles bilaterally.
16. *Ramus of the mandible*: two mandibular rami are present in this radiograph. Each of them includes the mandibular nerve canal and has two processes, the condylar and coronoid process.
17. *Gonial angle of the mandible*: it is also called mandibular angle and it describes the angle formed by the lower border of the mandibular body with the posterior border of the ramus.
18. *Antegonial notch*: it is a concavity of the lower border of the mandible, anteriorly to the gonial angle.
19. *Condyle*: it is the part of the mandible that articulates with the skull in the temporomandibular junction. Two condyles can be seen on the posteroanterior radiograph.
20. *Coronoid process*: it is the process of the mandible, which is located mesially to the condyle. On the posteroanterior radiograph two coronoid processes can be identified adjacent to the condyles, however, it is difficult to discern them.
21. *Symphysis*: it is radiographically located in the midline of the mandible.
22. *Mandibular midpoint*: it is the midline of the mandible.

- Dental anatomic structures.

23. *Upper dentition*: it describes the teeth of the upper jaw.
24. *Lower dentition*: it describes the teeth of the lower jaw.

6.2.2.2 Sinuses, Cavities, and Foramina

The non-hard tissue elements figured on a posteroanterior cephalogram (Fig. 6.3b) include mainly sinuses, cavities, and foramina and are described below:

- Paranasal sinuses.

25. *Frontal sinuses*: there are two frontal sinuses within the frontal bone, which are separated by a vertical line called septum.
26. *Ethmoid sinuses*: there are two ethmoid sinuses external to the nasal bone bilaterally and between the two orbits.
27. *Maxillary sinuses*: They are located laterally and slightly inferiorly to the nasal cavities.

- Cavities.

28. *Nasal cavity*: it is an air chamber in the middle of the face, which is divided in two cavities by the nasal septum.
29. *Mastoid air cells*: these are tiny air cavities within the mastoid process of the cranium.
30. *Orbit*: it is a bony cavity (socket) of elliptical shape, where the eyeball is enclosed.

- Foramina.

31. *Cribriform plate*: it is a structure pierced with small foramina between the cranial base and the nasal cavity.
32. *Mental foramen*: it is a foramen in the body of the mandible in proximity to the second premolar and is the terminal of the mandibular nerve canal.

6.2.3 Other Cephalometric Radiographic Views

Apart from the above standard cephalometric radiographs, which are being used for many years in the orthodontic and orthognathic field, various other cephalometric images have been used to examine the bones of the head from different views. Example of such views are the submentovertex and the occipitomental views of the skull, which are applied on specific occasions and mostly when fractures of craniofacial bones are suspected. Ideal head positioning for submentovertex cephalometric radiographs (SMV) involves the central X-ray starting from below the chin and being perpendicular to the midsagittal and coronal planes, while the head angulation is aimed upwards and backwards at 10-degrees angle [23]. For the occipitomental view a 30-degree angle is applied.

The main applications of submentovertex and occipitomental view in orthodontics include:

1. The determination of the long axis of the condyle. This facilitates the corrected tomography of the temporomandibular joint.
2. The measurement of mandibular length.
3. The assessment of skeletal asymmetry.
4. The evaluation of the imaged paranasal sinuses.
5. The evaluation of fractures of the imaged bones.

As seen in Fig. 6.4a, b, depending on head orientation, the following anatomic parts, most of which have been already analyzed above, can be identified on these radiographs:

1. *Frontal sinuses.*
2. *Sphenoid sinuses.*
3. *Maxillary sinuses.*
4. *Nasal cavity.*
5. *Nasal septum.*
6. *Lower orbital rim (6a) and lateral orbital wall (6b).*
7. *Zygomatic arches.*
8. *Upper dentition.*
9. *Mandible.*
10. *Body of the mandible.*
11. *Gonial angle.*
12. *Ramus of the mandible.*
13. *Condyle.*

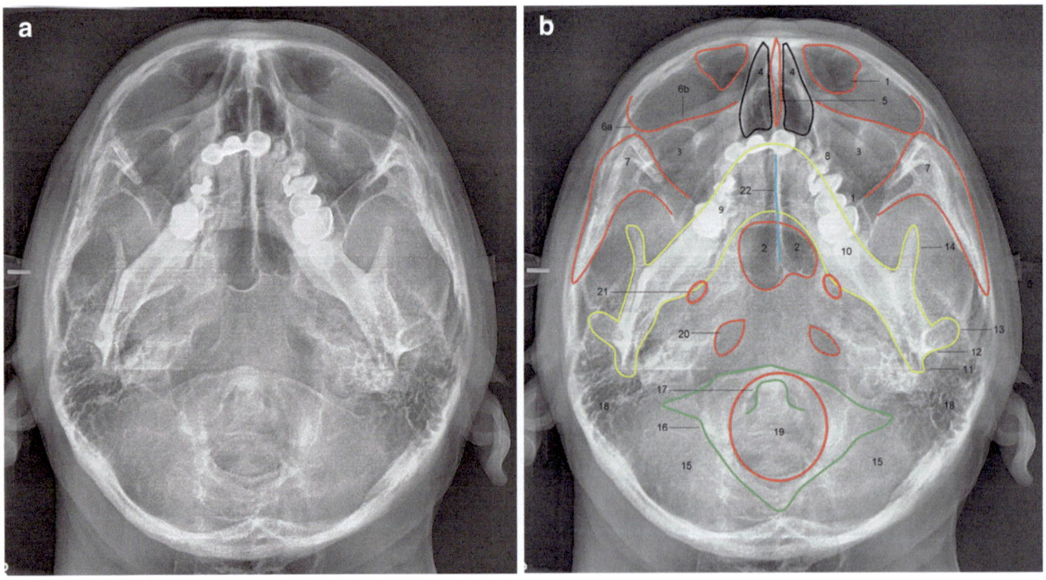

Fig. 6.4 (**a**) Example of submentovertex/occipitomental cephalometric view and (**b**) depiction of the most important anatomic elements. Numbering corresponds to the text. (Images were created by Dr. Athina Chatzigianni with the use of Viewbox 4 Software (dHAL Software, Kifissia, Greece) [28])

14. *Coronoid process.*
15. *Base of skull.*
16. *first cervical vertebra (atlas).*
17. *Odontoid process (dens) of second cervical vertebra.*
18. *Mastoid air cells.*
19. *Foramen magnum.*
20. *Foramen lacerum.*
21. *Foramen oval.*
22. *Intermaxillary suture*: it is the suture in the midline between the two maxillary bones. In this view it is superimposed with the projection of the nasal septum.

6.2.4 Three-Dimensional Cephalometric Imaging

To overcome the limitations of 2D cephalometric radiographic methods, the use of 2D cephalometric radiographs is being gradually replaced by three-dimensional (3D) radiographic images of the craniofacial bones in an attempt to describe craniofacial discrepancies in a 3D manner.

For this purpose, the medical CT, which was introduced in 1972 by G. Hounsfield, who received a Nobel prize in 1979 [24], quickly gained popularity for dental and orthodontic imaging, diagnosis, and treatment planning. However, due to its major drawbacks, such as high cost and high patient radiation dose, the alternative of CBCT was introduced in dentistry and has been since then the method of choice for a 3D hard tissue reconstruction and imaging [25]. Recently, high-resolution 3D magnetic resonance imaging (MRI) has been examined as an even more favorable alternative for 3D imaging of the head and neck region and as a tool for 3D treatment planning in orthodontics and orthognathic surgery with favorable results [26].

In the field of orthodontics, the 3D rendering of the craniofacial structures and the 3D anatomic landmarks acquisition and identification gave rise to the 3D cephalometric analysis of the craniofacial complex and face and new software for 3D orthodontic assessment have been developed. Despite the fact that the reliability of 3D cephalometric landmarks is still questionable and further research is required in the field [27], the 3D image modality of the craniofacial region is a new path on cephalometric analysis and treatment planning.

In general, the main clinical uses of 3D cephalometric imaging are described below:

1. Study of the 3D craniofacial shape and growth.
2. Study of the 3D skeletal asymmetries.
3. Study of the 3D soft tissue.
4. Study of the 3D upper airways.
5. Establishment of 3D cephalometric norms specific for a group of people.
6. Study of the 3D craniofacial differences between genders or between people of different racial/ethnic origin.
7. Study on the ageing of the 3D craniofacial skeleton and the 3D soft tissue.
8. Diagnosis of malocclusions, craniofacial anomalies, and skeletal deformities in a three-dimensional manner.
9. Orthodontic treatment planning.
10. 3D virtual orthognathic-surgical treatment planning.
11. Evaluation of orthodontic treatment results on the 3D hard and soft tissue.
12. Detections of abnormalities of the 3D skull and3D spine.

The hard tissue anatomic parts that can be recognized on a rendered 3D cephalometric image are listed below (Fig. 6.5a, b):

- 3D cranial and upper facial anatomic structures.

1. *Frontal bone.*
2. *Nasal bones.*
3. *Nasal cavity.*
4. *Nasal septum.*
5. *Sphenoid bone.*
6. *Ethmoid bone.*
7. *Orbital roof.*
8. *Lateral wall of orbit.*
9. *Inferior orbital rim.*

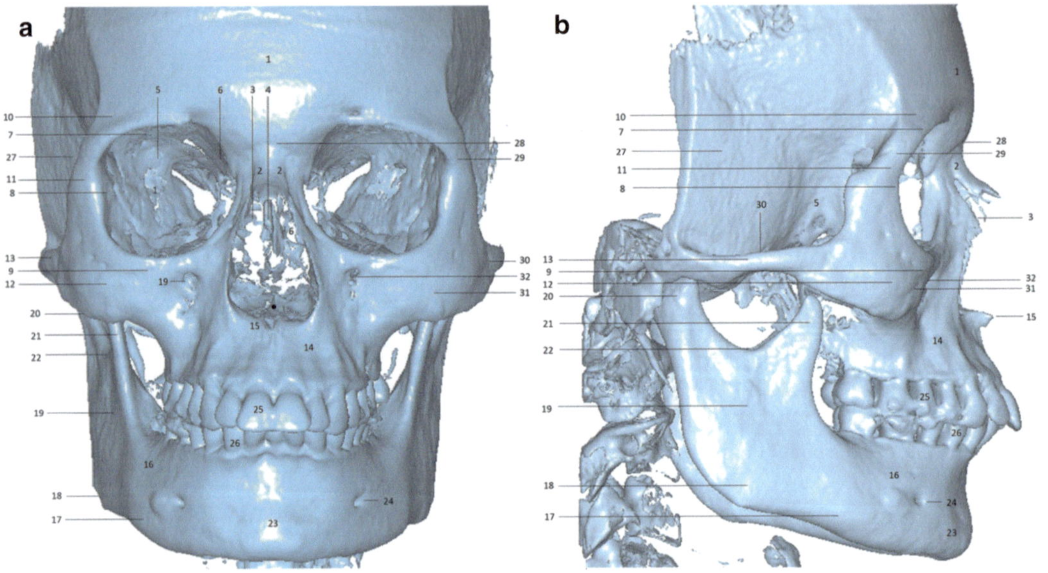

Fig. 6.5 Three-dimensional cephalometric image created by CBCT together with the numbering of the most important anatomic parts: (**a**) frontal view and (**b**) lateral view. Numbering corresponds to the text. (Images were created by Dr. Athina Chatzigianni with the use of Viewbox 4 Software (dHAL Software, Kifissia, Greece) [28])

10. *Zygomatic process of frontal bone.*
11. *Frontal process of zygomatic bone.*
12. *Maxillary process of zygomatic bone.*
13. *Zygomatic arch.*

- 3D Maxillary anatomic structures.

14. *Maxilla.*
15. *Anterior nasal spine.*

- 3D Mandibular anatomic structures

16. *Mandible.*
17. *Body of the mandible.*
18. *Gonial angle of the mandible.*
19. *Ramus of the mandible.*
20. *Condyle.*
21. *Coronoid process.*
22. *Antegonial notch.*
23. *Symphysis.*
24. *Mental foramen.*

- 3D Dental anatomic structures

25. *Upper dentition.*
26. *Lower dentition.*

- Additional anatomic parts identified on a 3D craniofacial image, which were not clearly discerned in the previous 2D images:

27. *Temporal bone*: it is situated at the side of the cranium and base of the skull. It articulates with the zygomatic bone, the mandible, the sphenoid bone, the parietal bone, and the occipital bone.
28. *Frontonasal suture*: it is the suture between the frontal bone and the two nasal bones.
29. *Frontozygomatic suture*: it is the suture connecting the frontal bone and the zygomatic bone.
30. *Zygomaticotemporal suture*: it is the suture connecting the temporal bone and the zygomatic bone.

31. *Zygomaticomaxillary suture*: it is the suture connecting the zygomatic process of the maxillary bone and the maxillary process of zygomatic bone.
32. *Infraorbital foramen*: it is situated in the maxillary bone, below the infraorbital margin. The infraorbital nerve, artery, and vein are transmitted through this foramen.

6.3 Summary

In conclusion, the aim of this chapter was neither to delve into technical aspects of cephalometric radiographic examination nor to present cephalometric landmarks or cephalometric analysis. The purpose was to feature the main cephalometric views, which can be utilized to image the bones, the sinuses, the nerve canals, and other important anatomic parts of the craniofacial skeleton. The deep knowledge of the cephalometric radiographic anatomy is essential for the correct identification of all the anatomic elements of the craniofacial region. The proper recognition of these anatomic structures is required for infallible cephalometric analysis in orthodontics and orthognathic surgery. The cephalometric analysis is based on the identification and use of anatomic landmarks of different craniofacial structures and possible errors on landmark placement may lead to measurement errors and diagnostics mistakes. Despite the inevitable limitations of 2D cephalometric radiographic images, they remain a valuable imaging tool for the clinicians. The transition to 3D cephalometric radiography not only has started, but has already shown great progress, nevertheless more research and technological advances are needed to fully adopt this imaging method in everyday clinical practice.

References

1. Pacini AJ, Carrera. First X-ray picture of skull: roentgen ray anthropometry of the skull. J Radiol. 1922;3:230–8.
2. Broadbent BH. A new X ray technique and its application to orthodontia. Angle Orthod. 1931;1:45–66.
3. Hofrath H. Bedeuting der rontgenfern und abstands aufnahme fur die diagnostic der kieferanomalien. Fortschr Orthod. 1931;1:232–58.
4. Bjork A. Prediction of mandibular growth rotation. Am J Orthod. 1969;55:585–99.
5. Moyers RE, Bookstein FL, Hunter WS. Analysis of the craniofacial skeleton: cephalometrics. In: Moyers RE, editor. Handbook of orthodontics. Chicago: Year Book Medical; 1988. p. 247–309.
6. Ingerslev CH, Solow B. Sex differences in craniofacial morphology. Acta Odontol Scand. 1975;33:85–94.
7. Broadbent BH Sr, Broadbent BH Jr, Golden WH. Bolton standards of dentofacial developmental growth. St. Louis, MO: CV Mosby; 1975.
8. Houston WJB. The analysis of errors in orthodontic measurements. Am J Orthod. 1983;83:382–90.
9. Baumrind S, Frantz RC. The reliability of head film measurements. I: landmark identification. Am J Orthod. 1971;60:111–27.
10. Na KC, Yoon YJ, Kim KW. A study on the errors in the cephalometric measurements. Korean J Orthod. 1998;28:75–84.
11. Malkoc S, Sari Z, Usumez S, Koyuturk AE. The effect of head rotation on cephalometric radiographs. Eur J Orthod. 2005;27:315–21.
12. Athanasiou AE, Miethke RR, Van De Meij AJW. Random errors in localization of landmarks in postero-anterior cephalograms. Br J Orthod. 1999;26:273–84.
13. Scarfe WC, Farman AG. What is cone-beam CT and how does it work? Dent Clin N Am. 2008;52:707–30.
14. Durão AR, Pittayapat, Rockenbach MIB, Olszewski R, Ng S, Ferreira AP, Jacobs R. Validity of 2D lateral cephalometry in orthodontics: a systematic review. Prog Orthod. 2013;14:31.
15. Grayson B, Cutting C, Bookstein FL, Kim H, McCarthy JG. The three-dimensional cephalograms: theory, technique, and clinical application. Am J Orthod Dentofacial Orthop. 1988;94:327–37.
16. Zhu M, Cai Z, Zhang LY, et al. Establishment of 3D analysis system of craniomaxillofacial skeleton. Chin J Oral Maxillofac Surg. 1998;8:15.
17. Athanasiou AE. Orthodontic cephalometry. London: Mosby-Wolf; 1995.
18. Proffit WR, Fields HW Jr, Sarver DM. Contemporary orthodontics. 4th ed. St. Louis, MO: Mosby Elsevier; 2007.
19. Bergensen EO. Enlargement and distortion in cephalometric radiography: compensation tables for linear measurements. Angle Orthod. 1980;50:230–44.
20. Weems RA. Radiographic cephalometric technique. In: Jacobson A, editor. Radiographic cephalometry from basics to video imaging. Carol Stream: Quintessence; 1995. p. 39–52.
21. Richardson ME. Reproducibility of depressed posterioranterior cephalometric radiographs. Angle Orthod. 1967;37:48–51.
22. Ricketts RM. Perspectives in the clinical application of cephalometrics: the first fifty years. Angle Orthod. 1981;51:115–50.

23. Tetradis S, Kantor ML. Extraoral radiographic examinations. In: White SC, Fharoah MJ, editors. Oral radiology: principles and interpretation. 6th ed. St. Louis, MO: Mosby, Elsevier; 2009. p. 191–206.
24. Hounsfield GN. Computed medical imaging. Nobel lecture, 1979. J Comput Assist Tomogr. 1980;4:665–74.
25. Mozzo P, Procacci C, Tacconi A, Martini PT, Andreis IA. A new volumetric CT machine for dental imaging based on the cone-beam technique: preliminary results. Eur Radiol. 1998;8:1558–64.
26. Juerchott A, Saleem MA, Hilgenfeld T, Freudlsperger C, Zingler S, Lux CJ, Bendszus M, Heiland S. 3D cephalometric analysis using magnetic resonance imaging: validation of accuracy and reproducibility. Sci Rep. 2018;8:13029.
27. Sam A, Currie K, Oh H, Flores-Mir C, Lagravere-Vich M. Reliability of different three-dimensional cephalometric landmarks in cone-beam computed tomography: a systematic review. Angle Orthod. 2019;89:317–32.
28. Halazonetis DJ. Computer-assisted cephalometric analysis. Am J Orthod Dentofacial Orthop. 1994;105:517–21.

Basic Principles of Computer Tomography (MDCT/CBCT). The Use of MDCT and CBCT in Dentomaxillofacial Imaging

7

Antigoni Delantoni and Alexandros Sapountzis

7.1 Conventional Tomography

Conventional tomography is an imaging modality in which the production of the radiographic image is achieved by the combined movement of an X-ray tube and an X-ray receptor around an imaginary axis or point that constitutes the tomographic center. In the frame of the tomograph, the X-ray tube is joined by a fixed arm to the X-ray receiver so that a smooth, simultaneous movement between them is achieved in the opposing directions. The space between the X-ray tube and the X-ray receptor constitutes the tomographic field [1], within which the scanner produces sections of the anatomical structures of interest. The generation of the various sections is achieved by intentionally blurring all structures outside the tomographic field, while in contrast, structures within the tomographic field are projected sharply at a fixed position on the X-ray receptor. A prerequisite for avoiding distortions in the resulting tomographic images is the positioning of the anatomical structures under examination as perpendicular as possible to the source of the rays [2].

The major factors that affect the quality of the resulting tomographic images are the type of movement of the X-ray tube, the thickness of the sections, and the degree of magnification [3].

The X-ray tube can move in a linear, circular, ellipsoidal, sub-cyclical or spiral trajectory. With the exception of the linear type of movement in which the X-ray tube moves in a horizontal or vertical straight line, in all other types of movements mentioned beforetake place in more than one plane. Complex-nonlinear motion types produce more uniform ambiguity in the tomographic image [3–5]. An advantage of the complex motion types mentioned before is that images are produced without unwanted projections and shadows [6].

The thickness of the tomographic slice produced depends on the tomographic angle. Wide angles of 50–60° produce thin tomographic sections of 1–2 mm, whereas as the velocity of the X-ray tube decreases the radiographic angle is blunted and the sections increase in thickness.

Finally, the degree of magnification in conventional tomography varies, depending on the scanner, from 10% to 30% and is constant and comparable for all anatomical structures within the same scanning field [7].

The authors state that the chapter does not contain any information or images or other third party material that is not copyrighted by the authors.

A. Delantoni (✉)
Department of Dentoalveolar Surgery, Implant Surgery and Radiology, Faculty of Dentistry, Aristotle University of Thessaloniki, Thessaloniki, Greece
e-mail: andelant@dent.auth.gr

A. Sapountzis
Department of Dentoalveolar Surgery, Implant Surgery and Radiology, Aristotle University of Thessaloniki, Thessaloniki, Greece

A. Delantoni, K. Orhan (eds.), *Atlas of Dentomaxillofacial Anatomical Imaging*,
https://doi.org/10.1007/978-3-030-96840-3_7

Conventional tomography has the disadvantages of increased patient exposure to radiation, magnification of the image, reduced resolution of details in the areas of similar density due to overlap and radiolucencies, and lack of features in each generated section to facilitate identification of the acquisition area [8].

7.2 Computed Tomography

7.2.1 Principles of Operation and Parts of the Tomograph

Computed tomography or CT is a digital imaging modality, which was first applied for brain tumor diagnosis in 1971 in the UK [9]. The main creators of computed tomography, Hounsfield and Cormack, were awarded the Nobel Prize in 1979.

A computed or CT tomographic scanner reconstructs images from various projections obtained using a rotating X-ray beam and software that uses complex mathematical algorithms. This enables it to produce sections of varying thicknesses of the anatomical structure under examination without the typical lack of definition and the overlap effect caused by neighboring anatomical structures of similar or higher density found in conventional tomography.

All CT scanners consist of the scanning system, the computing system, and the image display and recording system.

The scanning system of the CT scanner includes an X-ray tube, the radiation detector array and the examination table. The X-ray tube emits a confined fan-shaped X-ray beam while rotating 360° running on a ring approximately 1.5 m in diameter. The radiation detectors are attached to the same ring in an opposite position to the tube and collect the attenuated X-rays as they exit the structures of interest. The radiation detectors are mounted in rows and are usually either fluorescence or ionization chamber type. The movement of the X-ray tube is usually helical or spiral and continues until the area of interest is covered without interrupting the irradiation as was the case with older scanners where irradiation was interrupted and the examination table moved [4]. Finally, the examination table is constructed so that it can be moved along its axis and is positioned perpendicular to the plane defined by the tube and the radiation detectors.

The calculation system measures the attenuation of the X-ray beam after its passing through the structures under examination. The attenuation of the beam is not uniform but depends on the composition and density of the tissues it passes through. The computer of the tomograph receives the attenuation values from the array of detectors and then converts them into images. To create the image, the computer forms a matrix composed of a large number of pixels (elementary voxels). Each matrix is characterized by its size, i.e. by a certain number of pixels in each row and column. The computer first records the various linear attenuation coefficients of the X-rays as they exit the structures of interest. The linear attenuation coefficient is shown in the following formula, often referred to as Beer–Lambert's law.

$$I = I_0 e - \mu\chi$$

where I represents the intensity of the rays as they exit the structure of interest, I_0 is the intensity of the rays as they enter the structure of interest, e is Euler's constant equal to 2.718, μ is the linear attenuation coefficient or absorption coefficient, and χ is the thickness of the structure through which the rays pass. The resulting values of the linear coefficient are corresponded by the computer to grey color tones according to the Hounsfield scale and are called Hounsfield units (HU). Hounsfield units usually take values from −1000 which translates to zero attenuation of the rays to +1000 which translates to full absorption of the radiation [5]. In general, structures that exhibit high absorption of rays correspond to bright regions of the scale, while conversely structures that do not absorb rays to a large extent correspond to dark regions. The sum of Hounsfield's numbers from white to black constitute the window range which affects the contrast of the imaging. In reference, water has been defined as a value of 0, air −1000, adipose tissue from −50 to −100, parenchymal organs from +40 to +80, spongy bone from +300 to +800, and cortical bone values greater than +800.

These resulting values are included as tones of grey now within each of the matrix's generated volume cells.

The recording and display system, once the area of interest and the section have been selected, converts the 3D matrix into a two-dimensional representation on the computer screen. In the resulting image, the pixels of the selected section are now presented as small squares called pixels. Each pixel corresponds to the cross-sectional surface of the cross-sectional area of the matrix [5].

An important feature of computed tomography is that the original cross-sections taken during the movement of the tube are stored and can be reconstructed by the computer of the scanner in a different plane and direction (multi-planar reformatting), thus enabling the imaging of the structures of interest in different sections depending on the diagnostic need. Although the images resulting from multi-planar reformatting do not have the quality of the original CT images they still have a high diagnostic value.

7.2.2 Image Characteristics

The image quality in any tomograph depends on the spatial resolution capability, contrast resolution capability, noise, and blurring [10].

Spatial resolution is the ability of the scanner to distinguish small objects or structures that are very close to each other and is measured by line pairs per millimeter (l/mm). The spatial resolution is inversely proportional to the thickness of the section.

Contrast resolution is the ability of the scanner to distinguish objects or structures with very small differences in density. Computed tomography scanners, because of their large window range (−1000 to +1000), have the ability to distinguish anatomical structures with a difference in density of $<1\%$ [5].

Noise is defined as all information contained in a tomographic image that has no diagnostic value, while the sum of diagnostically useful information in an image is called signal. The sharpness of a tomographic image also depends on the signal-to-noise ratio (SNR). Noise cannot be completely eliminated, but with the evolution of scanners and their software it can be greatly reduced. So by reducing the noise or increasing the signal we can increase the quality of the tomographic image.

The lack of sharpness of the tomographic image can be the result of various factors such as: patient movements (physical or breathing movements), non-cooperation of the patient during the examination, the thickness of the anatomical structures under examination, the thickness of the slice chosen, limitations of the electronic parts (detection system, etc.) and the software of the tomograph, as well as the active size of the focus of the X-ray tube.

7.2.3 Evolution of Computed Tomography

Computed tomography scanners have gone through several stages of evolution and have incorporated various technologies and improvements in both their electronic components and software.

The first-generation scanners had a radiation detector and used a thin well-focused pencil-like X-ray beam. The scanning of the structure of interest was done by successive projections, with the tube-detector system rotating by 1° to create each of them. To create a section, 180 consecutive projections were required, resulting in an average examination time of 25–30 min.

In the second-generation scanners, the number of detectors was increased to 30 in an arc arrangement and the shape of the X-rays emitted by the tube took the form of a fan, which made it possible to reduce the average examination time to less than 90 s.

In the third generation, the number of detectors initially reached 288, while in more sophisticated scanners it rose to 700 in an arc configuration. The range of the beams was increased and adapted to cover the entire object under examination and thus, together with the increase in the number of detectors, a further reduction in the average examination time to about 5 s was achieved.

In the fourth generation, which consists of the most modern CT scanners, the number of radiation detectors has increased to over 2000 and the detectors are now mounted on an outer ring and do not move during the examination allowing to overcome the problems caused to the image by the movement of the scanning system. The average examination time was reduced to a few seconds.

In the third and fourth generation CT scanners, various improvements have been made, such as the spiral Ct scan, whereby the patient is moved as the tube-detector system rotates. The collection of information from the detectors is continuous and is not interrupted during the examination and thus the examination time is significantly reduced resulting in an improved image due to the reduction of distortions caused by the patient's physical and respiratory movements [11, 12]. Another improvement introduced in modern scanners is dual energy computed tomography (Dect), in which depending on the scanner, single or dual beam sources are used, as well as detectors with the ability to detect data of different energies. The advantage of dual energy computed tomography is the reduction of the noise, increase the ability to characterize and distinguish tissues, reduce artefacts resulting from the hardening of the beams, and further reduce the dose of beams received by the patient without negatively affecting the quality of the images [13].

7.2.4 Applications of Computed Tomography in Dental Science

In dental science, computed tomography has found applications in the identification of lesions of the jaws and adjacent anatomical structures, the assessment of occlusion of teeth, the diagnosis of temporomandibular joint disorders, the preoperative study for the placement of implants and in the postoperative assessment of the health of peri-implant bone structures [14]. Also, due to the zero magnification and the ability to match each section with the acquisition area, it enables the measurement of height and thickness of the bone, the estimation of its density and being able to transfer and match the information to the bony structures of interest on the patient. Finally, the ability of tomographs to reconstruct images in different planes and directions overcame the anatomical peculiarities of the maxillofacial region and made the positioning of the patient more adjustable during the examination.

7.2.5 Disadvantages of Computed Tomography

Computed tomography has several disadvantages. The presence of high-density structures, especially metallic structures such as metallic fillings, metallic frameworks of fixed prostheses, dental implants, etc., causes the hardening of the beam of X-rays and as a result the appearance of black zones in the image [15]. These black zones are called linear artefacts or artifacts and reduce the diagnostic ability of tomographic images by obscuring parts of the anatomical structures of interest or by simulating radiolucent pathological lesions. The radiation dose received by the patient is increased compared to the imaging modalities mentioned above, although low-dose imaging protocols have been developed in recent years without significant reduction in diagnostic information [16]. Finally, the increased cost of the examination is a disadvantage compared to the previous imaging modalities.

7.3 Cone Beam Computed Tomography

7.3.1 Principles of Operation

Cone beam computed tomography (CBCT) is an evolution of computed tomography. It initially found applications in angiography, radiotherapy, and mammography, and its use was subsequently extended to dental science [17–19]. The first cone beam scanner for use in dental science was installed in Europe in 1998 and later in the USA in 2001. It is a modern and now widely used imaging modality that uses a rotating tube that produces a cone-shaped beam of X-rays and is fixed opposite to the radiation detector system, thus showing several similarities with an orthopantomograph. The tube-detector system rotates typically 180–360° around the patient's head and takes successive tomographic images. The conical shape of the generated rays, the size of the cone, and the position and size of the detection system allows the tomograph to collect all the rays as they exit the various tissues of the patient and thus achieve scanning of the area of interest in a single rotation [20] (Fig. 7.1).

During its rotation the scanner takes 120–1024 two-dimensional images similar to lateral cephalometric radiographs as opposed to the axial sections found in computed tomography [21]. Total examination time, depending on the manufacturer and protocol used, ranges from 5 to 40 s.

Changing the shape of the beam of X-rays from a fan to a cone has increased the efficiency and reduced the mechanical complexity of the cone beam CT scanner compared to the conventional CT scanner, which scans the structures of interest step by step, producing axial sections of preselected thickness, therefore using more mechanical parts as well as increased examination time [22] (Fig. 7.2).

The production of a cone-beam computed tomography image is achieved in four stages: generating the beam and passing it through the structures of interest, collecting the radiation by the detection system, reconstructing the images, and viewing them [23].

7.3.2 The Beam Generation System

The beam is produced by a fixed-anode X-ray tube, which has similarities to the tubes used in orthopantomographs. The main difference

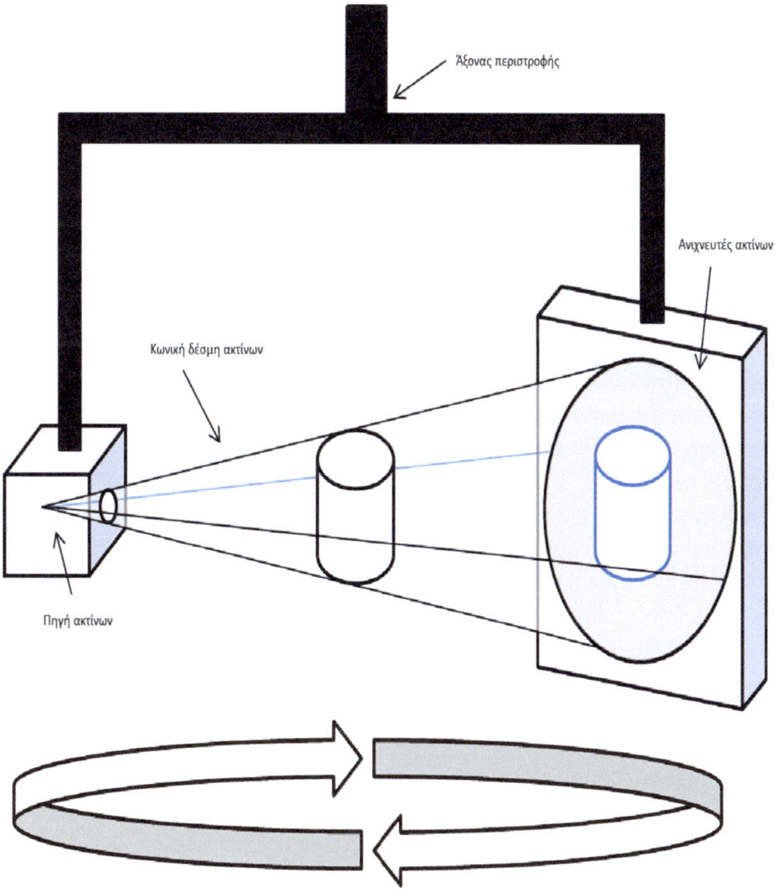

Fig. 7.1 The basic principle of rotation of the beam in CBCT machines

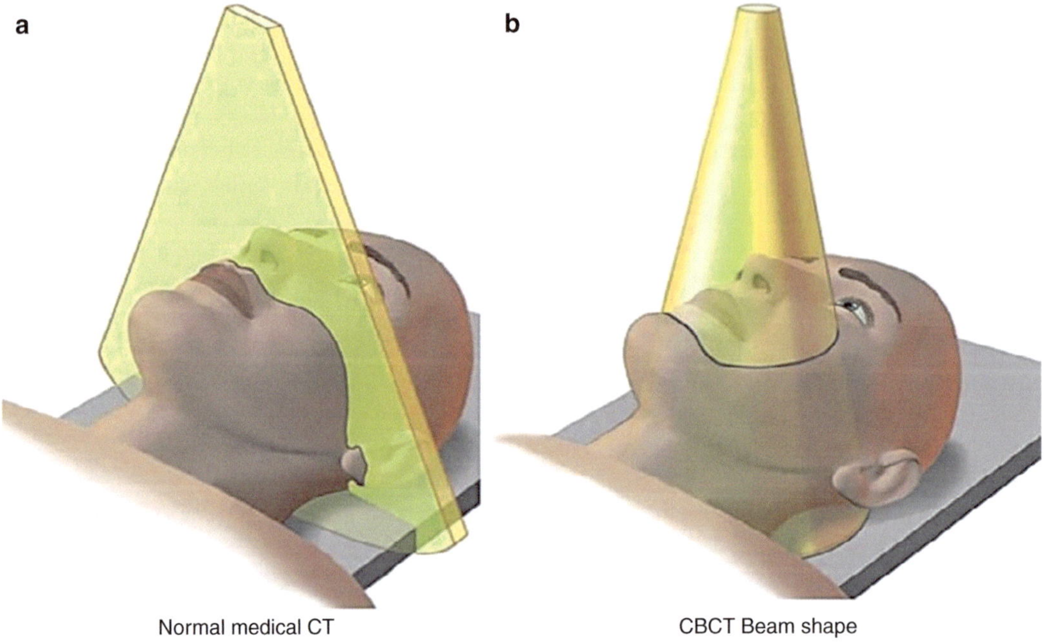

Fig. 7.2 The key difference of beam shape when compared to MDCT. (**a**) Normal medical CT and (**b**) CBCT beam shape

between the radiation system of the cone beam CT scanner and conventional CT is the introduction of beam confinement systems, which give the beam a cone shape with a base area approximately equal to that of the scanning system and limit the radiation exposure to the area of interest [24]. As the tube rotates around the patient, several images are produced, each corresponding to the projection of the structure of interest at the compared angle of irradiation. Due to the technical limitation of the detection system to receive the signal continuously, the beam emitted from the tube is not continuous but is interrupted (pulsed beam). The frequency of the pulsed beam is adjusted so that the interval between successive exposures coincides with the time required by the detection system of the scanner to process the data resulting from each exposure. Because of the pulsed beam, the patient's exposure time to radiation is much shorter than the total examination time [23, 24]. Each pulse produces a single projection image called the basal or structural image. As noted above, the basal images in cone-beam computed tomography are more similar to lateral cephalometric images than to basic axial sections generated by conventional CT. In most modern CT scanners the number of structural images produced is constant. A larger number of structural images in a cone-beam computed tomography scan results in an increase in the signal received by the detection system and consequently an improvement in the quality and sharpness of the final tomographic images due to an improvement in the signal-to-noise ratio (SNR). However, increasing the number of structural images, as long as the acquisition rate remains constant, leads to increased patient irradiation time.

7.3.3 The Radiation Detection System

The collection of the attenuated rays after they exit from the structures of interest is performed by the detection system of the cone-beam CT scanner. The detection system may consist of image intensifier tubes or the more modern and less bulky flat panel detectors [23].

Image intensifier tubes usually consist of an array of scintillation screens, two cesium iodide intensifier plates, corrective lenses, and a charge coupled device (CCD) sensor array [23–25]. In a detection system of this type, the attenuated beam enters the vacuum tube and is converted into light using an amplifying "input phosphor." The bright signal is then converted in the photocathode into an electron beam which is accelerated through an electric field and converted back into a light signal by the use of a second output phosphor. The intensity of the final light signal is adjusted by a series of lenses and an optical iris. The now corrected light signal is converted in the CCD sensor array into an electrical signal [25]. The intensity of the electrical signal generated by the CCD sensor is proportional to the intensity of the beam incident on the input intensifying plate. Tubular image intensifiers cause geometric distortion in tomographic reconstruction due to the shape of the vacuum tube and the many steps involved in acquiring the image, as well as increase the production of artefacts. The increase in noise in this type of scanning system is addressed by corrective mathematical algorithms in the scanner software [23–25]. Additional disadvantages of tubular image intensifiers include their increased volume, the need for more frequent calibration due to their sensitivity to magnetic fields and the fading of the intensification plates over time and use [26].

The flat plate detection system also uses an iodide cesium iodide amplifier plate to convert incident radiation into a light signal which is then captured and converted into an electrical signal by sensor arrays contained in a thin layer of amorphous silicon (a-si). The electrical signal produced by the sensors has an intensity proportional to that of the light signal, which in turn is proportional to the intensity of the radiation incident on the amplifying plate. These systems do not cause the geometric distortion and some of the artefacts found in tubular image intensifiers [5] and consequently reduce noise levels in tomographic images. The disadvantages of these systems are their non-linear sensitivity to low or high radiation intensities, the attenuation of the enhancement plate, and the uneven performance of their radiation detection capability exhibited at different points on their surface.

In both types of detectors, the dimensions and number of cells collecting the signal have a very large role in the analytical capability of the detection system. As the area of the sensitive cells is reduced, the analytical capability (resolution in space) of the detection system increases but at the same time the signal-to-noise ratio (SNR) decreases. The need for signal transport subsystems on the surface of the detectors limits the number of cells and therefore reduces the analytical capability of the system. In a comparison of the two types of detection systems, tomographic images produced with flat plate systems had higher resolution [24]. Finally, in contrast to computed tomography, the size of the voxel and therefore the resolution of the image in cone-beam computed tomography depends on the size of the sensitive cells of the detection system and not on the section thickness selected.

7.3.4 Reconstruction of the Tomographic Images

The process of converting the electrical signal generated by the detector system into an image is a complex process performed by the scanner's computer. First, a pre-correction of the inhomogeneity of the structural images produced is performed. This lack of homogeneity is the result of the different sensitivity levels of the cells included in various parts of the surface of the detection system and on of the inhomogeneity of the efficiency of the intensifying plate. After pre-correction, the computer, using complex mathematical algorithms, the most common being Feldkamp's algorithm or Feldkamp–Davis–Kress (FDK) method [27], sorts and corrects the data from the original structural images and finally displays them with a pixel brightness diametrically opposite to the original one. This technique is called a back projection technique.

7.3.5 Viewing the Scan Images

The cone-beam CT scanners project the tomographic images reconstructed from the original structural images in the axial, frontal, or ocular plane. These images are called secondary reconstructed images. The user can select the slice thickness of each reconstruction, enhance the resulting images with a number of tools available in the scanner software, as well as perform measurements and pre-operative planning. Particularly useful is the ability of cone-beam scanners to store and use all the scan data and to reconstruct images in other planes beyond the three basic ones depending on the user's diagnostic needs (multi-planar reformatting). Finally, as in conventional computed tomography, using specific algorithms, the scanner's computer creates shadows by illuminating the projected volumes in such a way as to give a three-dimensional appearance to the resulting image.

7.3.6 Advantages of Cone Beam Tomography

Cone beam computed tomography has a number of advantages compared to other imaging modalities. The scanning and data acquisition time is short (5–40 s), reducing the possibility of image distortion due to physical or respiratory movements of the patient. In modern cone-beam scanners the isotropic voxel size ranges from 80 to 400 μm and depicting the structures of the maxillofacial region with sufficient resolution, and thus allowing the operator to obtain measurements accurately. When compared to conventional computed tomography, cone beam computed tomography shows significantly fewer artifacts due to metallic structures in the region of interest [28] and the radiation dose to the patient (effective dose), depending always on the scanner, protocol and field size, is lower [28]. An important advantage is also the interactivity, i.e. the ability of modern systems to allow the transfer of tomographic data for study in other computer systems. Finally, the size and the cost of a cone beam computed tomography scanner is significantly reduced compared to conventional computed tomography scanners.

7.3.7 Limitations: Disadvantages of Cone Beam Tomography

In cone beam computed tomography a large part of the patient's head is irradiated due to the conical nature of the beam of X-rays produced. This fact statistically increases the probability of photon scattering and consequently the production of secondary radiation, which is recorded in the scanner's detection system as noise.

As a result of this phenomenon there is a reduction in the resolution and diagnostic capability of the resulting tomographic images. In conventional CT scanners, the fan-shaped beam improves the secondary (scatter radiation) to primary radiation ratio (SPR), compared to cone beam scanners. The SPR fraction has a value of 0.01 for single beam computed tomographs, 0.05–0.15 for fan-beam computed tomographs with helical scanning, and 0.4–2 for cone beam computed tomographs [23]. Finally, increasing the angular range of the cone beam leads to a larger area of the cone base, a larger imaging field, and consequently increased secondary radiation and noise generation.

As mentioned before, the production of artifacts is reduced compared to conventional computed tomography, yet their presence continues to affect the diagnostic ability of tomographic reconstructions despite the efforts of manufacturers to reduce them using improved mathematical algorithms. Artifacts are produced by differences between the mathematical model used by the scanner for the 3D image reconstruction and the physical properties of the various elements (detection system, object to be examined) involved in it. In cone beam computed tomography, the relevant artifacts are those caused by beam hardening, the partial volume averaging artifacts, the patient motion artifacts, the extinction artifacts, and the ring and aliasing artifacts.

7.3.8 Applications of Cone Beam Tomography

Cone beam computed tomography has a multitude of uses in dental science. In the surgery of the maxillofacial region it provides information for diagnosis and surgical planning needed to treat fractures and deformities, surgical extraction of impacted teeth and their relationship to structures of interest (maxillary canal, sinus, roots of adjacent teeth) and identification and determination of the location of foreign bodies [24–27]. In implantology, cone-beam computed tomography contributes to 3D preoperative planning and assessment of implant sites, assessment of peri-implant tissue health and planning of possible corrective procedures after the prosthetic rehabilitation stage, as well as the construction of surgical guides for guided implant placement.

In recent years, the usefulness of cone beam computed tomography in orthodontics as well as in endodontics has been studied.

7.3.9 Guidelines in Cone Beam Computed Tomography

Cone beam computed tomography, like any form of imaging examination using ionizing radiation, should follow a set of guidelines aimed at protecting the patient. A recent study speculates that in the USA up to 2% of recorded cases of malignancy may be due to radiation exposure from CT scans. The increase in the number of cone-beam CT scanners and their uses in more and more fields in dental science has led to efforts, both in the United States and Europe, to establish guidelines for indications for use, protocols and the conduct of examinations with cone-beam technology.

Initially, the American Academy of Oral and Maxillofacial Radiology in 2008, based on the ALARA (as low as reasonably achievable) principle, proposed in a related article a series of recommendations on how to use cone beam computed tomography, the responsibilities of the examiner, the basic principles of radiation protection and equipment quality assurance, and finally the justification of each scan. Similarly, in Europe, the SEDENTEXCT project (Safety and Efficacy of a new and emerging Dental X-ray modality) was developed with the contribution of the European Atomic Energy Commission (EURATOM) and the European Association of Dental Radiology (EADMFR). The project has published a set of guidelines including the basic principles of using cone beam computed tomography, suggested modalities for its application in the maxillofacial region, radiation dosage, and radiation protection for patients and medical staff.

SEDENTEXCT expired in 2011 and in May 2012 the guidelines published in a related article (Radiation Protection: Cone beam CT for Dental and Maxillofacial Radiology. Evidence based guidelines) were incorporated with the European Union radiation protection series.

References

1. Coin CG. Tomography of the temporomandibular joint. Med Radiogr Photogr. 1974;2:26–39.
2. Curry TS, Dowdey JE, Murry RC. Christensen's physics of diagnostic radiology. 4th ed. Philadelphia, PA: Lea & Febiger; 1990. p. 243–56, 289–322.
3. Misch CE. Contemporary implant dentistry. 2nd ed. St. Louis, MO: Mosby; 1999. p. 73–87.
4. Bushong SC. Radiologic science for technologists: physics, biology and protection. 5th ed. St. Louis, MO: Mosby; 1993. p. 325–35.
5. White SC, Pharoah M. Oral radiology: principles and interpretation. 6th ed. St. Louis, MO: Mosby; 2008. p. 79–99, 207–224.

6. Yune HY. Two-dimensional-three-dimensional reconstruction computed tomography techniques. Dent Clin N Am. 1993;4:613–26.
7. Grondahl K, Ekestubbe A, Grondahl HG. Radiography in oral endosseous prosthetics. Goteborg: Nobel Biocare; 1996.
8. Eckerdal O, Kvint S. Presurgical planning for osseointegrated implants in the maxilla: a tomographic evaluation of available alveolar bone and morphological 145 relations in the maxilla. Int J Oral Maxillofac Surg. 1986;15(6):722–6.
9. Beckmann EC. CT scanning the early days. Br J Radiol. 2006;79(937):5–8.
10. Jurik AG, Jessen KA, Hansen J. Image quality and dose in computed tomography. Eur Radiol. 1997;7(1):77–81.
11. Brink JA, Wang G, Mcfarland EG. Technical developments optimal section spacing in single-detector helical CT. Radiology. 2000;214(4):575–8.
12. Hanazawa T, Sano T, Seki K, Okano T. Radiologic measurements of the mandible: a comparison between CT-reformatted and conventional tomographic images. Clin Oral Implants Res. 2004;15(2):226–32.
13. Grajo JR, Patino M, Prochowski A, Sahani DV. Dual energy CT in practice: basic principles and applications. Appl Radiol. 2016;45(7):6–12.
14. Abrahams JJ. Dental CT imaging: a look at the jaw. Radiology. 2001;2:334–45.
15. Draenert FG, Coppenrath E, Herzog P, Müller S, Mueller-Lisse UG. Beam hardening artefacts occur in dental implant scans with the NewTom® cone beam CT but not with the dental 4-row multidetector CT. Dentomaxillofac Radiol. 2007;36(4):198–203.
16. Rustemeyer P, Sireubühr U, Suttmoeller J. Low-dose dental computed tomography: significant dose reduction without loss of image quality. Acta Radiol. 2004;45(8):847–53.
17. Robb RA. The dynamic spatial reconstructor: an X-ray video-fluoroscopic CT scanner for dynamic volume imaging of moving organs. IEEE Trans Med Imaging. 1982;1(1):22–33.
18. Chen B, Ning R. Cone-beam volume CT breast imaging: feasibility study. Med Phys. 2002;29(5):755–70.
19. Cho PS, Johnson RH, Griffin TW. Cone-beam CT for radiotherapy applications. Phys Med Biol. 1995;40(11):1863–83. Detection PU. 154/Pulmonary Disease. 2007; 154–5.
20. Araki K, Maki K, Seki K, Sakamaki K, Harata Y, Sakaino R, et al. Characteristics of a newly developed dentomaxillofacial X-ray cone beam CT scanner (CB MercuRayTM): system configuration and physical properties. Dentomaxillofac Radiol. 2004;33(1):51–9.
21. Venkatesh E, Elluru SV. CBCT: basics and applications in dentistry. J Istanbul Univ Fac Dent. 2017;51:102–21.
22. Yamamoto K, Ueno K, Seo K, Shinohara D. Development of dento-maxillofacial cone beam X-ray computed tomography system. Orthod Craniofac Res. 2003;6:160–2.
23. Scarfe WC, Farman AG. What is cone-beam CT and how does it work? Dent Clin N Am. 2008;52(4):707–30.
24. Scarfe WC, Farman AG, Sukovic P. Clinical applications of cone-beam computed tomography in dental practice. J Can Dent Assoc (Tor). 2006;72(1):75–80.
25. Baba R, Konno Y, Ueda K, Ikeda S. Comparison of flat-panel detector and image intensifier detector for cone-beam CT. Comput Med Imaging Graph. 2002;26(3):153–8.
26. Abramovitch K, Rice DD. Basic principles of cone beam computed tomography. Dent Clin N Am. 2014;58(3):463–84.
27. Feldkamp LA, Davis LC, Kress JW. Practical cone-beam algorithm. J Opt Soc Am. 1984;1(6):612–9.
28. Ritter L, Elger MC, Rothamel D, Fienitz T, Zinser M, Schwarz F, et al. Accuracy of peri-implant bone evaluation using cone beam CT, digital intra-oral radiographs and histology. Dentomaxillofac Radiol. 2014;43(6):20130088.

CBCT Anatomical Imaging

8

Spyros Damaskos and Antigoni Delantoni

8.1 Introduction

It is now known that cone beam computed tomography has revolutionized imaging in dentistry [1, 2]. Due to the ability of CBCT imaging to provide reconstructed images of high-contrast structures, in the head and neck as well as throughout the dentomaxillofacial region, this technic introduced dentistry in the cross-sectional era [3]. Reasonably, it now has extensive applications in the evaluation, and treatment plan of the head and neck pathology. It is also worth noting that the radiation dose required for CBCT imaging is significantly lower than that of MDCT [3, 4].

Based on the above, the multiplanar CBCT reformatted images are particularly useful for assessing the anatomy of the maxillofacial complex, as well as the anatomy of the skull base, temporal bone, and sinonasal cavities [5–8].

This radiological atlas demonstrates the normal anatomy seen in routine CBCT scans of the craniomaxillofacial complex [3, 4, 6–15]. Please note that prior to each individual image, the direction in which the cross-sectional images obtained and processed is indicated. In the Ist part, axial, coronal, and sagittal images of the cranio-maxillofacial complex are included. Specifically for the temporal bone (IInd part) [10–12, 16–19], reformatted images were used to display Pöschl projection and Stenvers plane (part III).

This radiological atlas is intended to be used as a learning/introductory object of the complex bone anatomy of the oral and maxillofacial region, as well as a "tool" that will assist both dentists and maxillofacial surgeons in the diagnosis and rehabilitation of the stomatognathic and craniomaxillofacial diseases. A "tool" that may also be useful to other medical professionals (e.g. ENT).

8.2 Part I

Note

- The interslice interval of the axial images is approximately 2 mm, in a cephalic/caudal orientation. This is indicated in the reference image on the left (surrounded by a blue line).
- The reconstruction level of the coronary images, in anteroposterior orientation, is indicated in the reference image on the left (surrounded by a red line).
- The reconstruction level of the sagittal images, in lateromedial orientation, is indicated in the

S. Damaskos (✉)
Oral Diagnosis and Radiology Department, School of Dentistry, National and Kapodistrian University of Athens, Athens, Greece
e-mail: sdamask@dent.uoa.gr

A. Delantoni
Department of Dentoalveolar Surgery, Implant Surgery and Radiology, Faculty of Dentistry, Aristotle University of Thessaloniki, Thessaloniki, Greece
e-mail: andelant@dent.auth.gr

A. Delantoni, K. Orhan (eds.), *Atlas of Dentomaxillofacial Anatomical Imaging*,
https://doi.org/10.1007/978-3-030-96840-3_8

reference images on the left (surrounded by a green line).

The CBCT volumetric data set was acquired with a NewTom™VGi CBCT imaging unit (QR S.r.l., Verona, Italy), and the volumetric reconstructions of the data set (FOV: 15 × 15 cm; voxel size of 0.2 mm) were created by using the manufacturer's proprietary software (NNT v6.2, Verona, Italy).

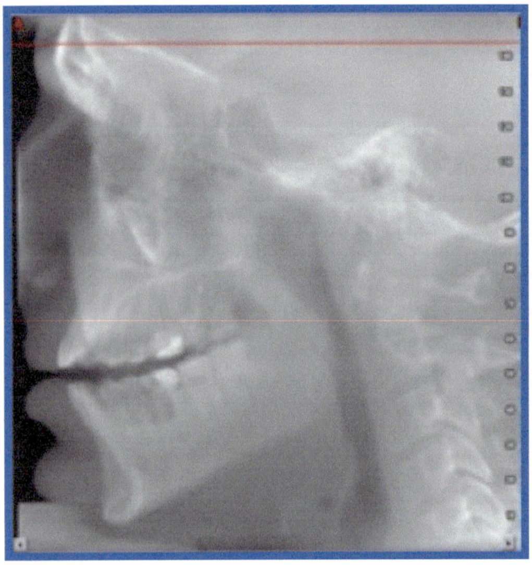

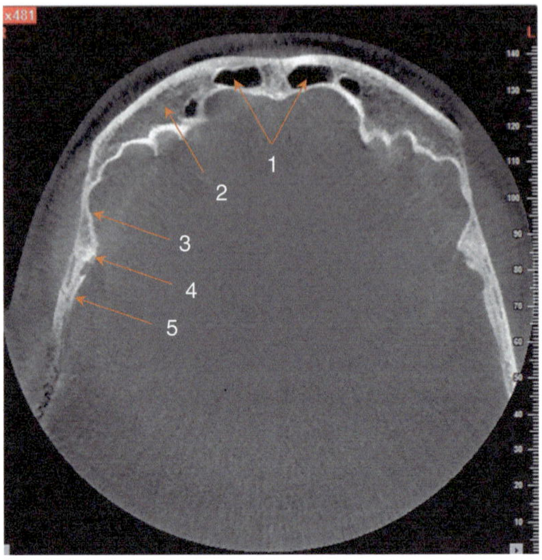

1. Frontal sinus.
2. Frontal bone.
3. Sphenoid bone.
4. Sphenosquamosal suture.
5. Temporal bone.

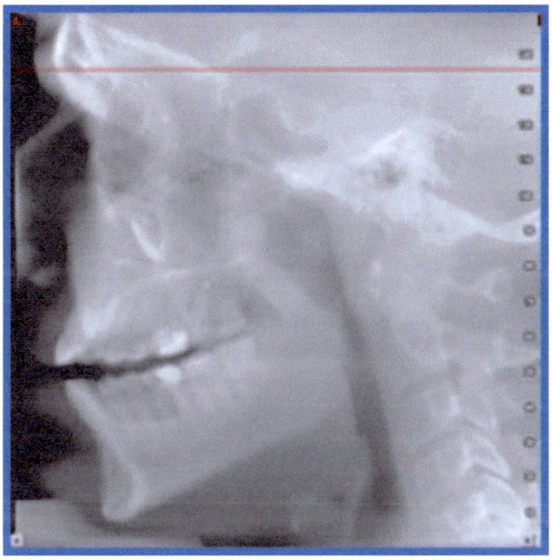

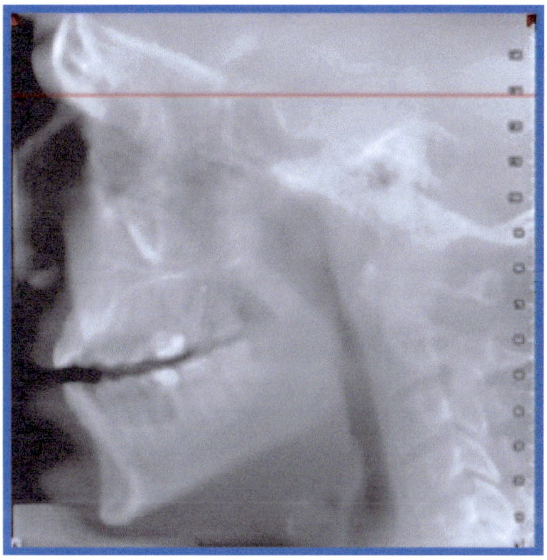

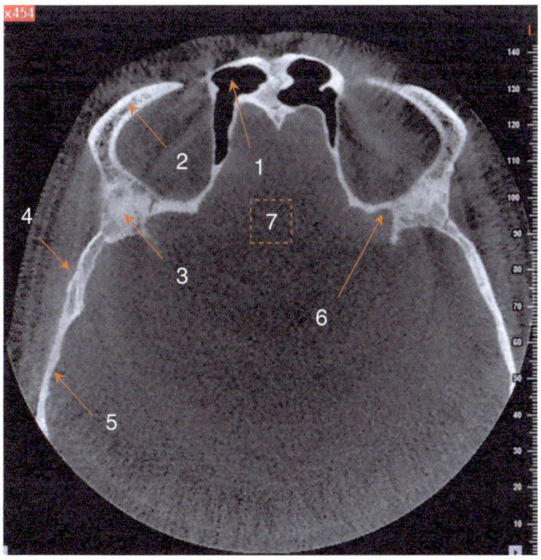

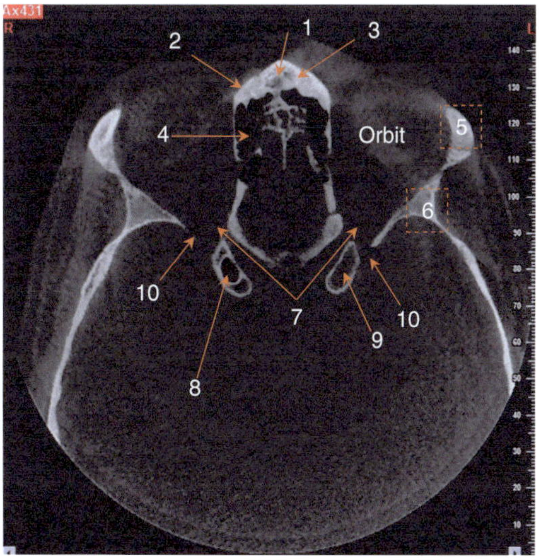

1. Frontal sinus.
2. Frontal bone.
3. Sphenoid bone.
4. Sphenosquamosal suture.
5. Temporal bone.
6. Optic canal.
7. Anterior Cranial Fossa.

1. Nasal bone.
2. Maxillary bone.
3. Nasomaxillary suture.
4. Ethmoid air cells.
5. Frontal bone.
6. Sphenoid bone.
7. Optic canal (Optic chiasma).
8. Sphenoid sinus.
9. Anterior clinoid process.
10. Superior orbital fissure.

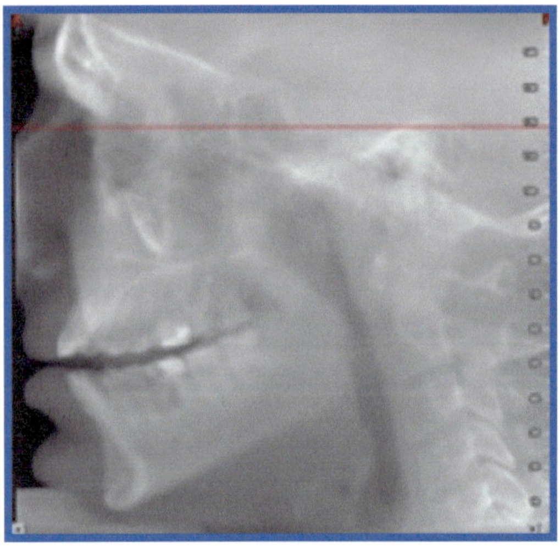

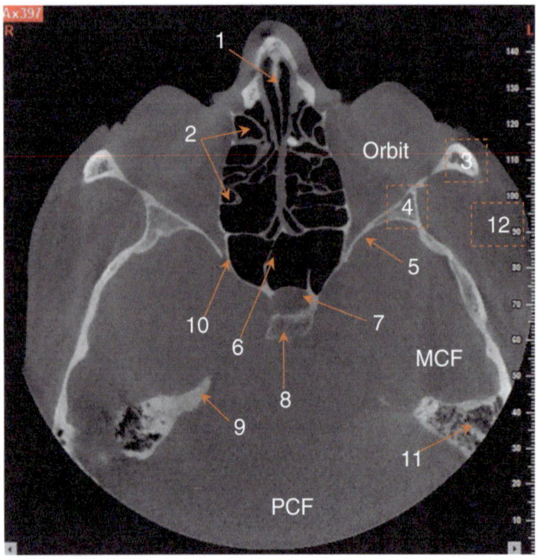

1. Nasal septum.
2. Ethmoid air cells.
3. Frontal bone.
4. Sphenoid bone.
5. Greater wing of the sphenoid.
6. Sphenoid sinus and septa.
7. Sellaturcica.
8. Dorsum sellae.
9. Internal acoustic meatus.
10. Superior orbital fissure.
11. Mastoid air cells.
12. Temporal fossa.

Posterior **C**ranial **F**ossa.
Middle **C**ranial **F**ossa.

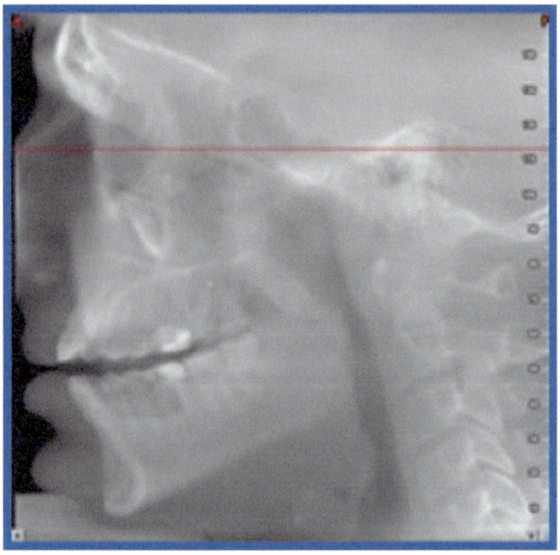

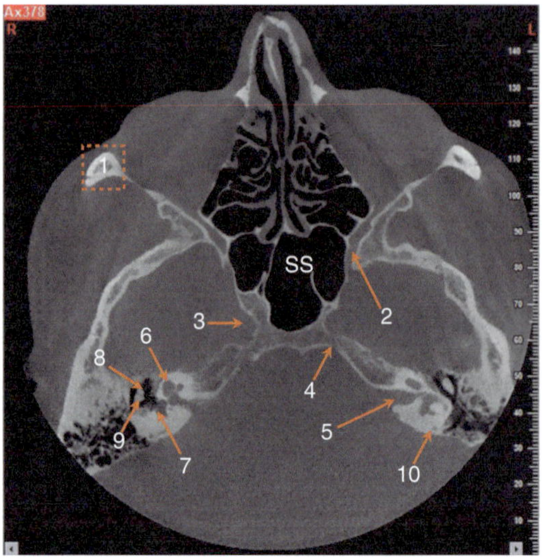

1. Zygomatic bone.
2. Foramen rotundum.
3. Carotid canal.
4. Petro-occipital fissure.
5. Internal auditory canal.
6. Cochlea.
7. Vestibule.
8. Malleus.
9. Incus.
10. Posterior semicircular canal.

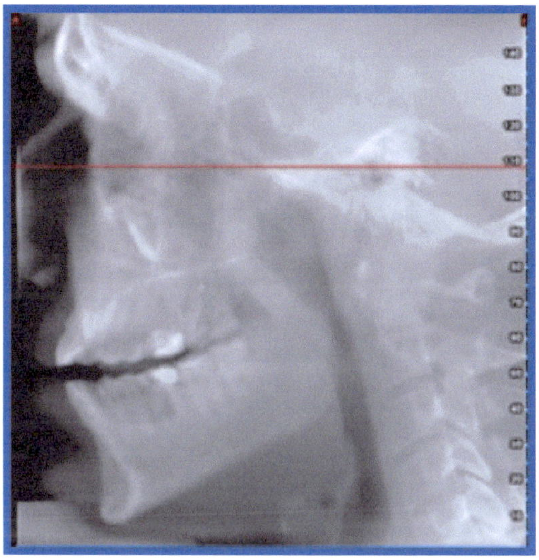

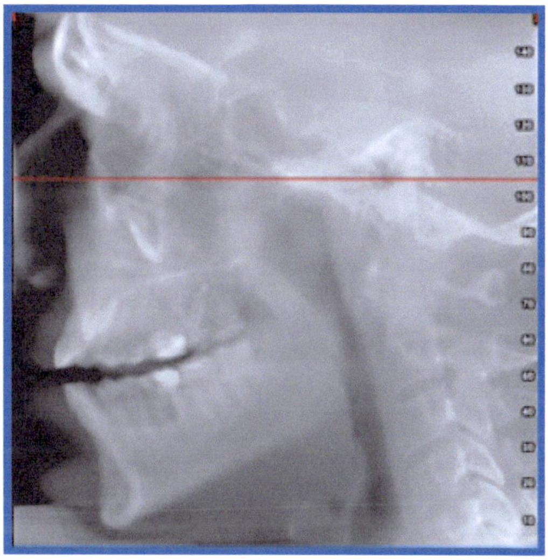

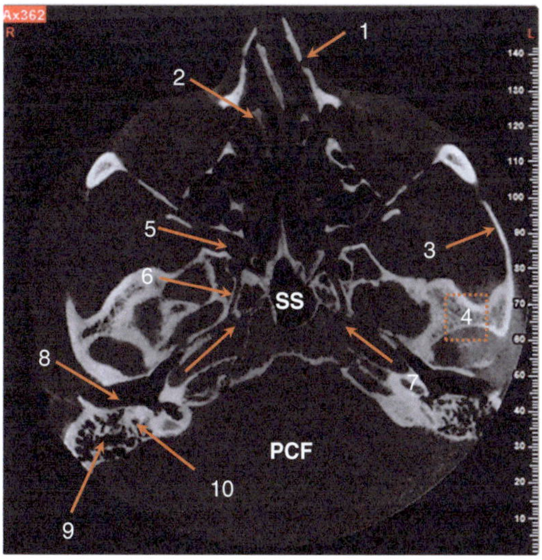

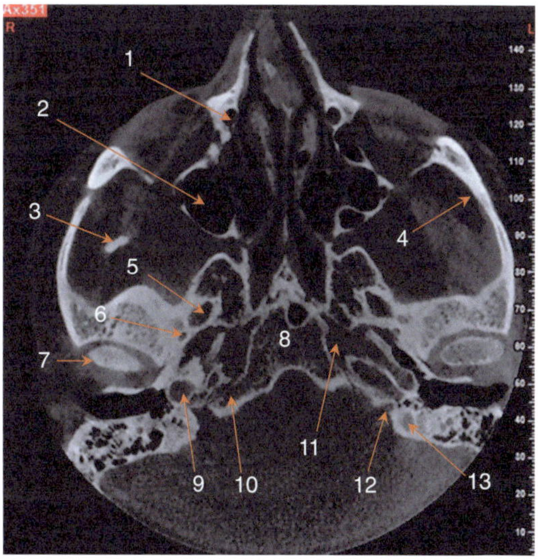

1. Nasomaxillary suture.
2. Middle nasal concha.
3. Zygomatic arch.
4. Temporal bone.
5. Pterygopalatine fossa.
6. Pterygoid (Vidian) canal.
7. Carotid canal.
8. External acoustic meatus, 5.
9. Mastoid air cells.
10. Facial nerve canal.

Sphenoid **S**inus.
Posterior **C**ranial **F**ossa.

1. Nasolacrimal duct,
2. Maxillary sinus.
3. Mandible's coronoid process.
4. Zygomaticomaxillary suture.
5. Foramen ovale.
6. Foramen spinosum.
7. Mandibular condyle.
8. Clivus.
9. Carotid canal (vertical p.).
10. Occipital bone.
11. Foramen lacerum.
12. Jugular foramen.
13. Jugular bulb.

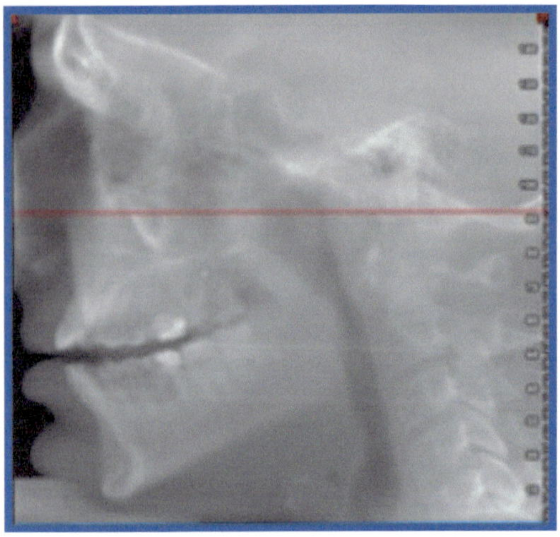

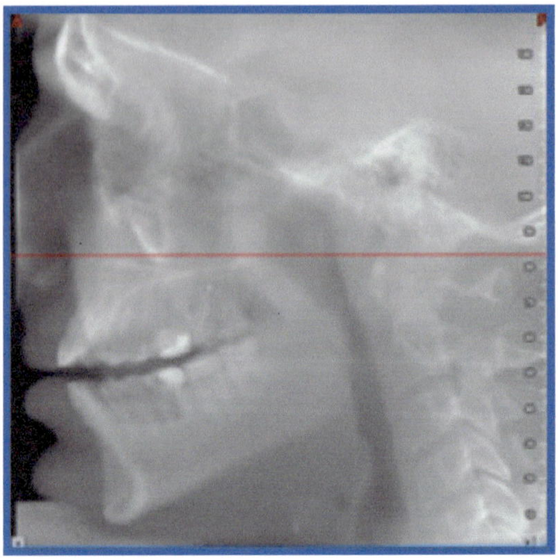

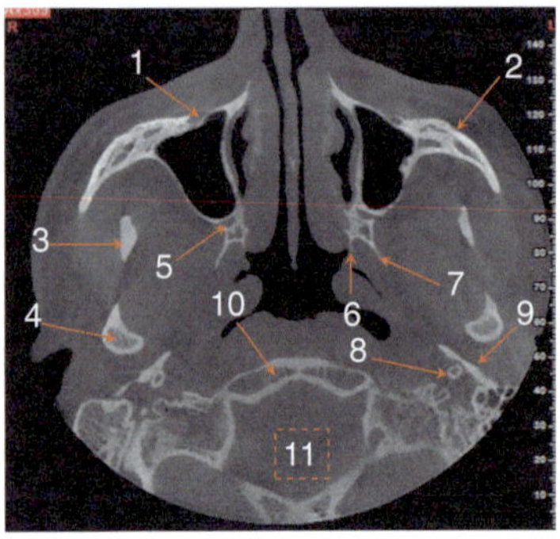

1. Infraorbital canal.
2. Zygomaticomaxillary suture.
3. Coronoid process of mandible.
4. Condylar process of m.
5. Pterygopalatine fossa.
6. Medial pterygoid process.
7. Lateral pterygoid process.
8. Styloid process.
9. Tympanic part of temporal bone (vaginal process).
10. Occipital condyle.
11. Foramen magnum.

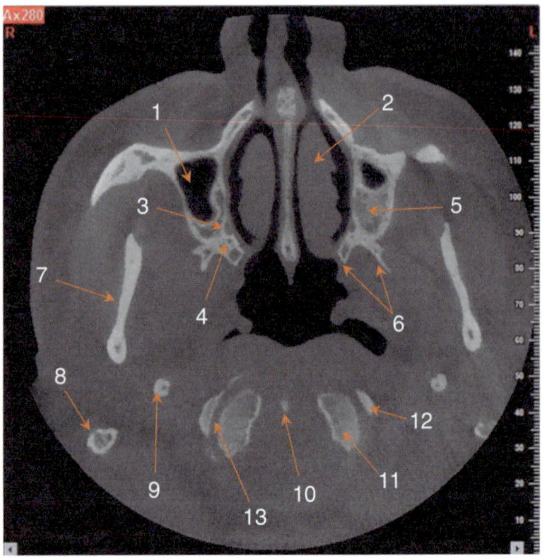

1. Maxillary sinus.
2. Inferior nasal concha.
3. Greater palatine foramina.
4. Lesser palatine foramina.
5. Maxilla.
6. Lateral and medial pterygoid plates.
7. Ramus of mandible.
8. Mastoid process.
9. Styloid process.
10. Axis – C2 Dens (odontoid process).
11. Occipital condyle.
12. Atlas – C1; Lateral mass.
13. Atlantooccipital joint.

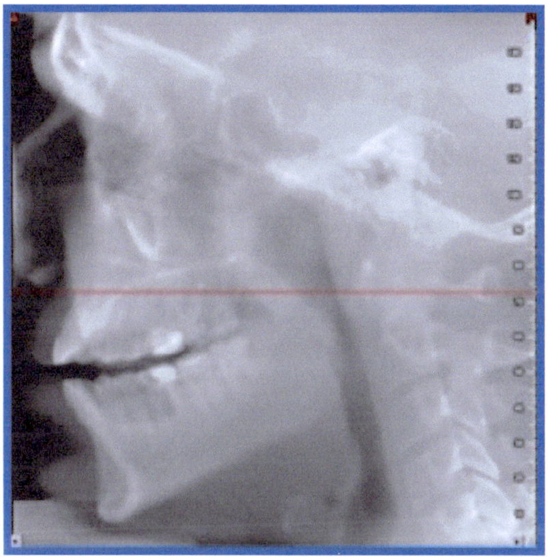

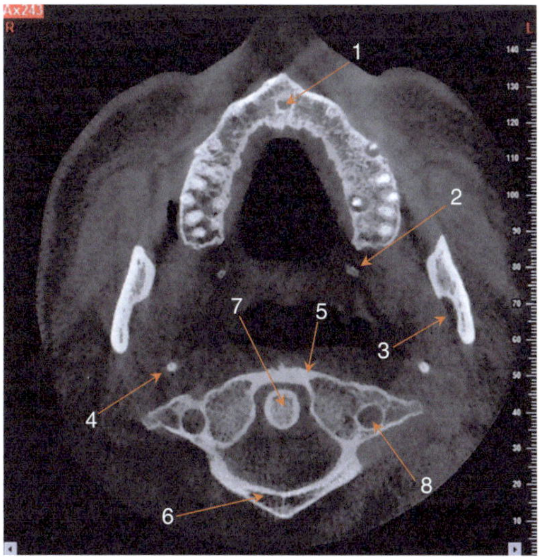

1. Incisive foramen.
2. Lateral pterygoid plate.
3. Mandibular canal.
4. Styloid process.
5. Atlas – C1; anterior arch.
6. Atlas – C1; posterior arch.
7. Axis – C2 Dens (odontoid process).
8. Transvers foramen.

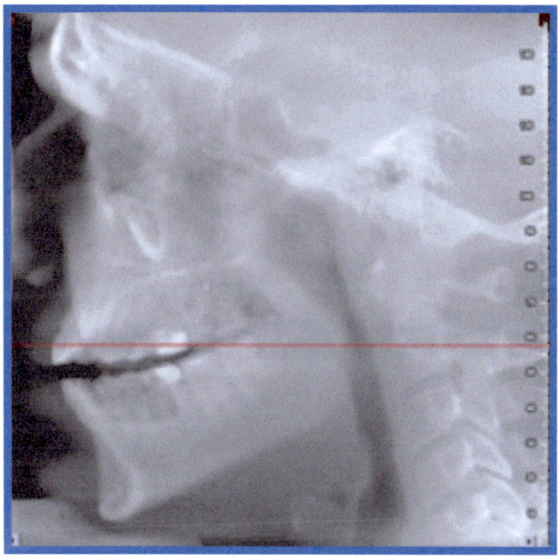

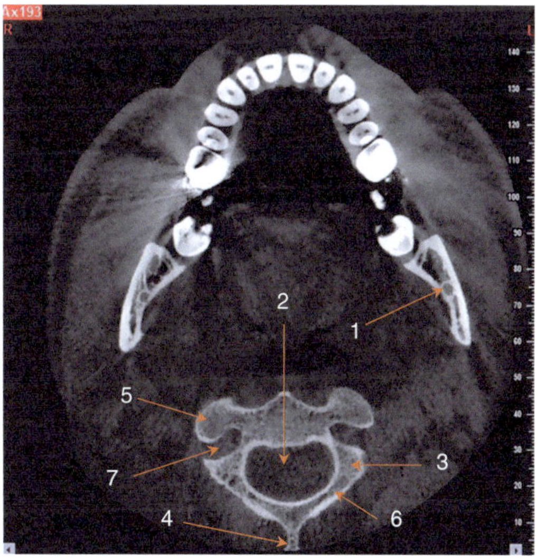

1. Mandibular canal.
2. Vertebral foramen.
3. Pedicle.
4. Spinous process – C2.
5. Transverse process – C2.
6. Lamina – C2.
7. Transverse foramen.

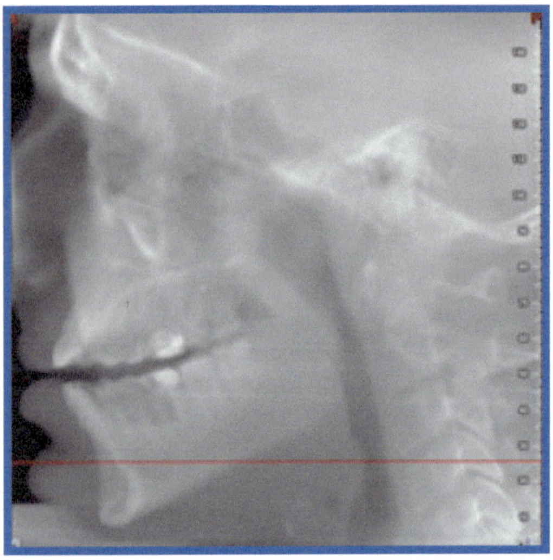

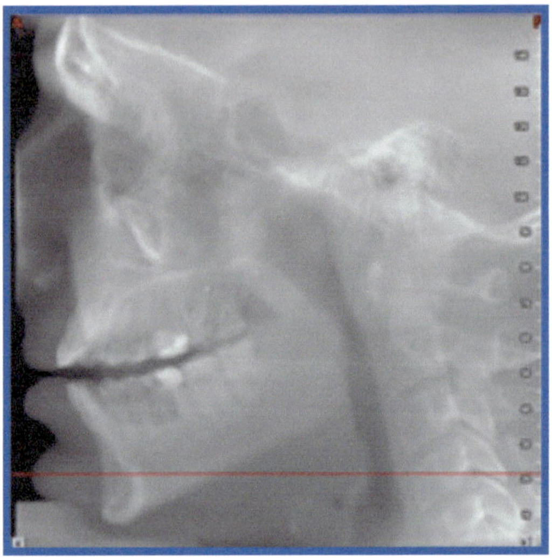

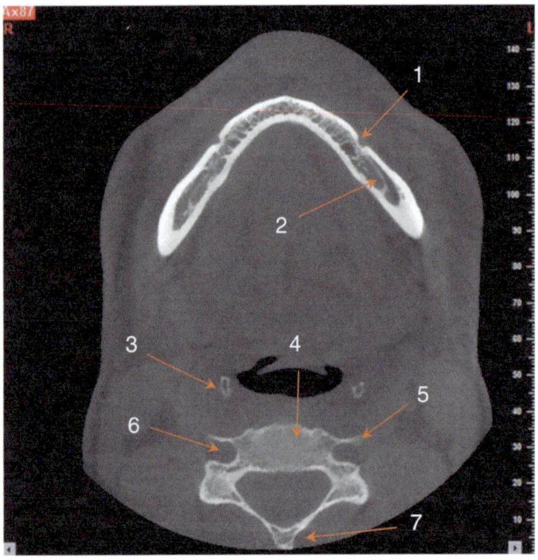

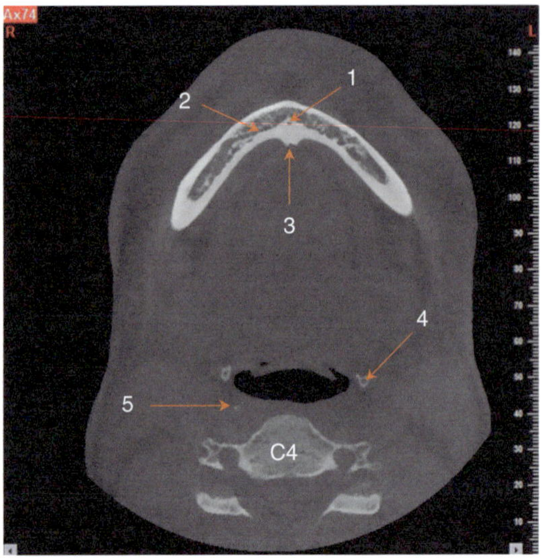

1. Mental foramen.
2. Mandibular canal.
3. Greater cornu of hyoid.
4. C4 – vertebral body.
5. C4 – transverse process.
6. C4 – transverse foramen.
7. Spinous process of C4.

1. Lingual foramen.
2. Mandibular incisive canal.
3. .Mental spines.
4. Greater cornu of hyoid bone.
5. Triticeous cartilage.

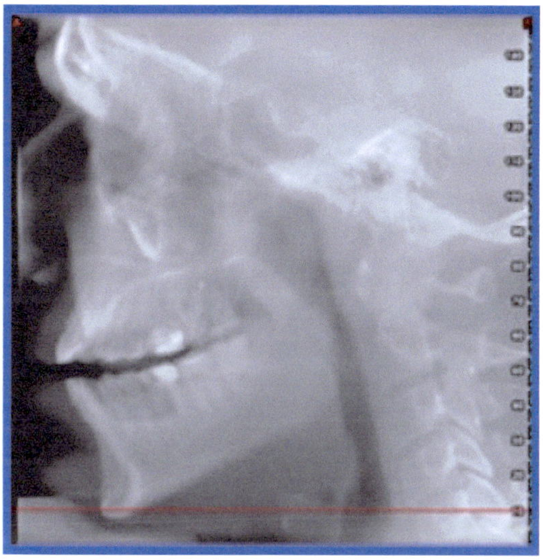

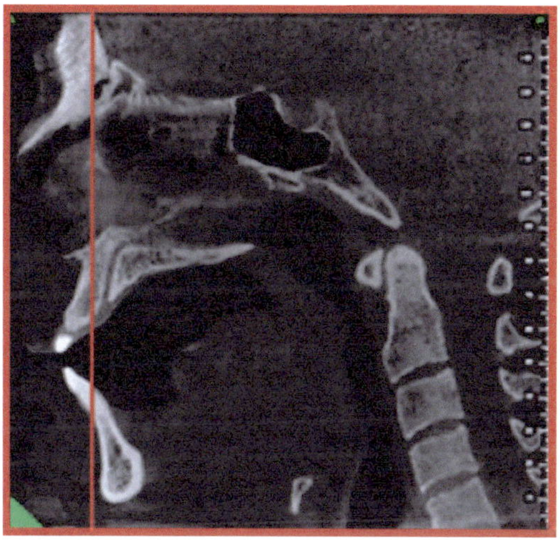

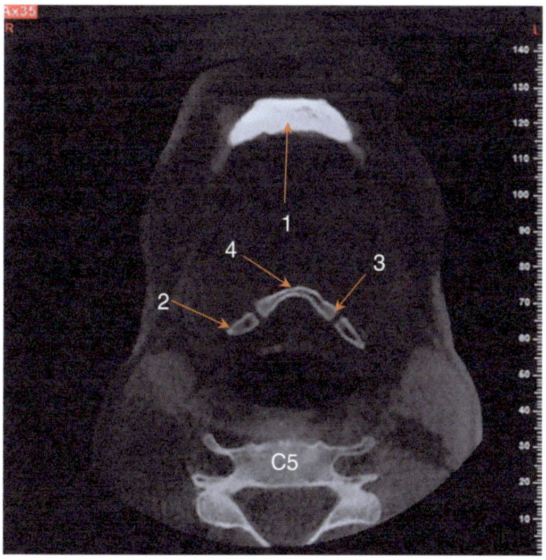

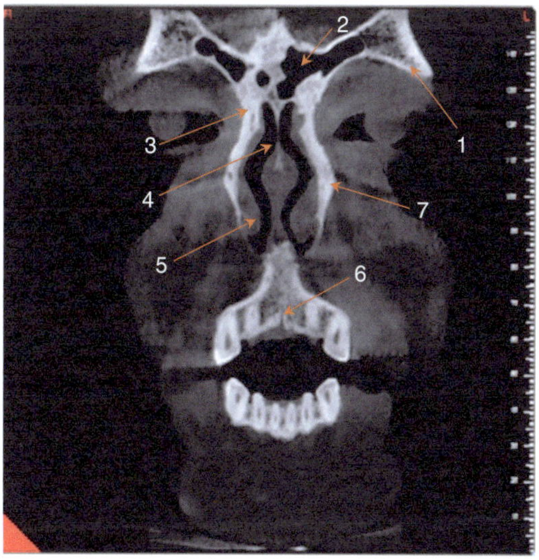

1. Lingual foramen.
2. Greater cornu of hyoid bone.
3. Lesser cornu of hyoid bone.
4. Body of hyoid bone.

1. Frontal bone.
2. Frontal sinus.
3. Nasal bone.
4. Nasal septum.
5. Inferior nasal concha.
6. Incisive canal.
7. Frontal process of maxilla.

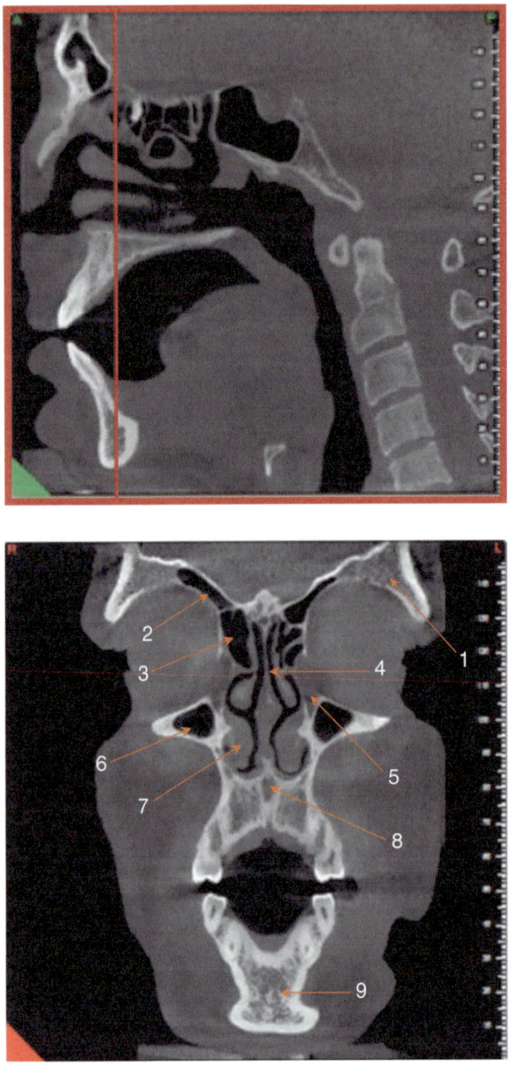

1. Frontal bone.
2. Frontal sinus.
3. Ethmoid air cells.
4. Nasal septum.
5. Nasolacrimal duct.
6. Maxillary sinus.
7. Inferior nasal concha.
8. Incisive canal.
9. Lingual foramen.

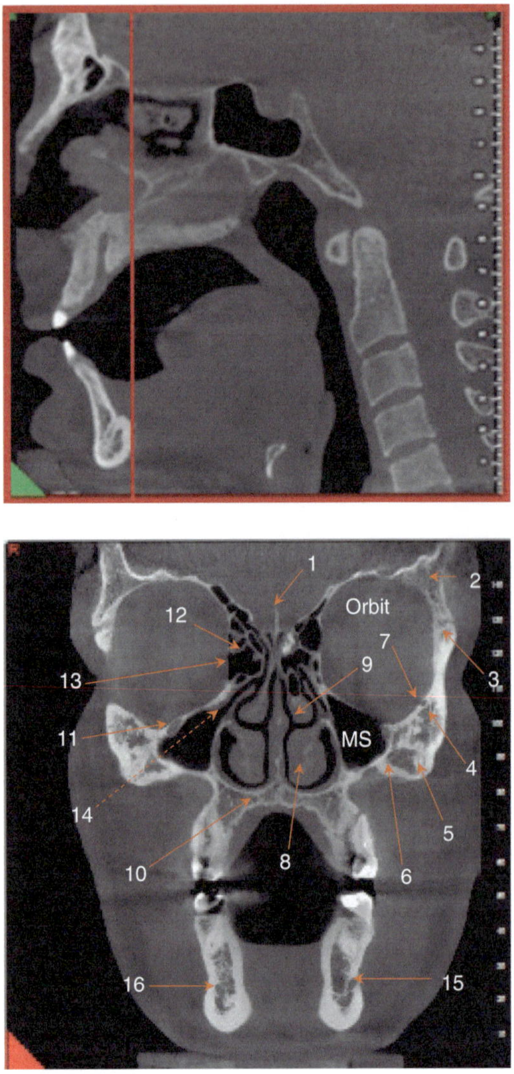

1. Crista galli.
2. Frontal bone.
3. Frontozygomatic suture.
4. Zygomatic bone.
5. Zygomaticomaxillary suture.
6. Maxilla.
7. Zygomaticofacial foramen.
8. Inferior nasal concha.
9. Middle nasal concha.
10. Hard palate.
11. Infraorbital canal.
12. Ethmoid air cells.
13. Ethmoid bone.
14. Ostia (Drainage channel to **M**axillary **S**inus).
15. Mental foramen.
16. Mandibular canal.

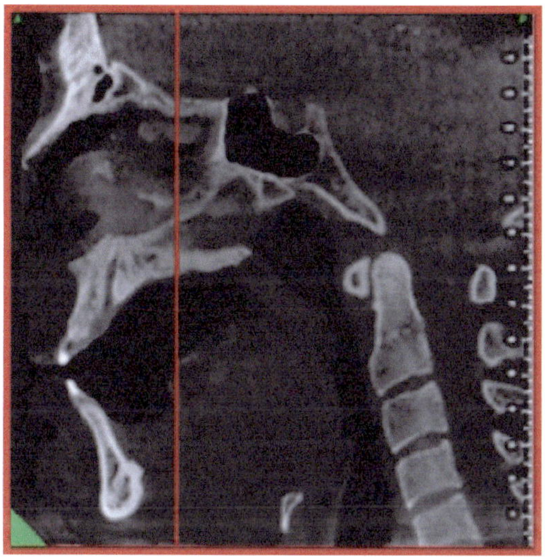

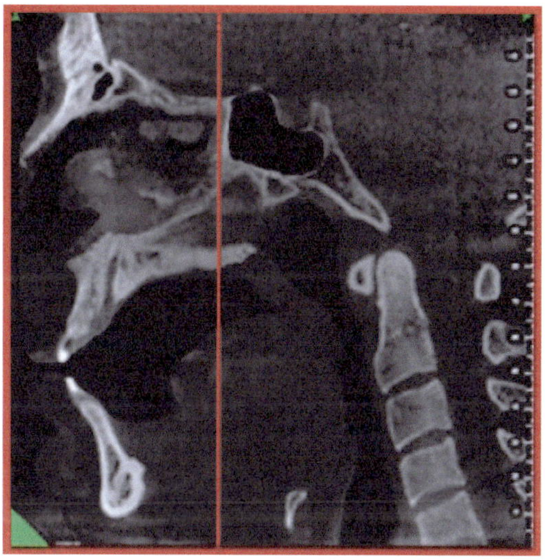

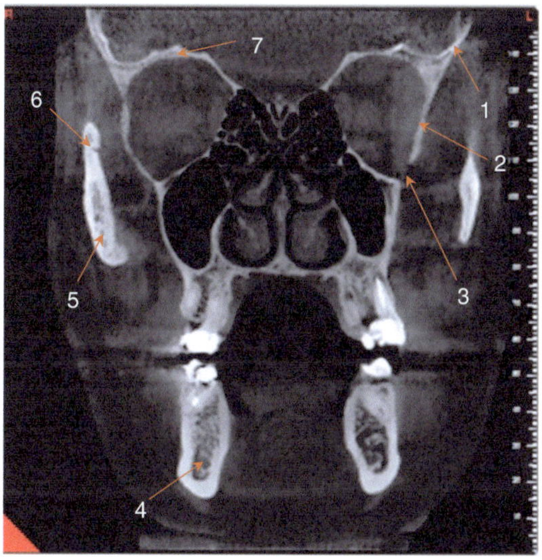

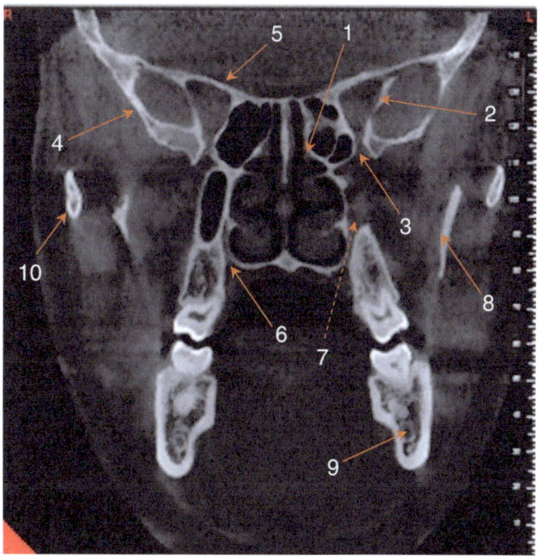

1. Frontal bone.
2. Greater wing of sphenoid b.
3. Inferior orbital fissure.
4. Mandibular canal.
5. Zygomatic bone.
6. Frontozygomatic suture.
7. Orbital roof.

1. Superior nasal concha.
2. Greater wing of sphenoid b.
3. Superior orbital fissure.
4. Sphenoid bone.
5. Lesser wing of sphenoid b.
6. Greater palatine foramina.
7. Pterygopalatine fossa.
8. Coronoid process of mandible.
9. Mandibular canal.
10. Zygomatic arch.

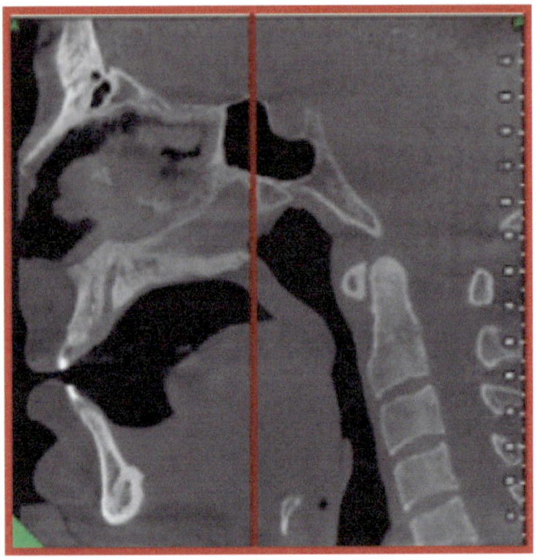

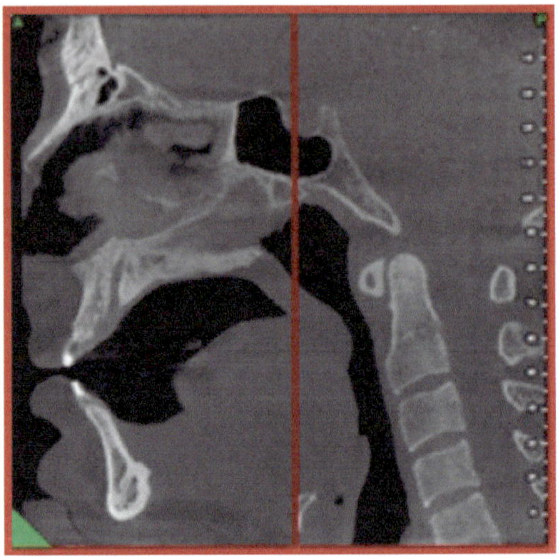

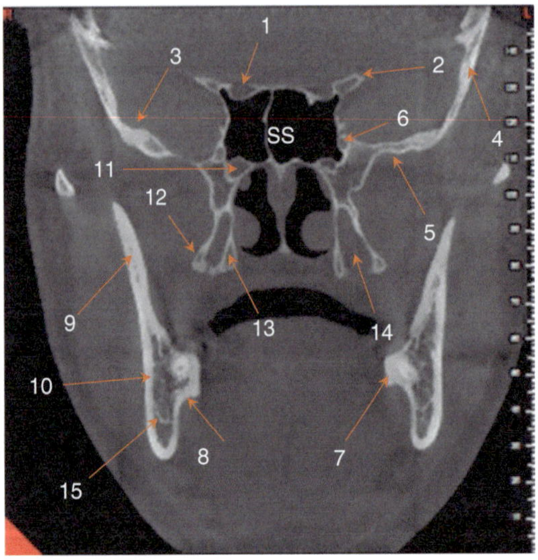

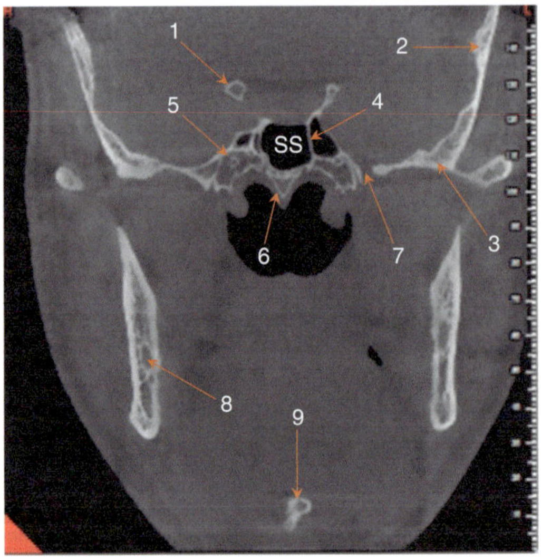

1. Optical canal.
2. Lesser wing of sphenoid b.
3. Sphenosquamosal suture.
4. Temporal bone.
5. Greater wing of sphenoid b.
6. Foramen rotondum.
7. Mylohyoid line.
8. Submandibular fossa.
9. Ramus.
10. Mandible.
11. Pterygopalatine fossa.
12. Lateral lamina of pterygoid process.
13. Medial lamina of p.p.
14. Pterygoid fossa.
15. Mandibular canal.

1. Anterior clinoid process.
2. Squamosal suture.
3. Sphenosquamosal suture.
4. Septum of SS.
5. Pterygoid (Vidian) canal.
6. Nasal septum.
7. Foramen ovale.
8. Mandibular canal.
9. Body of hyoid bone.

Sphenoid **S**inus.

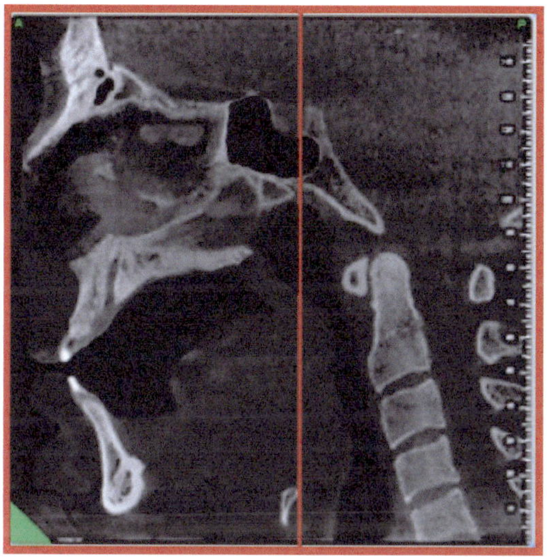

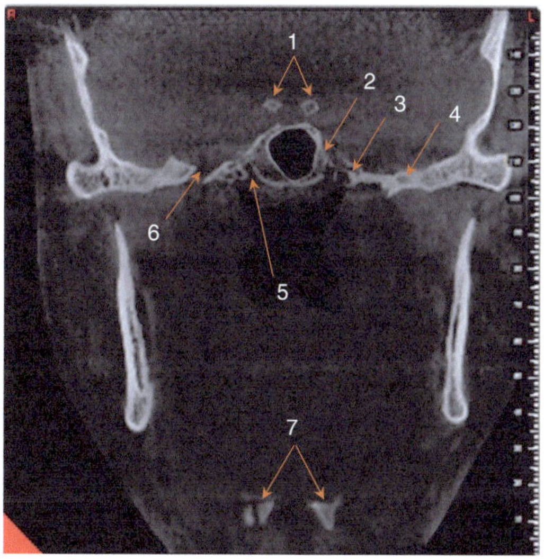

1. Posterior clinoid process.
2. Carotid sulcus.
3. Carotid canal.
4. Foramen spinosum.
5. Foramen lacerum.
6. Foramen ovale.
7. Body of hyoid bone.

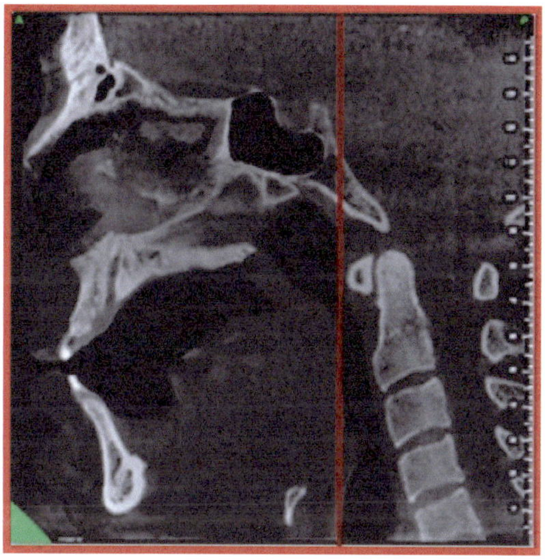

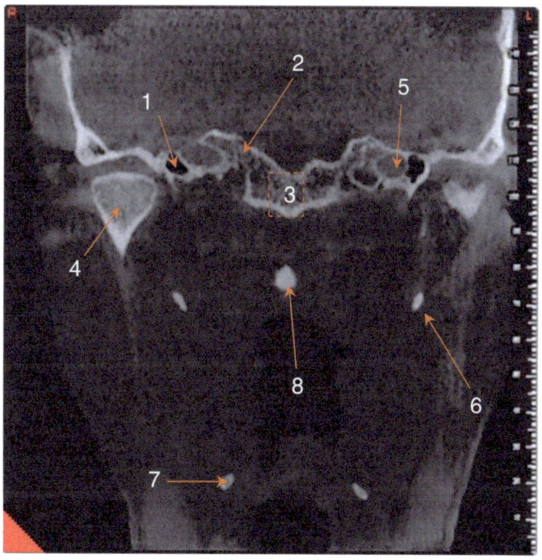

1. External acoustic meatus.
2. Petro-occipital fissure.
3. Occipital bone.
4. Mandibular condyle.
5. Carotid canal.
6. Styloid process.
7. Greater cornu of hyoid bone.
8. Atlas – C1; anterior arch.

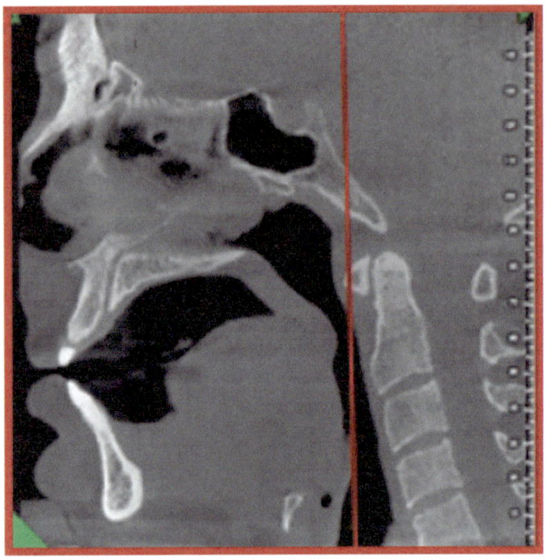

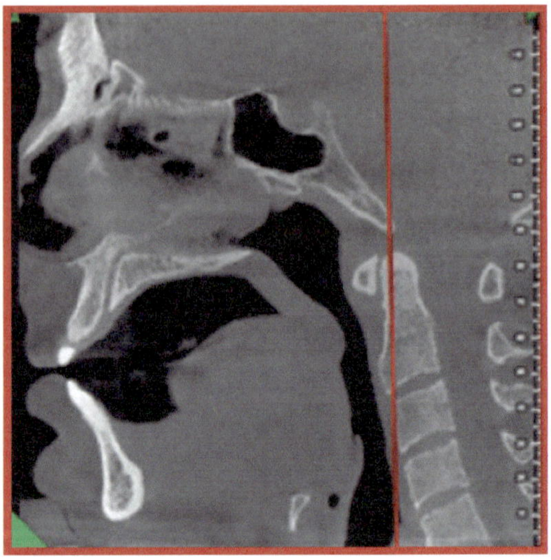

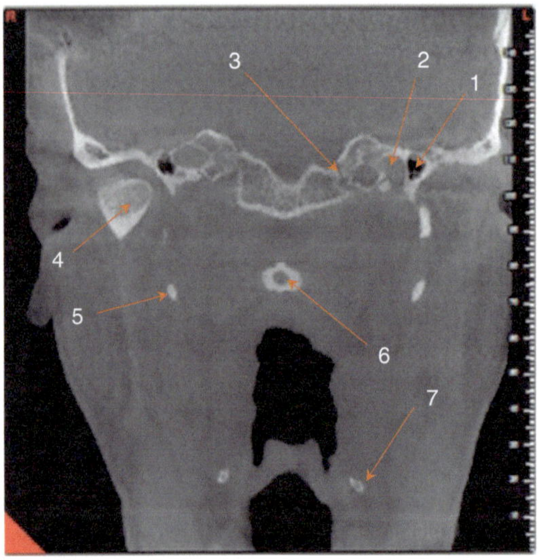

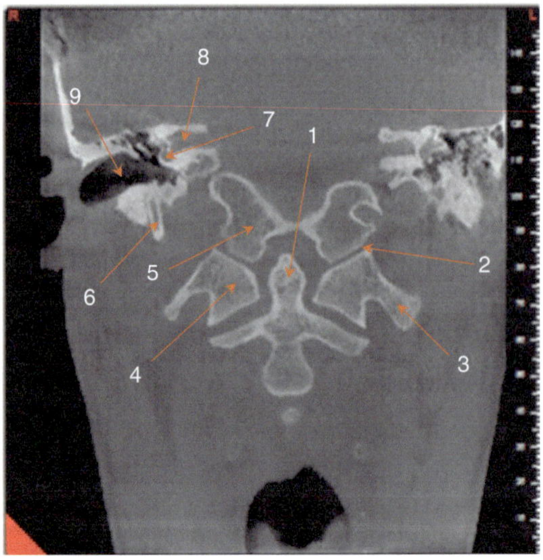

1. External acoustic meatus.
2. Carotid canal.
3. Petro-occipital fissure.
4. Mandibular condyle.
5. Styloid process.
6. Atlas – C1; anterior arch.
7. Greater cornu of hyoid bone.

1. Dens (Axis-C2).
2. Atlantooccipital joint.
3. Transverse process of C1.
4. Lateral mass of C1.
5. Occipital condyle.
6. Styloid process.
7. Round window.
8. Internal auditory canal.
9. External acoustic meatus.

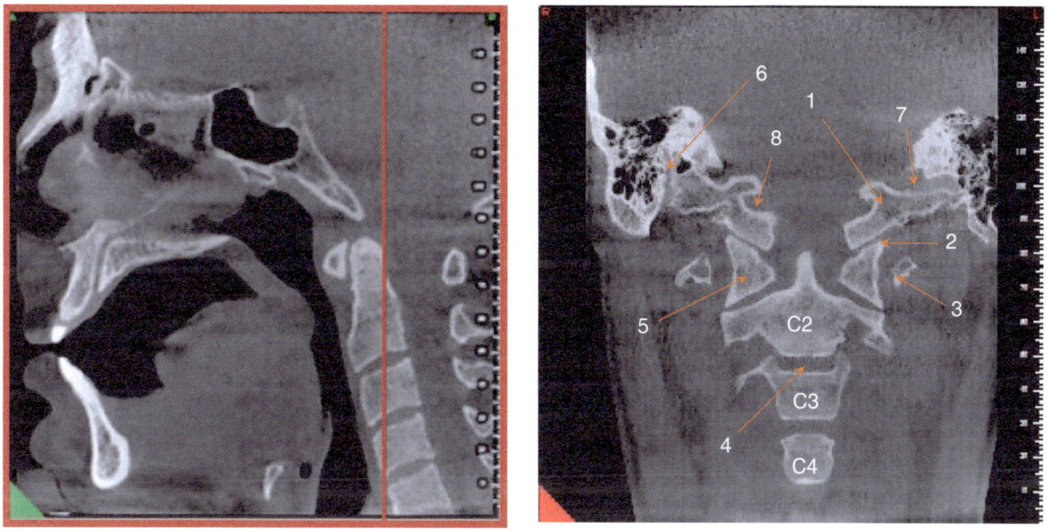

1. Occipital condyle.
2. Atlantooccipital joint.
3. Transverse process of C1.
4. Intervertebral space (C2–C3).
5. Lateral mass of C1.
6. Facial nerve canal.
7. Jugular foramen.
8. Hypoglossal canal.

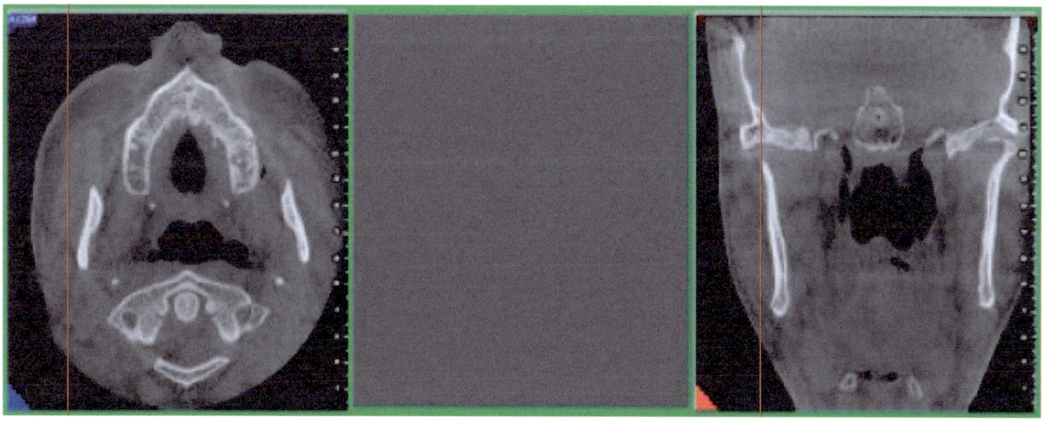

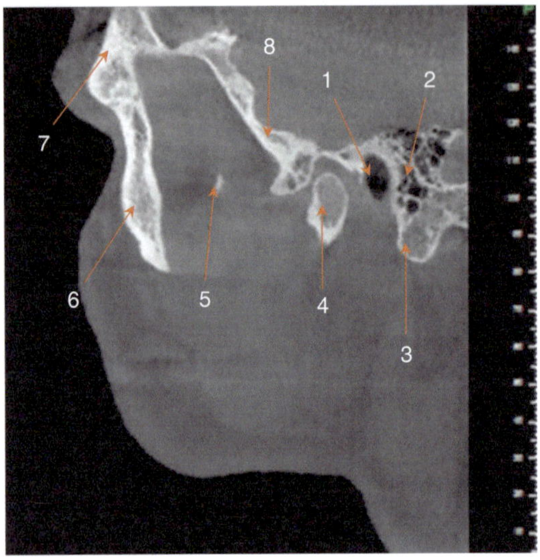

1. External acoustic meatus.
2. Mastoid air cells.
3. Mastoid process.
4. Condyle of mandible.
5. Coronoid process of mandible.
6. Zygomatic bone.
7. Frontal bone.
8. Temporal bone.

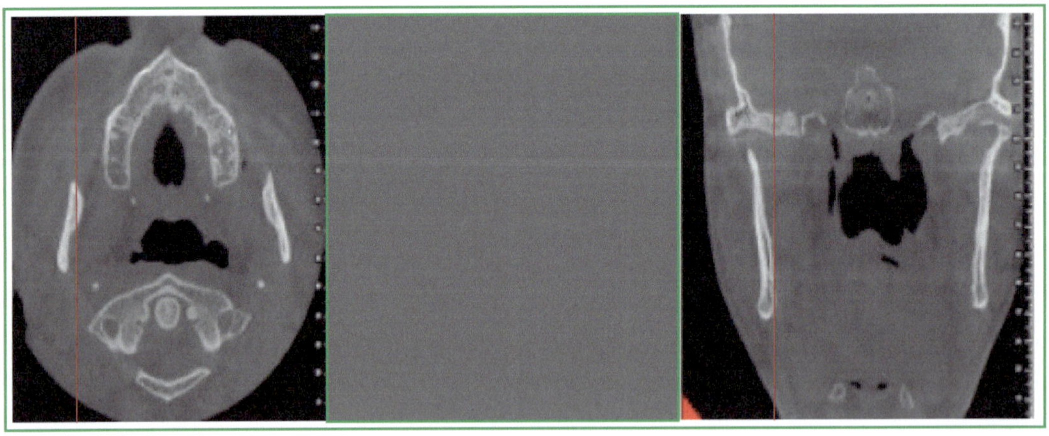

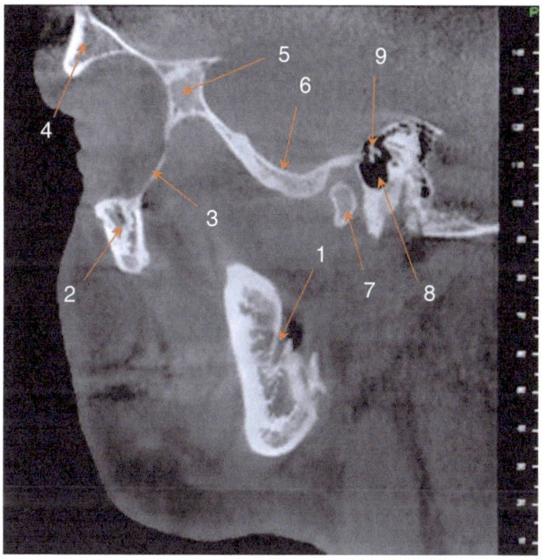

1. Mandibular canal.
2. Zygomatic bone.
3. Greater wing of sphenoid b.
4. Frontal bone.
5. Sphenoid bone.
6. Temporal bone.
7. Mandibular condyle.
8. External acoustic meatus.
9. Incus and Malleus.

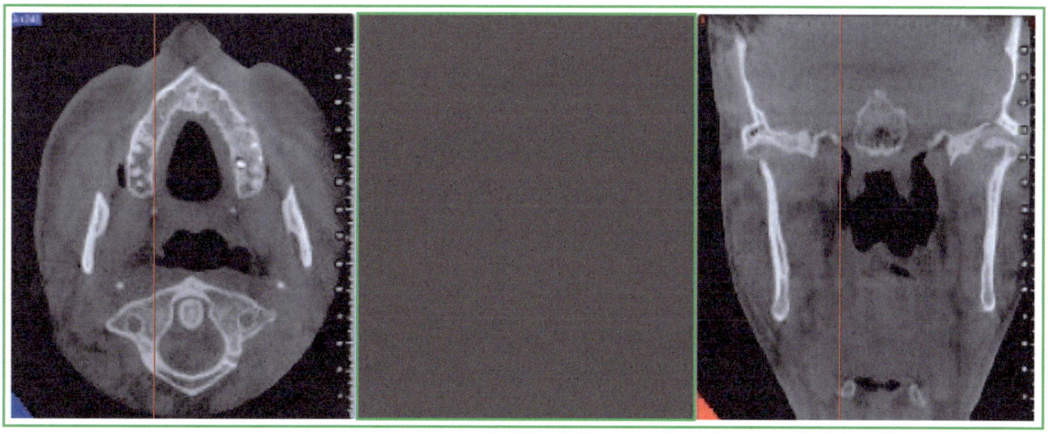

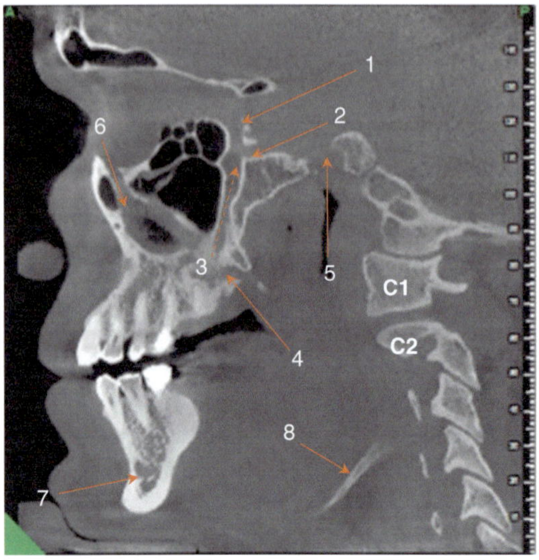

1. Superior orbital fissure.
2. Foramen rotondum.
3. Pterygopalatine fossa.
4. Greater palatine foramina.
5. Carotid canal.
6. Nasolacrimal duct.
7. Mental foramen.
8. Hyoid bone.

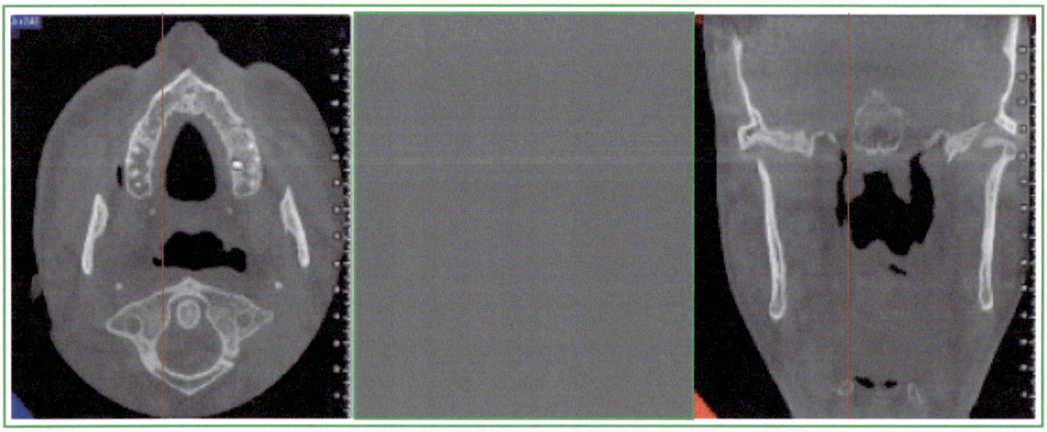

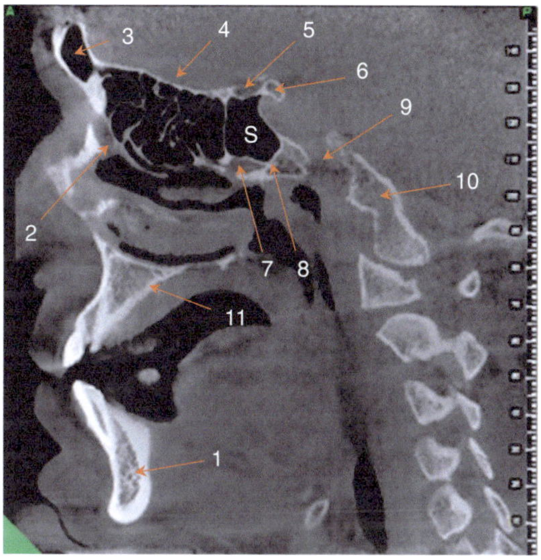

1. Mandibular canal.
2. Nasolacrimal duct.
3. Frontal sinus.
4. Cribriform plate of ethmoid canal.
5. Optic canal.
6. Anterior clinoid process.
7. Pterygo palatine fossa.
8. Pterygoid (Vidian) canal.
9. Foramen lacerum.
10. Clivus.
11. Palatine process of maxilla.

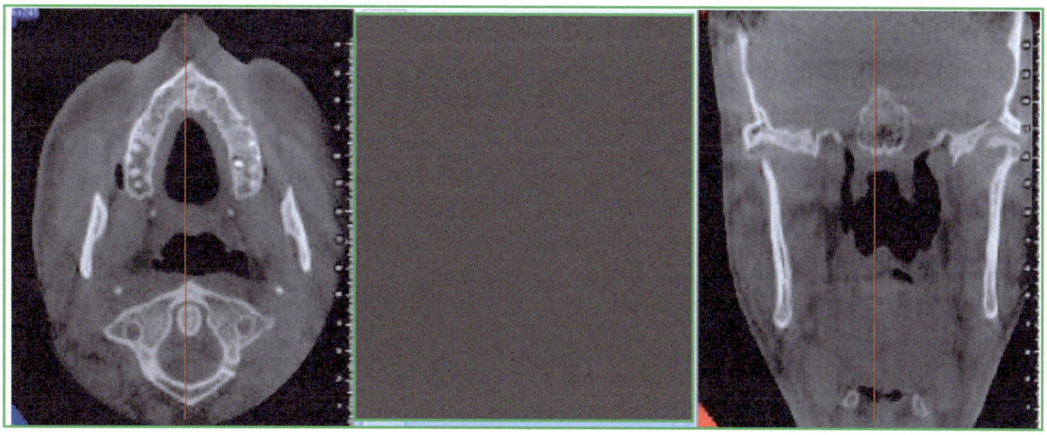

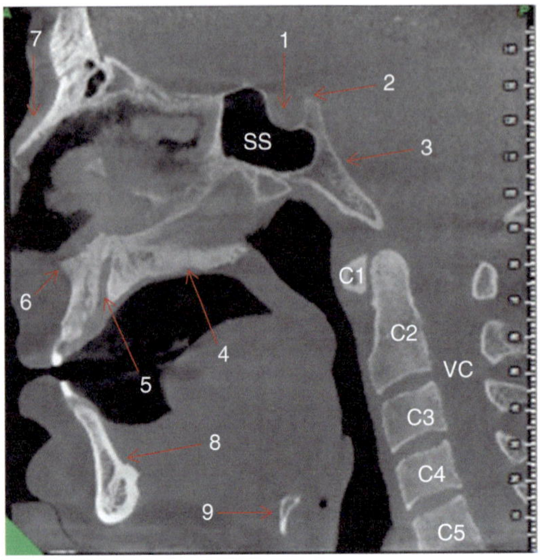

1. Hypophysial fossa.
2. Dorsum sellae.
3. Clivus.
4. Palatine process of maxilla.
5. Incisive canal.
6. Anterior nasal spine.
7. Nasal bone.
8. Lingual foramen.
9. Hyoid bone.

   Sphenoid **S**inus.

   Vertebral **C**anal.

8.3 Part II

Note

- The interslice interval of the axial images is approximately 2 mm, in a caudal/cephalic orientation. This is indicated in the reference image on the left (surrounded by a blue line).
- The reconstruction level of the coronary images, in anteroposterior orientation, is indicated in the reference image on the left (surrounded by a red line).
- The reconstruction level of the sagittal images, in lateromedial orientation, is indicated in the reference images on the left (surrounded by a green line).

The CBCT volumetric data set was acquired with a NewTom™ VGi CBCT imaging unit (QR S.r.l., Verona, Italy), and the volumetric reconstructions of the data set (FOV: 15 × 15 cm; voxel size of 0.2 mm) were created by using the manufacturer's proprietary software (NNT v6.2, Verona, Italy).

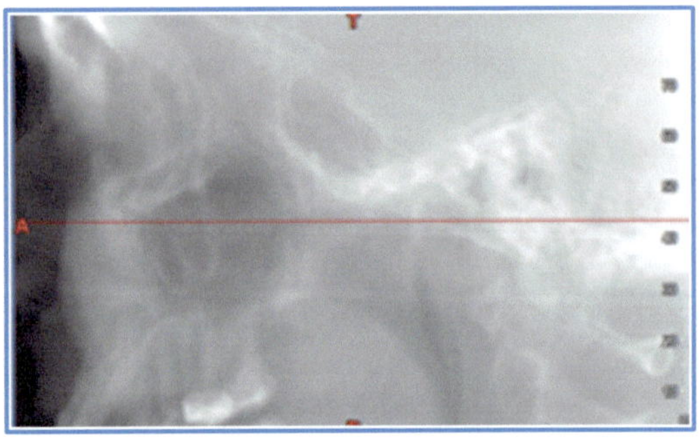

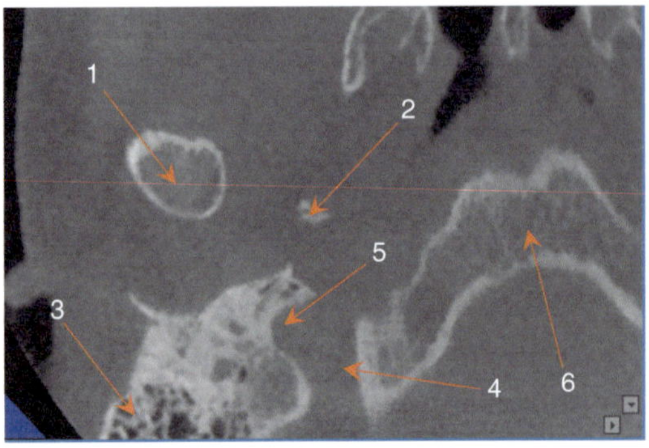

1. Condylar process of mandible.
2. Styloid process.
3. Mastoid process (mastoid air-cells).
4. Hypoglossal canal.
5. Jugular foramen.
6. Clivus.

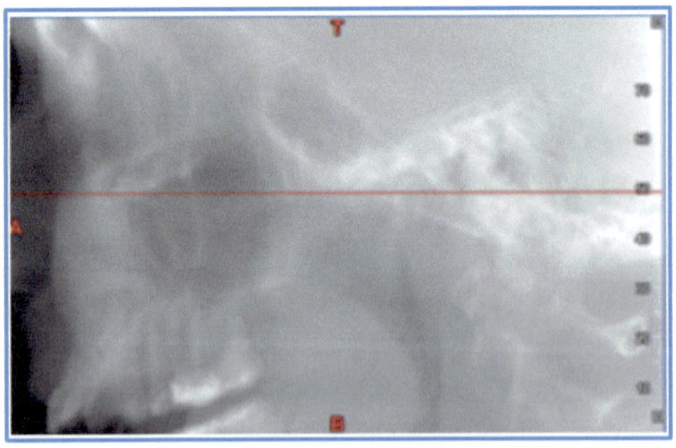

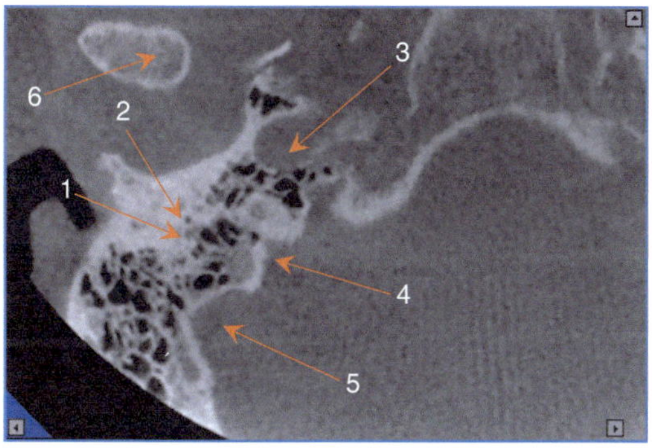

1. Facial nerve canal (mastoid segment).
2. Canal for the chorda tympani.
3. Carotid canal (petrous portion).
4. Jugular bulb.
5. Sigmoid sinus.
6. Mandibular condyle.

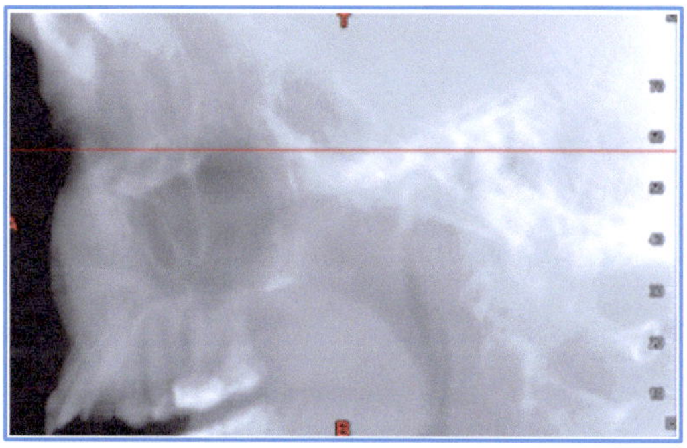

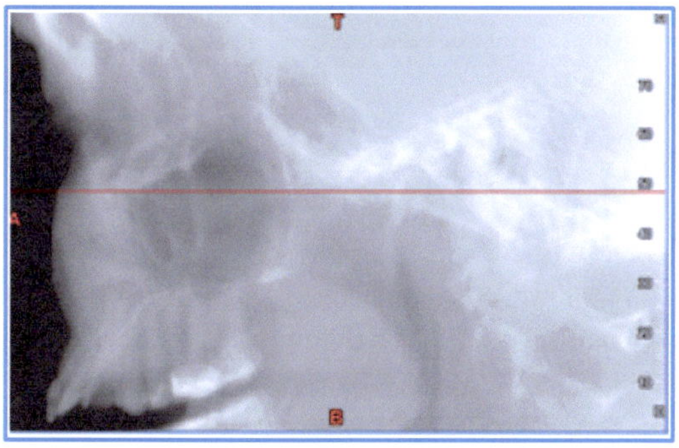

1. Facial nerve canal.
2. Canal for the chorda tympani.
3. Carotid canal (horizontal segment).
4. Jugular bulb.
5. Sigmoid sinus.
6. Jugular foramen.

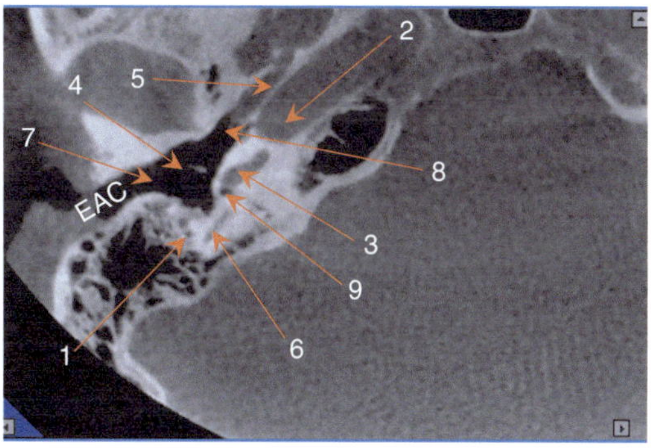

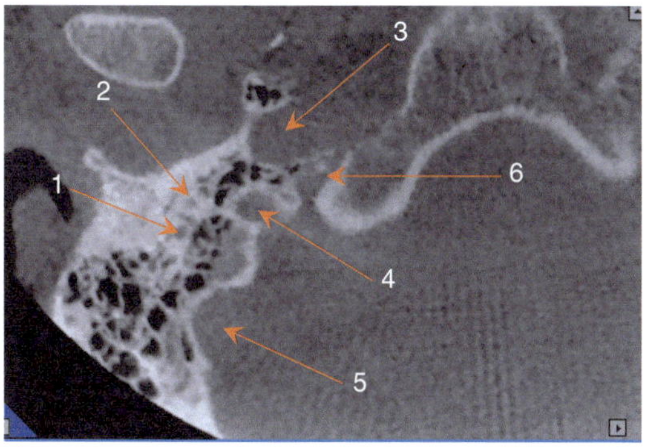

1. Facial nerve canal.
2. Carotid canal (horizontal segment).
3. Cochlea (basal turn).
4. Manubrium of malleus.
5. Canal for tensor tympani muscle.
6. Ampulla of posterior semicircular canal.
7. Tympanic membrane.
8. Eustachian tube opening.
9. Round window.

External **A**uditory **C**anal.

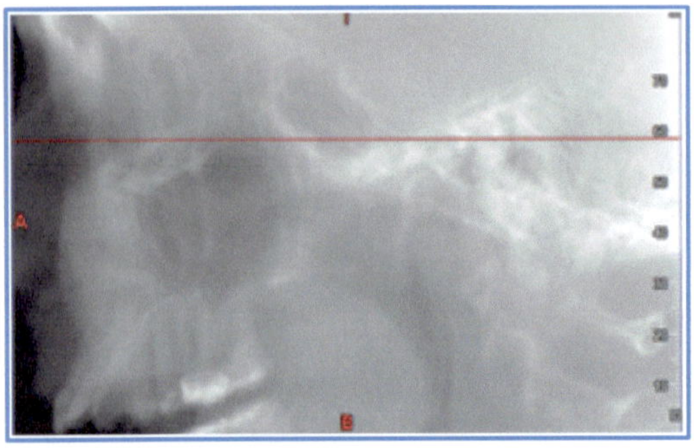

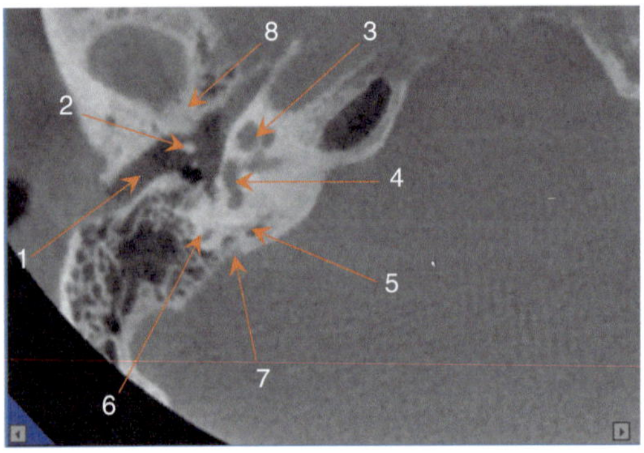

1. External auditory canal.
2. Maleus.
3. Cochlea (basal turn).
4. Vestibule.
5. Ampula of posterior semicircular canal.
6. Posterior semicircular canal.
7. Vestibular aqueduct.
8. Petrotympanic fissure.

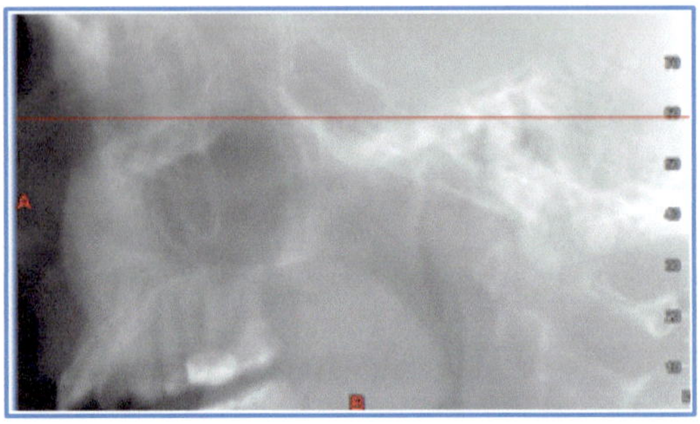

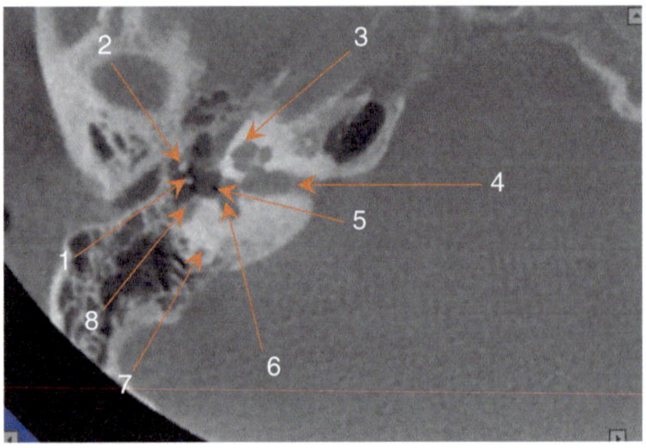

1. Incus.
2. Maleus.
3. Modiolus.
4. Internal auditory canal.
5. Oval window.
6. Vestibule.
7. Posterior semicircular canal.
8. Facial nerve canal.

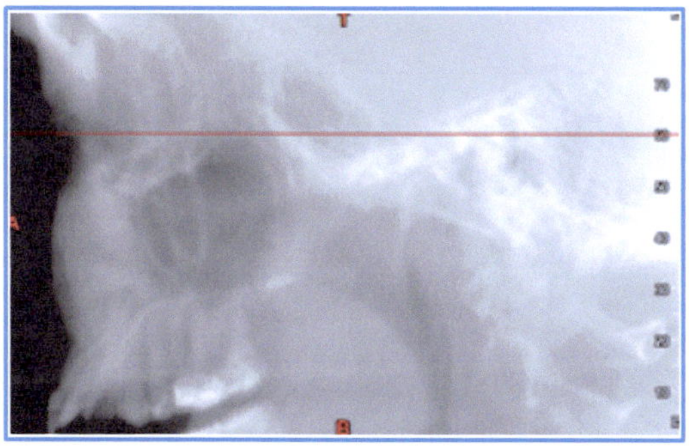

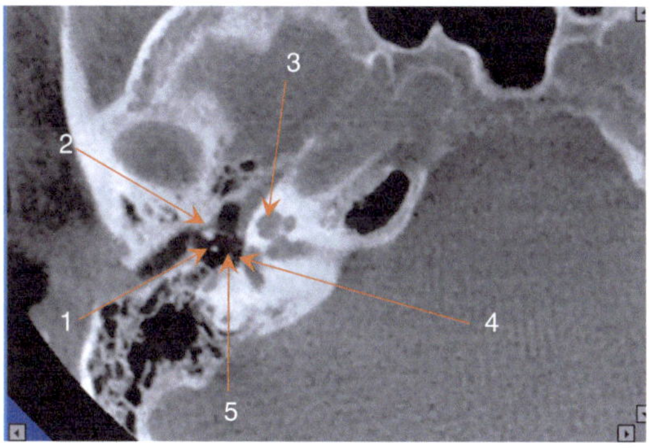

1. Incus (long process).
2. Maleus (long process).
3. Modiolus.
4. Oval window.
5. Stapes.

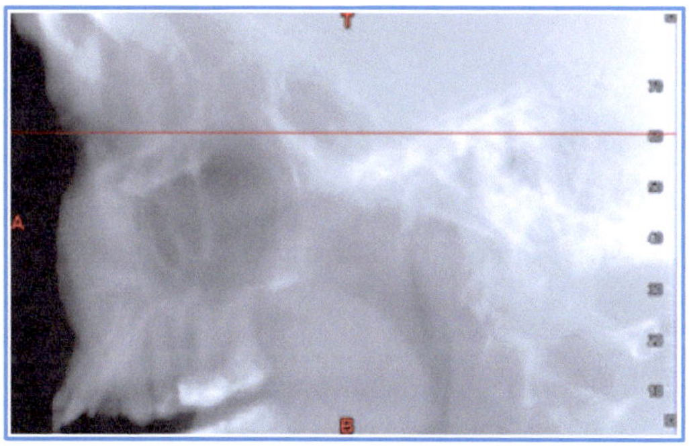

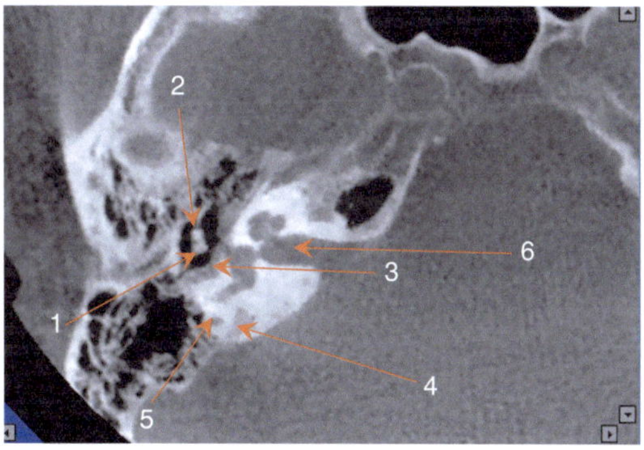

1. Incus.
2. Maleus.
3. Facial nerve canal.
4. Vestibular aqueduct.
5. Posterior semicircular canal.
6. **I**nternal **A**uditory **C**anal.

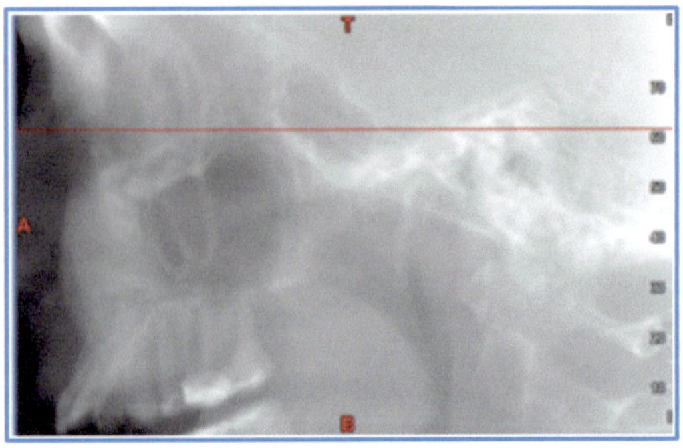

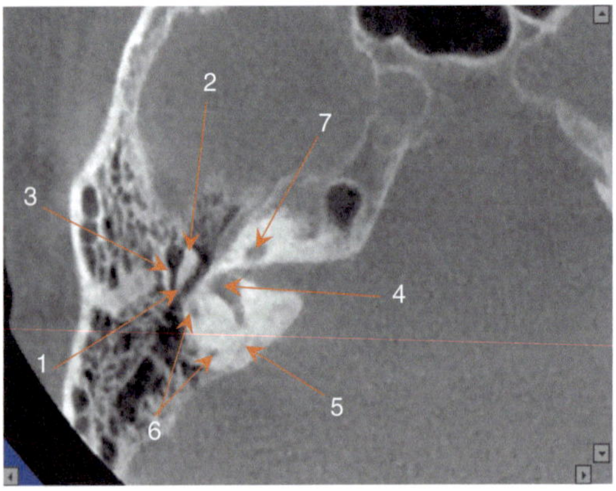

1. Incus body.
2. Maleus head.
3. Köerner's septum.
4. Vestibule.
5. Vestibular aqueduct.
6. Posterior semicircular canals.
7. Cochlea (apical turn).

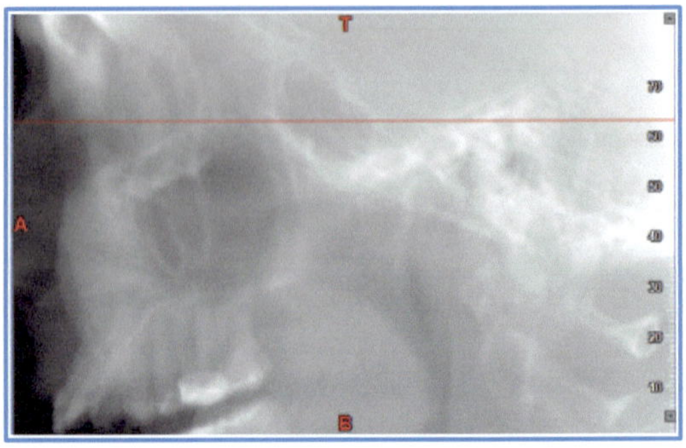

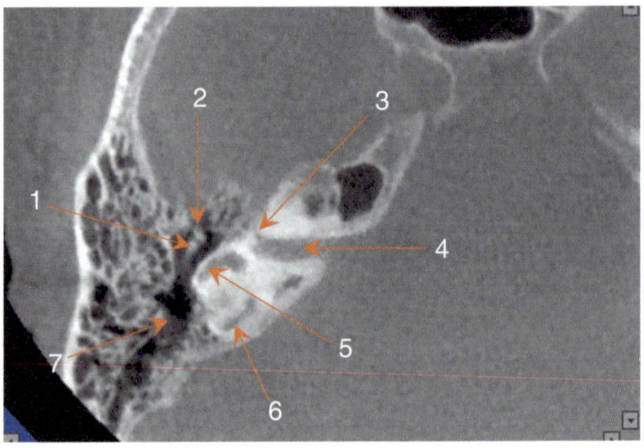

1. Incus body.
2. Maleus head.
3. Facial nerve canal.
4. Internal auditory canal.
5. Lateral semicircular canal.
6. Posterior semicircular canal.
7. Antrum.

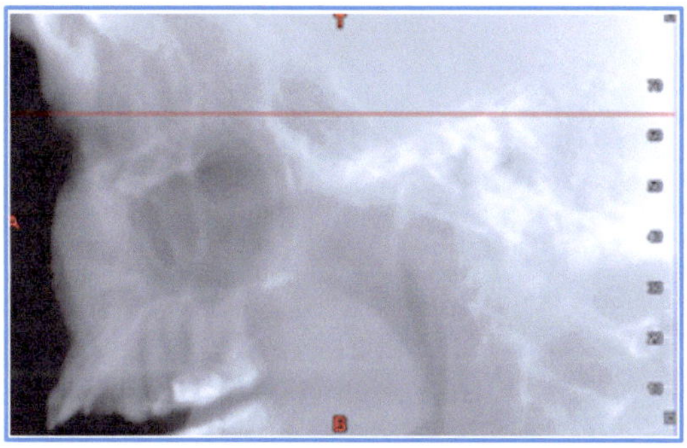

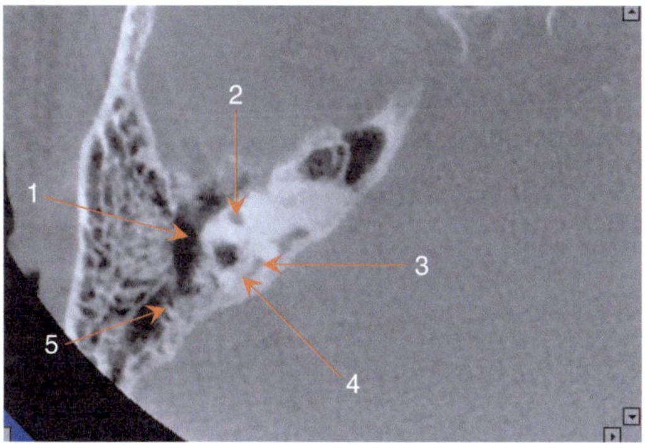

1. Tympanic cavity (epitympanum).
2. Superior semicircular canal (ant. limb).
3. Superior semicircular canal (pos. limb).
4. Lateral semicircular canal.
5. Antrum.

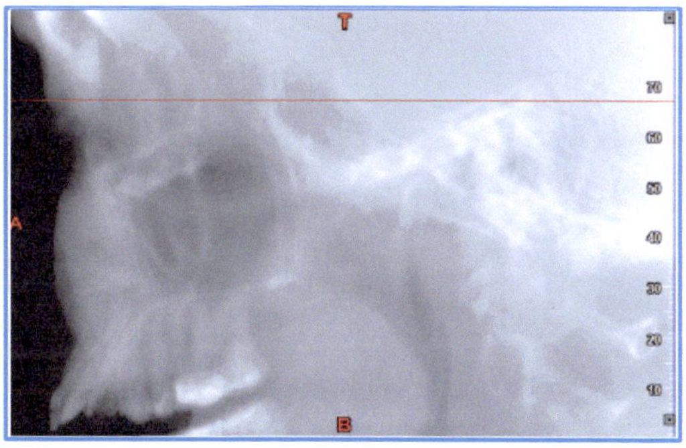

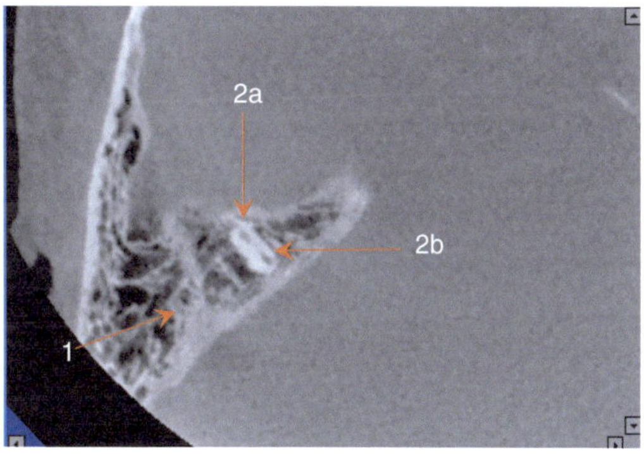

1. Mastoid air cells.
2. Superior semicircular canals
   [anterior (2a)—posterior (2b) limb].

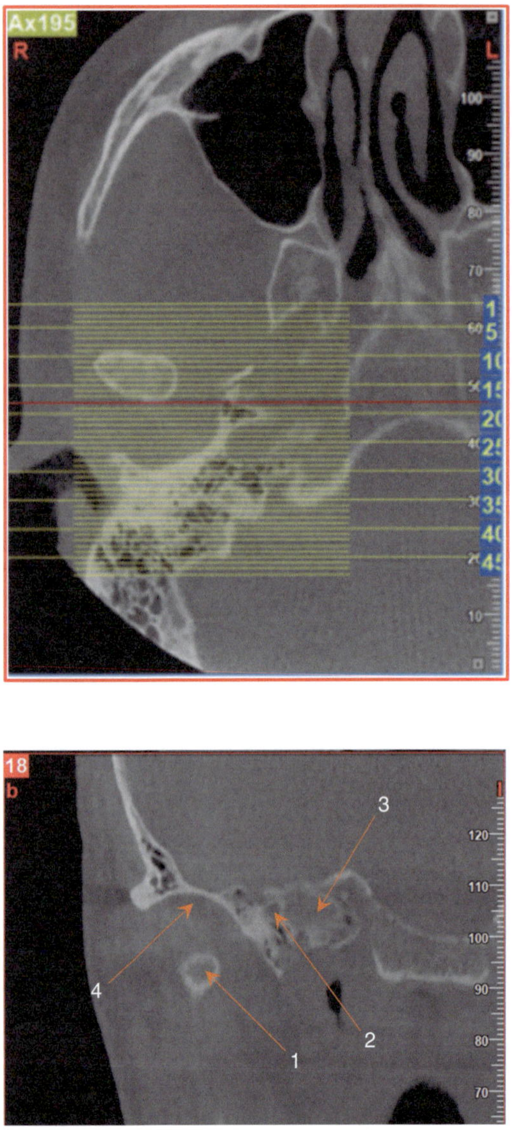

1. Mandibular condyle.
2. Auditory tube.
3. Carotid canal (horizontal segment).
4. Mandibular fossa.

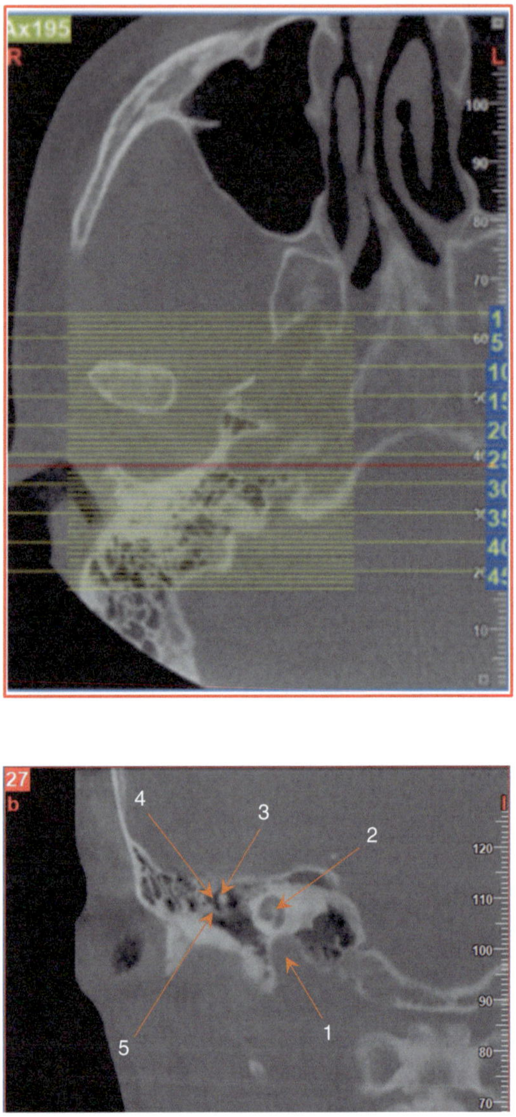

1. Carotid canal (vertical segment).
2. Basal turn of Cochlea.
3. Malleus head.
4. Prussak's space.
5. Scutum.

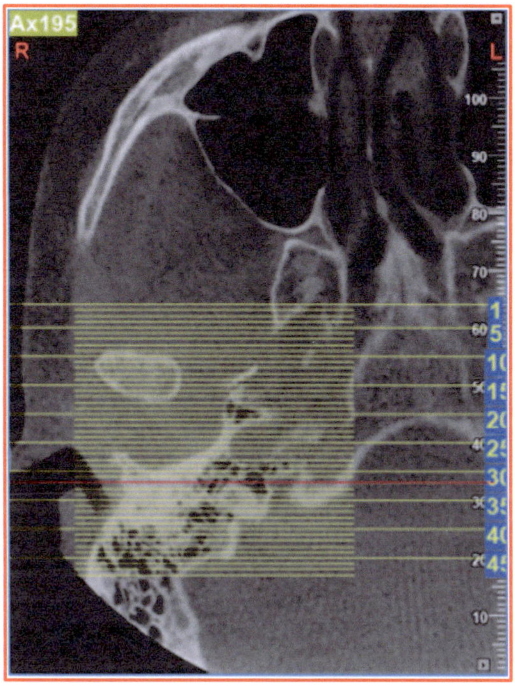

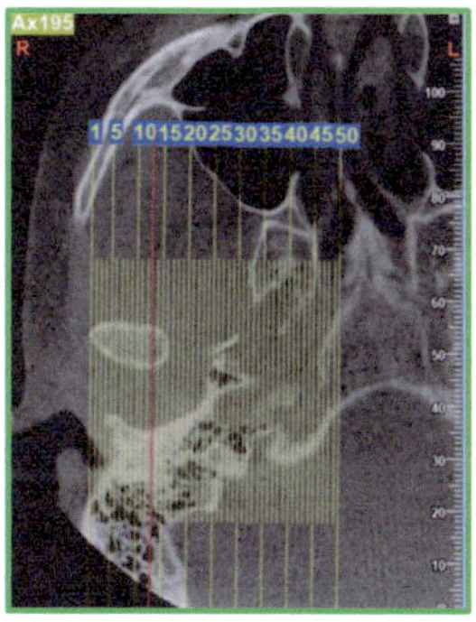

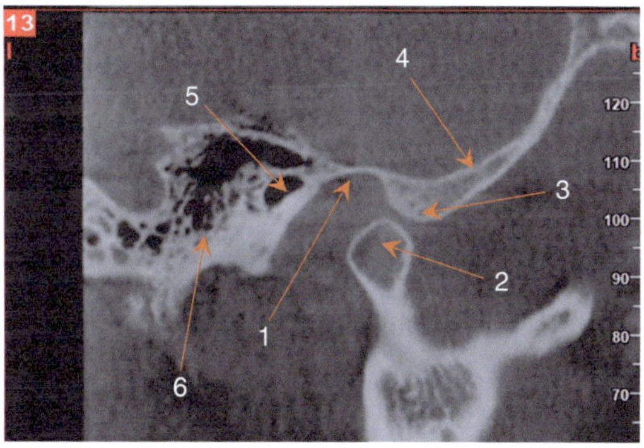

1. Mandibular fossa.
2. Mandibular condyle.
3. Articular tubercle.
4. Temporal bone.
5. **E**xternal **A**uditory **C**anal.
6. Mastoid air-cells.

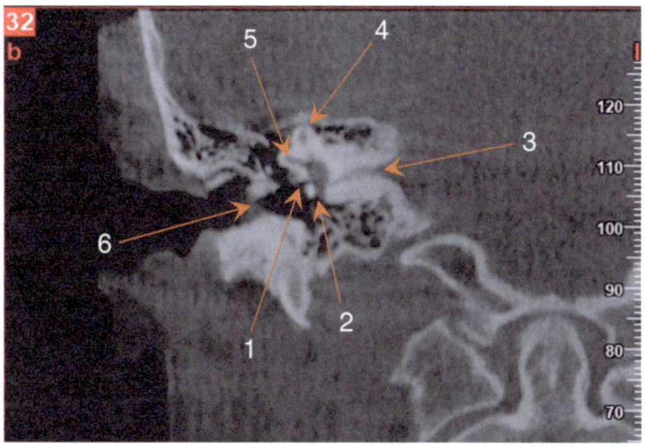

1. Oval window.
2. Round window.
3. Internal auditory canal.
4. Superior semicircular canal,
5. Posterior semicircular canal,
6. External auditory canal.

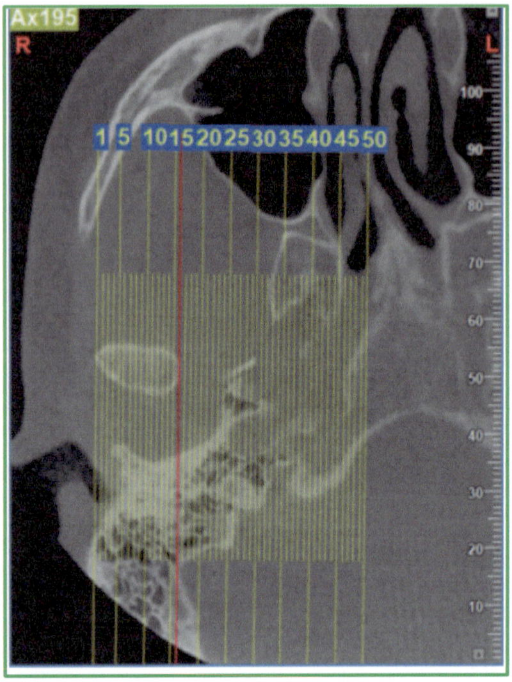

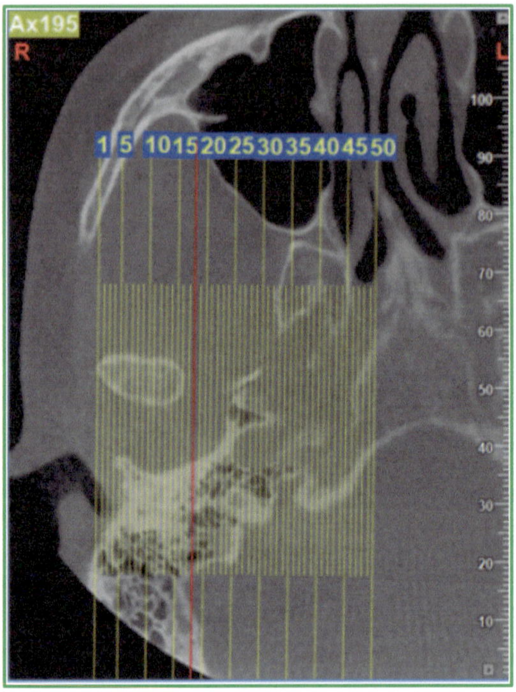

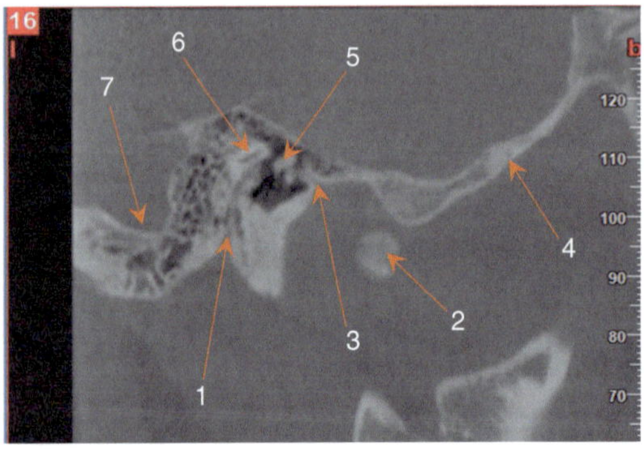

1. Stylomastoid foramen.
2. Mandibular condyle.
3. Petrotympanic fissure.
4. Sphenosquamosal suture.
5. Maleus.
6. Superior semicircular canal.
7. Sigmoid sinus.

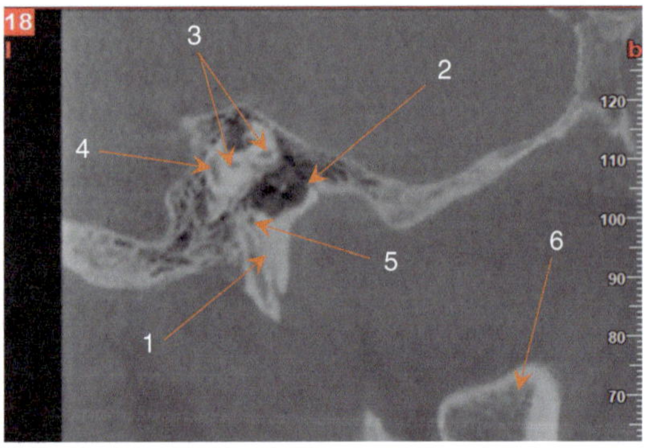

1. Facial nerve canal (mastoid segment).
2. Petrotympanic fissure.
3. Superior semicircular canal.
4. Posterior semicircular canal.
5. Canal for the chorda tympani.
6. Ramus of the mandible.

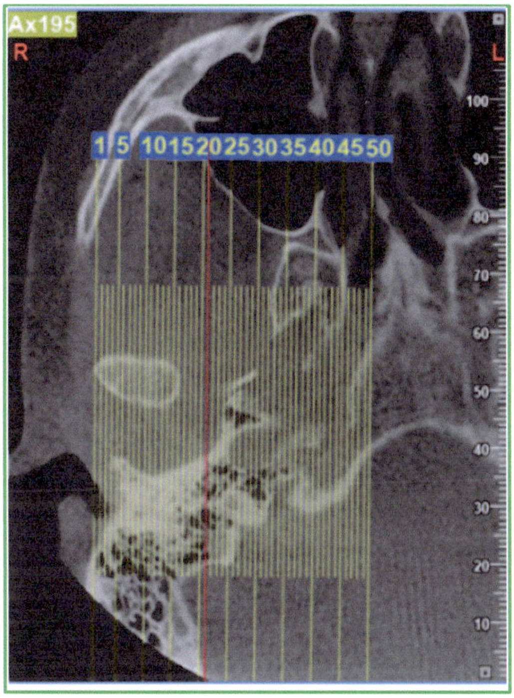

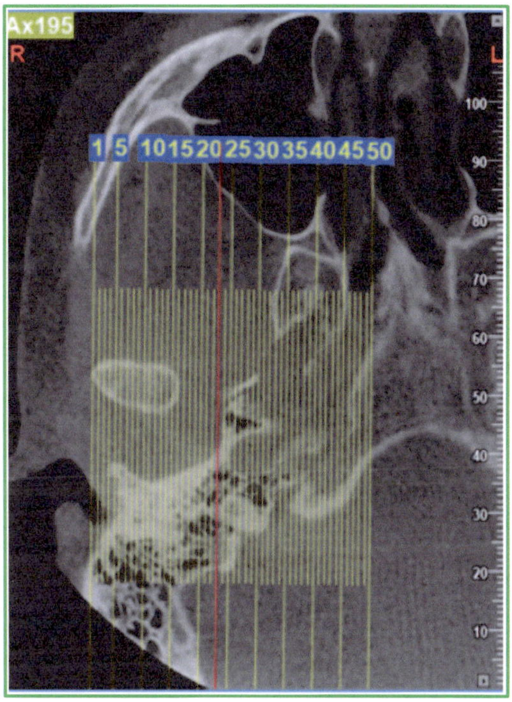

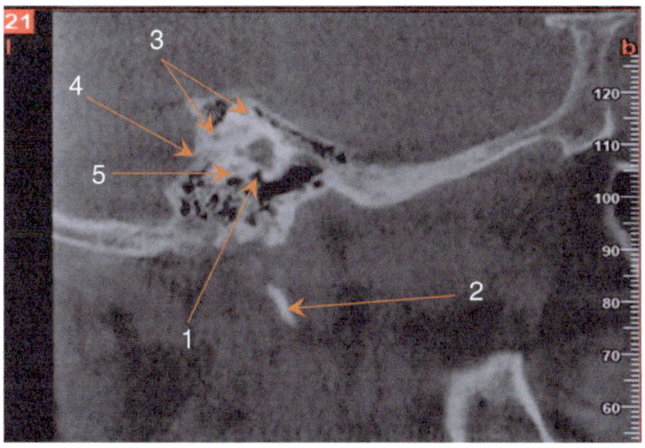

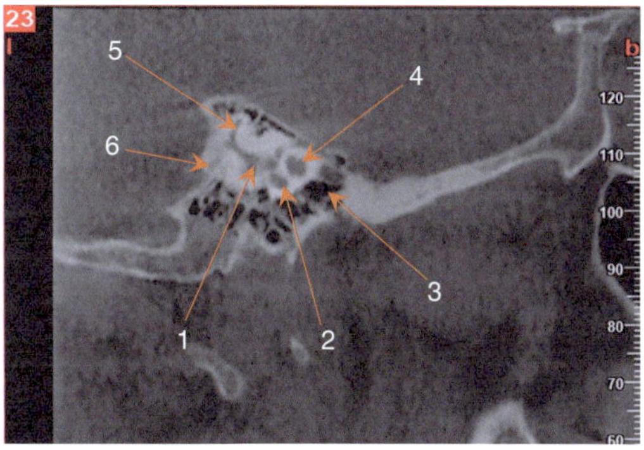

1. Round window.
2. Styloid process.
3. Superior semicircular canal.
4. Vestibular aqueduct.
5. Posterior semicircular canal.

1. Vestibule.
2. Cochlea (basal turn).
3. Hypotympanum-Auditory tube.
4. Cochlea.
5. Superior semicircular canal.
6. Vestibular aqueduct.

8.4 Part III

Note

- The CBCT images were created in a plane *perpendicular* to the long axis of the petrous bone and show the normal anatomy of the temporal bone from posterolateral to anteromedial orientation. This plane is also known as the ***Pöschl projection***. The interslice interval of these images is approximately 2 mm.
- The CBCT images were created in a plane *parallel* to the long axis of the petrous bone and show the normal anatomy of the temporal bone from oblique posterior to oblique anterior orientation. This plane is also known as the ***Stenvers projection***. The interslice interval of these images is approximately 2 mm.

The CBCT volumetric data set was acquired with a NewTom™ VGi CBCT imaging unit (QR S.r.l., Verona, Italy), and the volumetric reconstructions of the data set (FOV: 15 × 15 cm; voxel size of 0.2 mm) were created by using the manufacturer's proprietary software (NNT v6.2, Verona, Italy).

8.4.1 Pöschl Projection

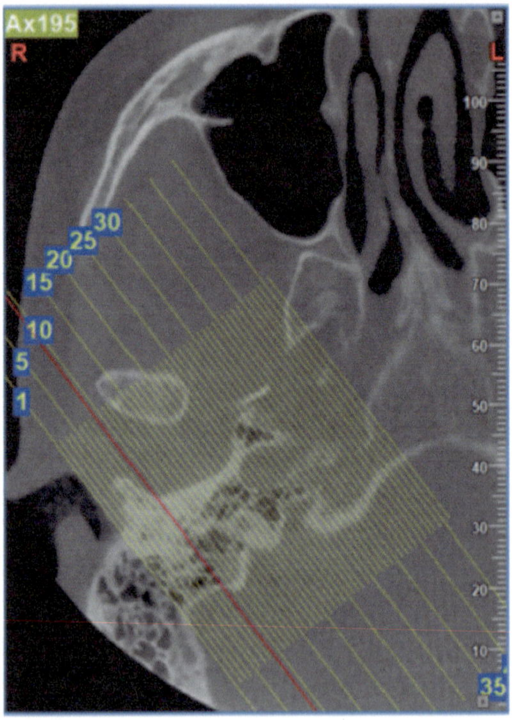

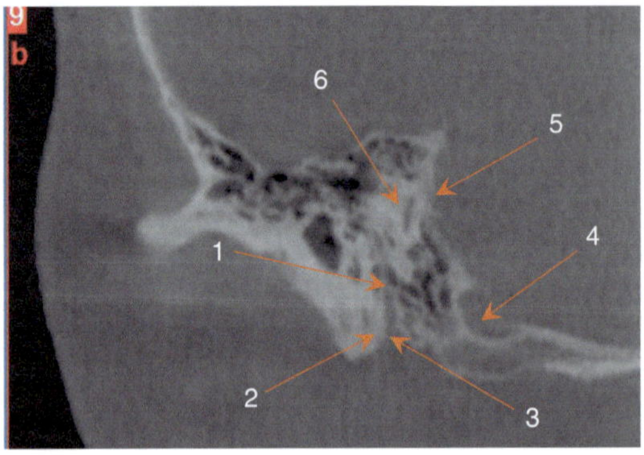

1. Mastoid segment of the facial nerve canal.
2. Canal for chorda tympani nerve.
3. Styloid-mastoid foramen.
4. Sigmoid sinus.
5. Vestibular aqueduct.
6. Posterior semicircular canal.

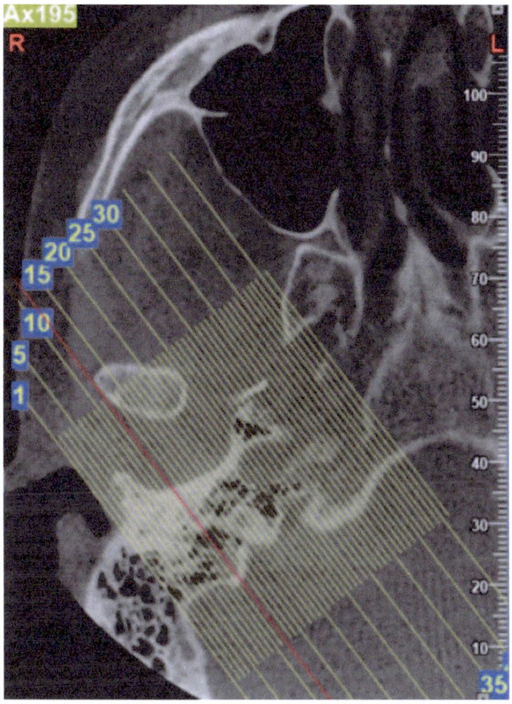

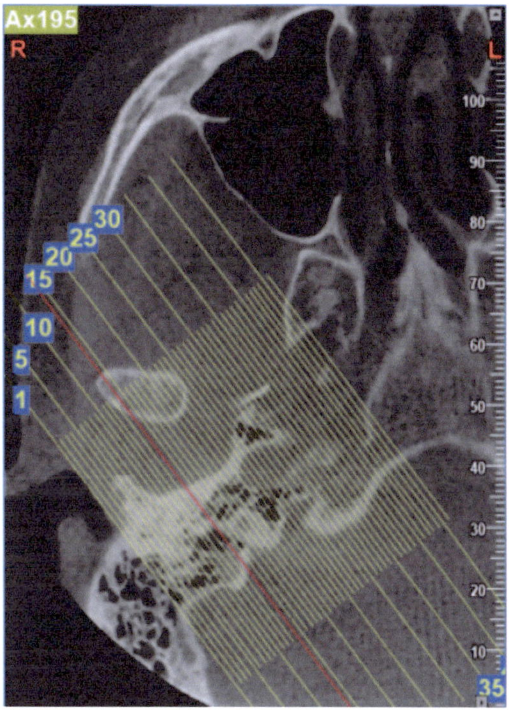

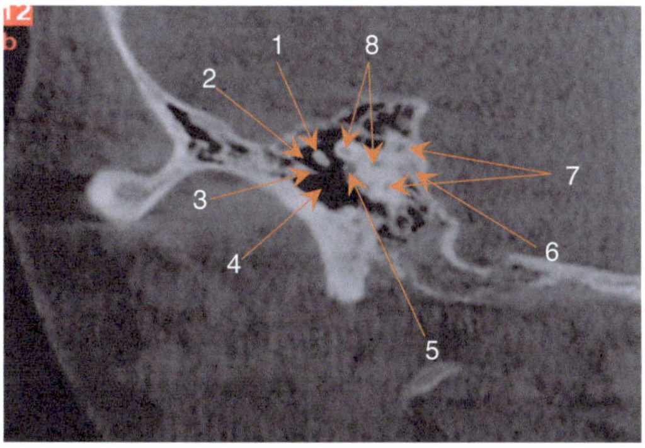

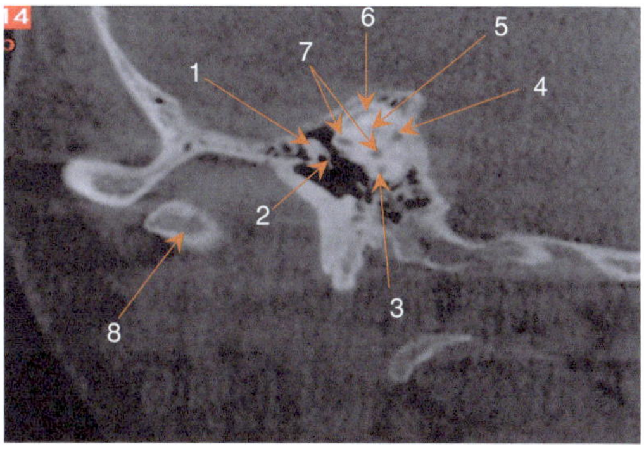

1. Body of incus.
2. Prussak's space.
3. Scutum.
4. External Acoustic Meatus.
5. Facial nerve canal (tympanic segment).
6. Vestibular aqueduct.
7. Posterior semicircular canals.
8. Lateral semicircular canals.

1. Maleus head.
2. Incus (long process).
3. Posterior semicircular canal.
4. Common crus.
5. Sudarcuate canal.
6. Superior semicircular canal.
7. Lateral semicircular canals.
8. Condylar head.

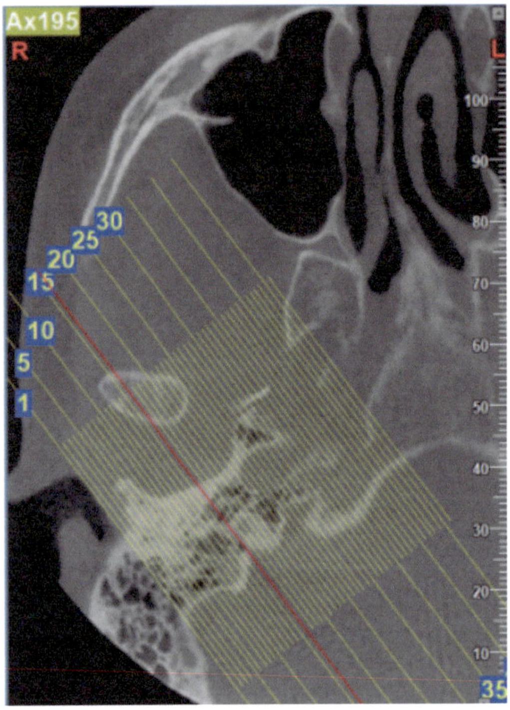

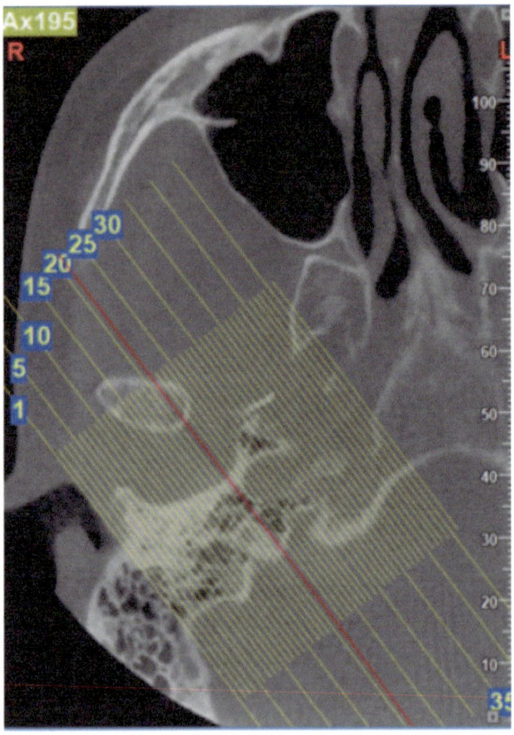

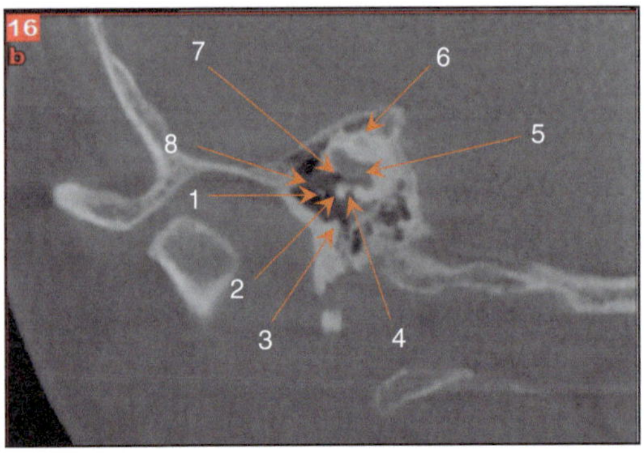

1. Incus (long process).
2. Cochlear promontory.
3. Tympanic membrane annulus.
4. Round window.
5. Vestibule.
6. Superior semicircular canal.
7. Oval window.
8. Tensor tympani tendon.

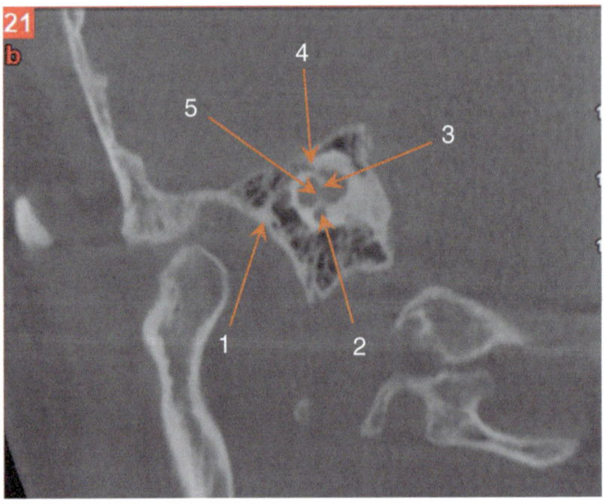

1. Glasserian fissure (for chorda tympani).
2. Cochlear promontory.
3. Cochlea (crista faciformis).
4. Facial nerve canal (labyrinthine segment).
5. Apical turn of cochlea.

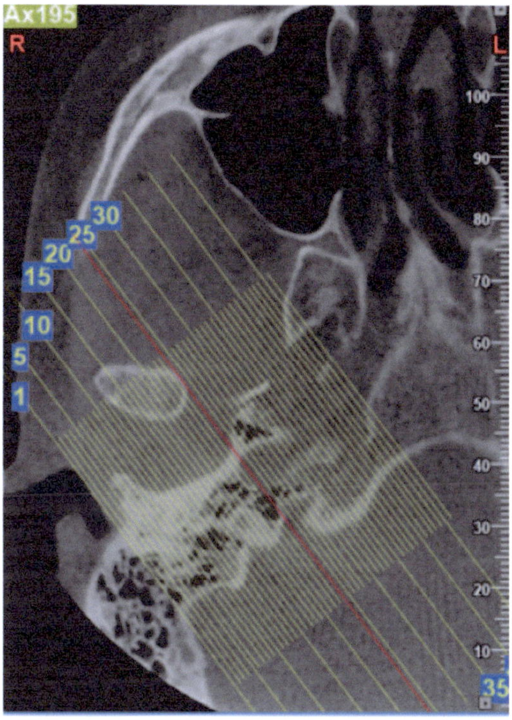

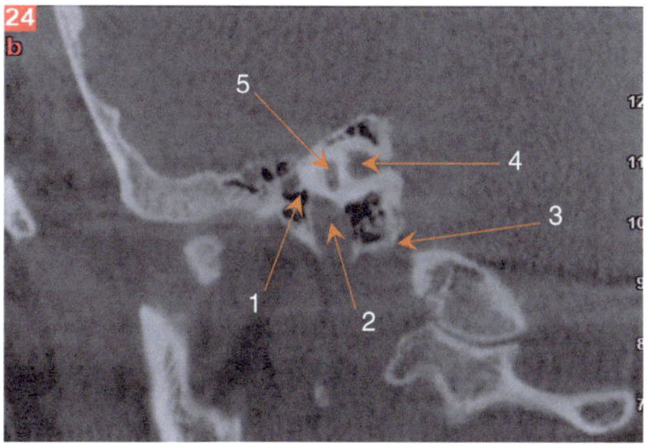

1. Auditory tube.
2. Carotid canal (petrous vertical portion).
3. Jugular foramen.
4. **I**nternal **A**uditory **C**anal.
5. Apical turn of cochlea.

8.4.2 Stenvers Plane

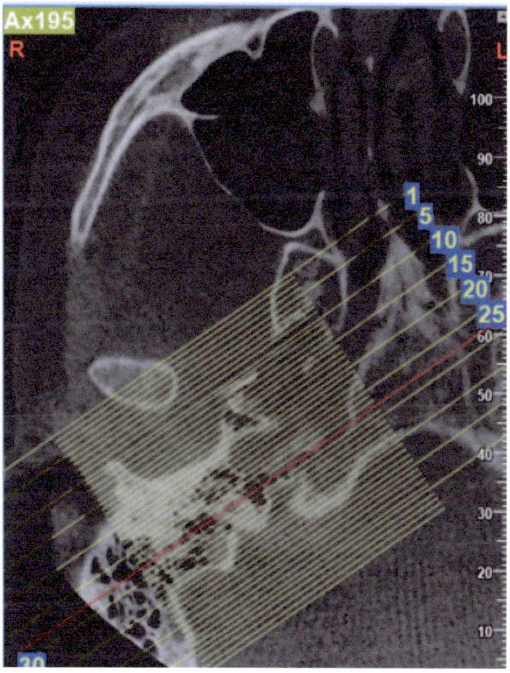

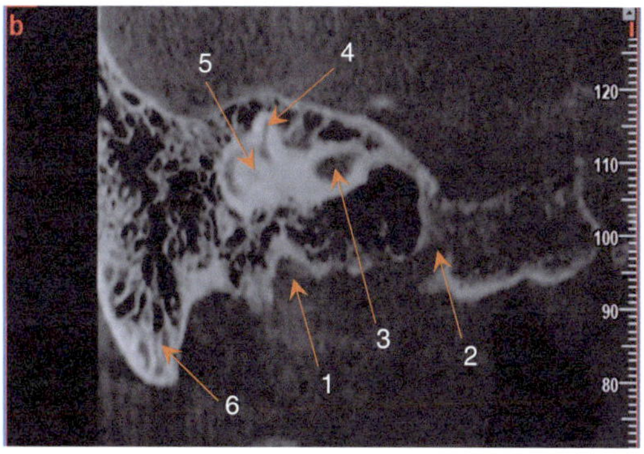

1. Jugular bulb.
2. Foramen lacerum.
3. **I**nternal **A**coustic **C**anal.
4. Superior semicircular canal.
5. Posterior semicircular canal.
6. Mastoid process (Mastoid air-cells).

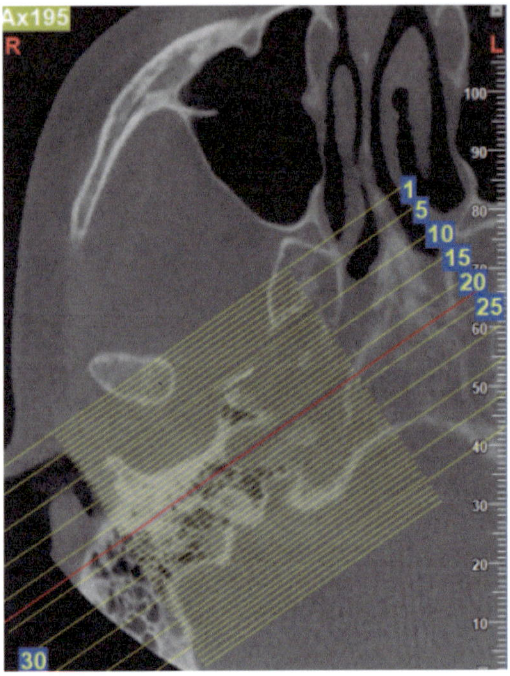

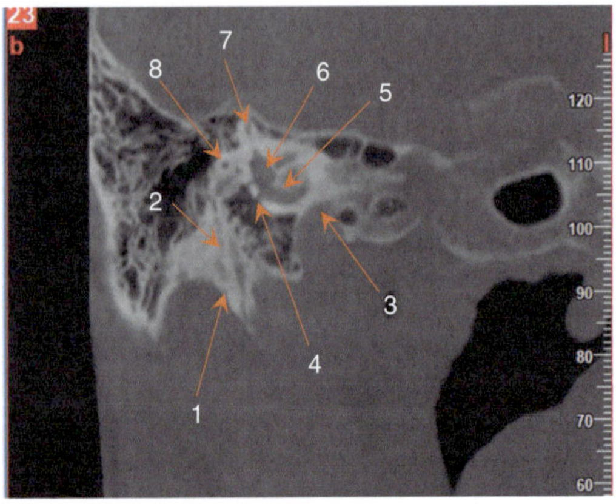

1. Stylomastoid foramen.
2. Facial nerve canal (mastoid segment).
3. Carotid canal.
4. Round window.
5. Basal turn of Cochlea.
6. Vestibule.
7. Superior semicircular canal.
8. Posterior semicircular canal.

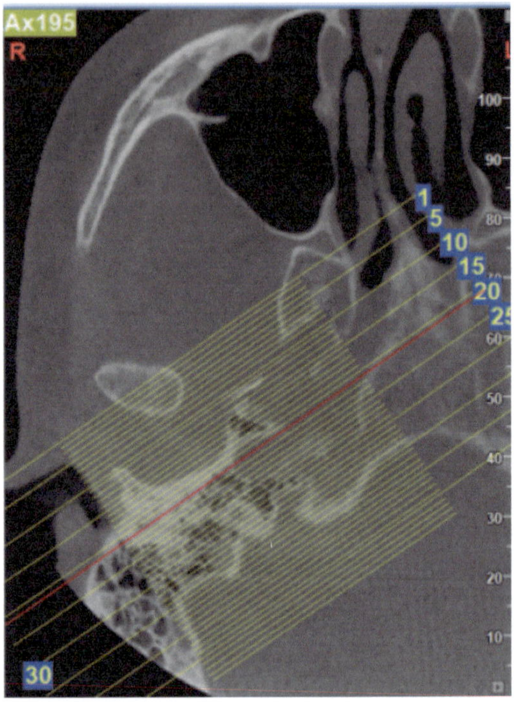

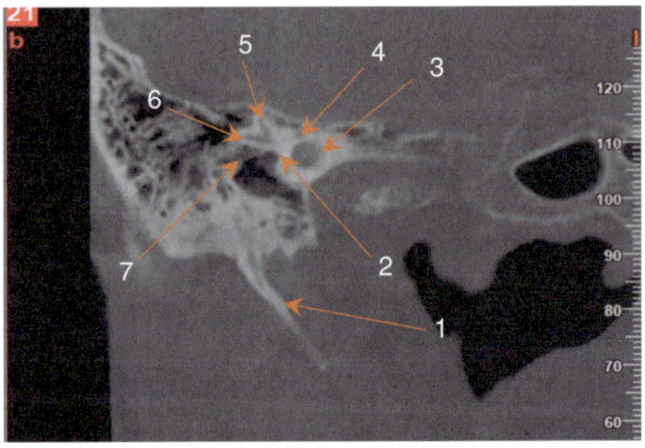

1. Styloid process.
2. Oval window.
3. Cochlea.
4. Facial nerve canal (labyrinthine segment).
5. Superior semicircular canal.
6. Posterior semicircular canal.
7. Facial nerve canal (posterior genu).

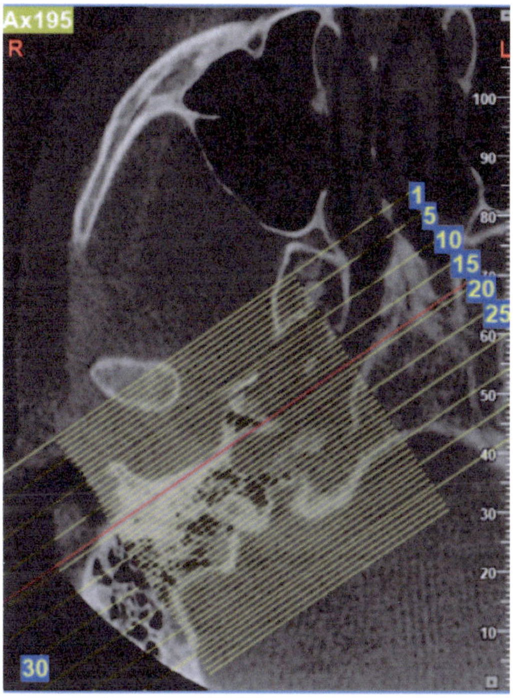

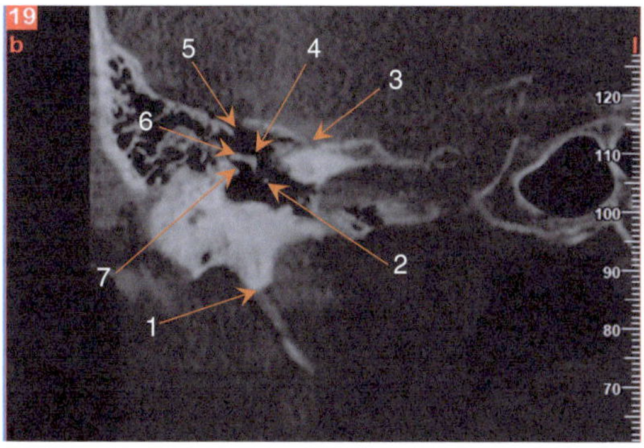

1. Styloid process.
2. Malleus (long process).
3. Geniculate ganglion.
4. Malleus (short process).
5. Köerner's septum.
6. Incus body.
7. Scutum.

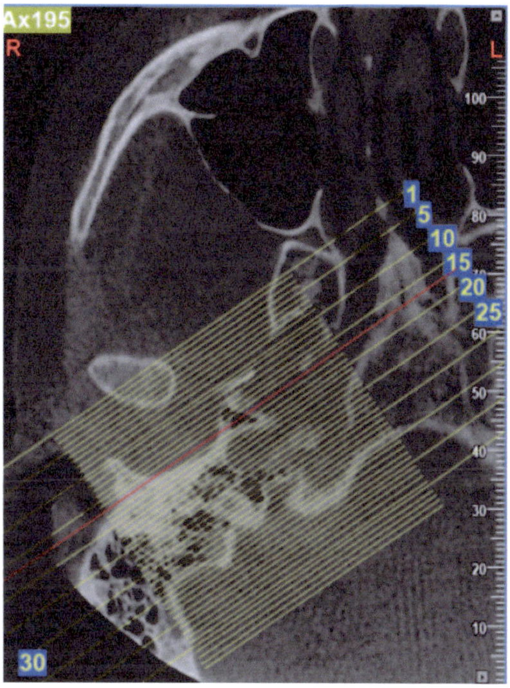

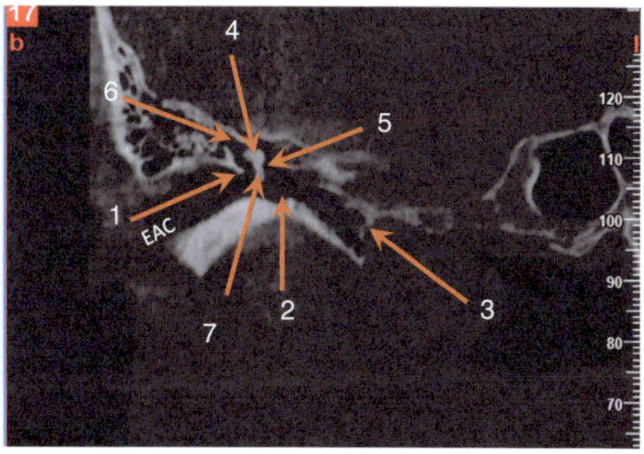

1. Scutum.
2. Mesotympanum.
3. Hypotympanum-Auditory tube.
4. Malleus.
5. Incudomalleolar joint.
6. Epitympanum.
7. Incus body.

External **A**uditory **C**anal.

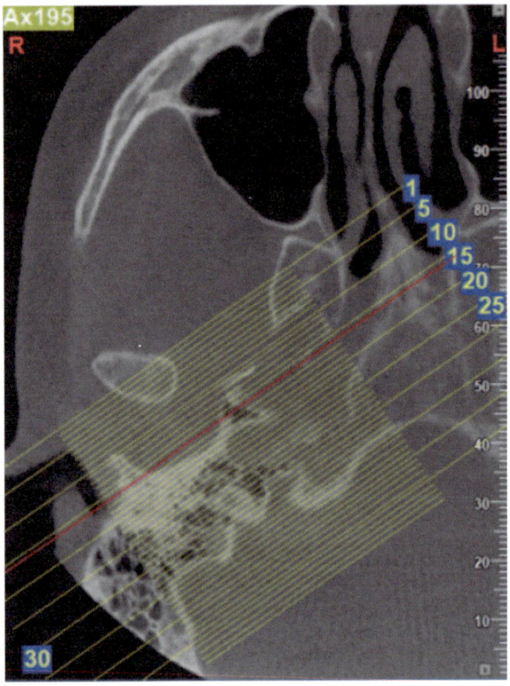

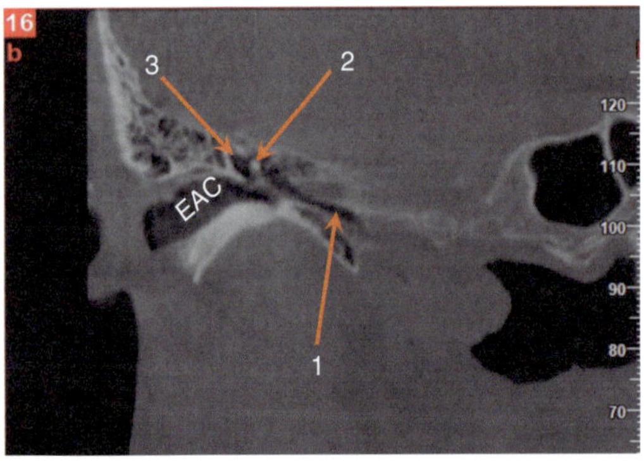

1. Auditory tube.
2. Malleus head.
3. Prussak's space.

External **A**uditory **C**anal.

References

1. Guyader E, Savéan J, Clodic C, Letellier P, Meriot P, Marianowski R. Three-dimensional reconstruction of the temporal bone: comparison of in situ, CT, and CBCT measurements. Eur Ann Otorhinolaryngol Head Neck Dis. 2018;135(6):393–8. https://doi.org/10.1016/j.anorl.2018.08.013.
2. Jain S, Choudhary K, Nagi R, Shukla S, Kaur N, Grover D. New evolution of cone-beam computed tomography in dentistry: combining digital technologies. Imaging Sci Dent. 2019;49(3):179–90. https://doi.org/10.5624/isd.2019.49.3.179.
3. Miracle AC, Mukherji SK. Conebeam CT of the head and neck, part 2: clinical applications. AJNR Am J Neuroradiol. 2009;30(7):1285–92. https://doi.org/10.3174/ajnr.A1654.
4. Dahmani-Causse M, Marx M, Deguine O, Fraysse B, Lepage B, Escudé B. Morphologic examination of the temporal bone by cone beam computed tomography: comparison with multislice helical computed tomography. Eur Ann Otorhinolaryngol Head Neck Dis. 2011;128(5):230–5. https://doi.org/10.1016/j.anorl.2011.02.016.
5. Zou J, Lähelmä J, Arnisalo A, Pyykkö I. Clinically relevant human temporal bone measurements using novel high-resolution cone-beam CT. J Otolaryngol. 2017;12(1):9–17. https://doi.org/10.1016/j.joto.2017.01.002.
6. von Arx T, Lozanoff S, Bornstein MM. Extraoral anatomy in CBCT—a literature review. Part 1: Nasoethmoidal region. Swiss Dent J. 2019;129(10):804–15.
7. von Arx T, Lozanoff S, Bornstein MM. Extraoral anatomy in CBCT—a literature review. Part 2: Zygomatico-orbital region. Swiss Dent J. 2020;130(2):126–38.
8. von Arx T, Lozanoff S, Bornstein MM. Extraoral anatomy in CBCT—a literature review. Part 3: Retromaxillary region. Swiss Dent J. 2020;130(3):216–28.
9. Juliano AF. Cross sectional imaging of the ear and temporal bone. Head Neck Pathol. 2018;12(3):302–20. https://doi.org/10.1007/s12105-018-0901-y.
10. Güldner C, Diogo I, Bernd E, Dräger S, Mandapathil M, Teymoortash A, Negm H, Wilhelm T. Visualization of anatomy in normal and pathologic middle ears by cone beam CT. Eur Arch Otorhinolaryngol. 2017;274(2):737–42. https://doi.org/10.1007/s00405-016-4345-2.

11. Juliano AF, Ginat DT, Moonis G. Imaging review of the temporal bone. Part I. anatomy and inflammatory and neoplastic processes. Radiology. 2013;269(1):17–33. https://doi.org/10.1148/radiol.13120733.
12. Phillips GS, LoGerfo SE, Richardson ML, Anzai Y. Interactive web-based learning module on CT of the temporal bone: anatomy and pathology. Radiographics. 2012;32(3):E85–105. https://doi.org/10.1148/rg.323115117.
13. Shumway CL, Motlagh M, Wade M. Anatomy, head and neck, orbit bones. In: StatPearls [Internet]. Treasure Island, FL: StatPearls; 2021.
14. https://radiopaedia.org/cases/normal-temporal-bone-ct-with-annotated-images
15. https://epos.myesr.org/posterimage/esr/ecr2016/131661/mediagallery/638091
16. McManus LJ, Dawes PJ, Stringer MD. Clinical anatomy of the chorda tympani: a systematic review. J Laryngol Otol. 2011;125(11):1101–8. https://doi.org/10.1017/S0022215111001873.
17. Singh D, Hsu CC, Kwan GN, Bhuta S, Skalski M, Jones R. High resolution CT study of the chorda tympani nerve and normal anatomical variation. Jpn J Radiol. 2015;33(5):279–86. https://doi.org/10.1007/s11604-015-0417-2.
18. Wojciechowski T, Skadorwa T, Drożdż A, Ciszek B, Szopiński K. The radioanatomical assessment of the Körner's septum. Surg Radiol Anat. 2019;41(6):669–73. https://doi.org/10.1007/s00276-018-2149-3.
19. Damaskos S, Syriopoulos K, Sens RL, Politis C. An investigation of the morphology of the petrotympanic fissure using cone-beam computed tomography. J Oral Maxillofac Res. 2018;9(1):e4. https://doi.org/10.5037/jomr.2018.9104.

9 MDCT Soft Tissue Anatomy

Antigoni Delantoni and Kaan Orhan

9.1 Introduction

A computed tomography scan (formerly known as computed axial tomography) is an imaging technique in radiology which enables radiologists to get detailed images of the body noninvasively for diagnostic purposes.

CT scanners use a rotating X-ray tube and a row of detectors placed in the gantry to measure X-ray absorption and attenuations by different tissues inside the body. The multiple X-ray measurements taken from different angles are then processed on a computer using reconstruction algorithms to produce Tomographic (cross-sectional) images of a body organ or section. The use of ionizing radiations sometimes restricts its use owing to its adverse effects.

Its main function is to serve as a supplementary and more detailed examination technique where conventional X-rays and ultrasonography do not provide adequate information to set the diagnosis.

A detailed description of the methodology is described in the previous chapter.

Since in dentistry, the vast majority of the lesions of the facial skeleton are located in the osseous structures of the facial skeleton, CBCT is the most frequently used imaging method for 3D imaging of the maxillofacial region. However, MDCT can in many cases be proven useful particularly where a more detailed diagnosis is required in the soft tissues of the area or in cases where there is both involvement of hard and soft tissues. Finally more complicated maxillofacial surgery cases are viewed with the use of MDCT to have a detailed imaging of both soft and hard structures.

The following is a series of medical CT images with emphasis on the soft tissue imaging. All images are sequences of slices every 5 mm so that no major elements of the maxillofacial region are omitted. Also the images in each level are of both soft tissue window and hard tissue imaging window.

A. Delantoni (✉)
Department of Dentoalveolar Surgery, Implant Surgery and Radiology, Faculty of Dentistry, Aristotle University of Thessaloniki, Thessaloniki, Greece
e-mail: andelant@dent.auth.gr

K. Orhan
Department of DentoMaxillofacial Radiology, Faculty of Dentistry, Ankara University, Ankara, Turkey
e-mail: knorhan@dentistry.ankara.edu.tr

A. Delantoni, K. Orhan (eds.), *Atlas of Dentomaxillofacial Anatomical Imaging*,
https://doi.org/10.1007/978-3-030-96840-3_9

9.2 Axial/Horizontal

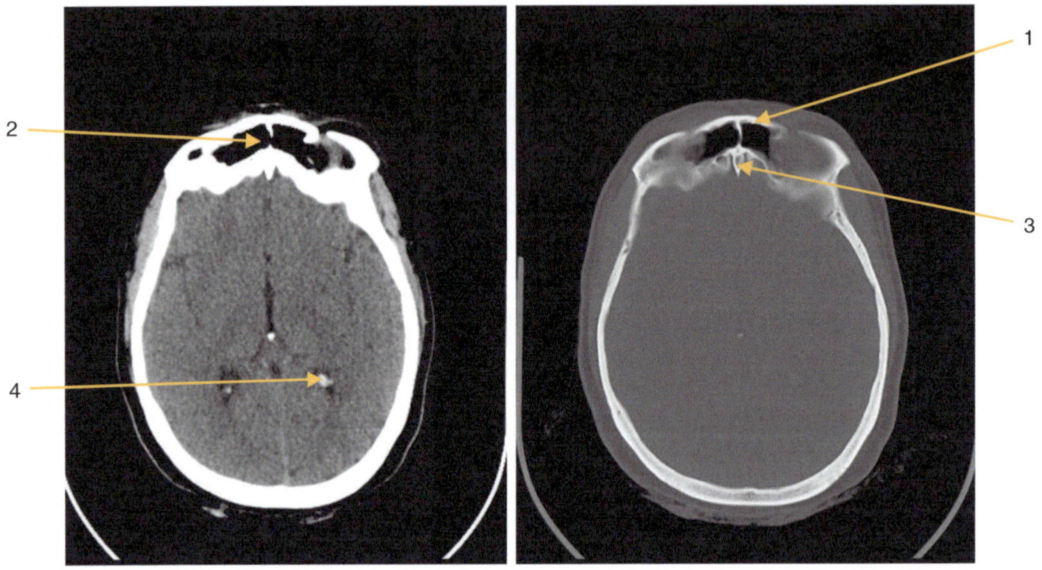

1. Frontal bone
2. Frontal Sinus
3. Crista Galli
4. Ventricular calcifications

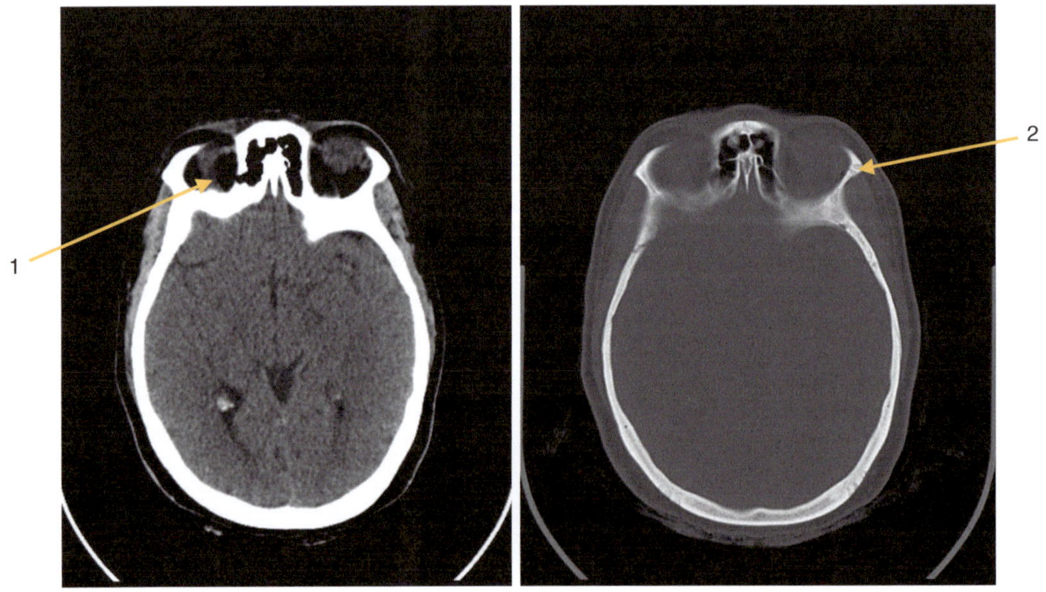

1. Superior rectus muscle
2. Zygomatic bone

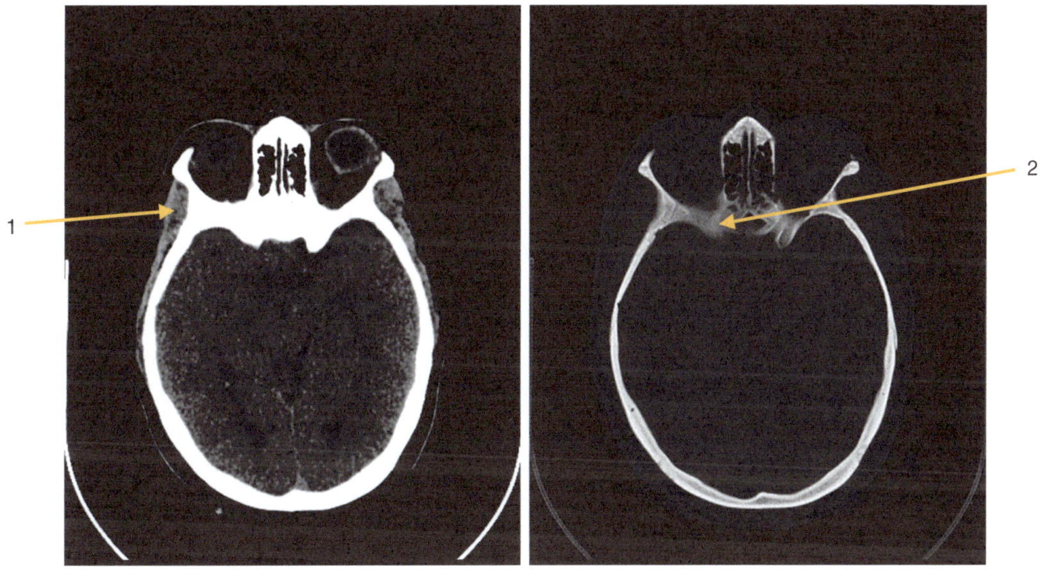

1. Temporalis muscle
2. Sphenoid bone

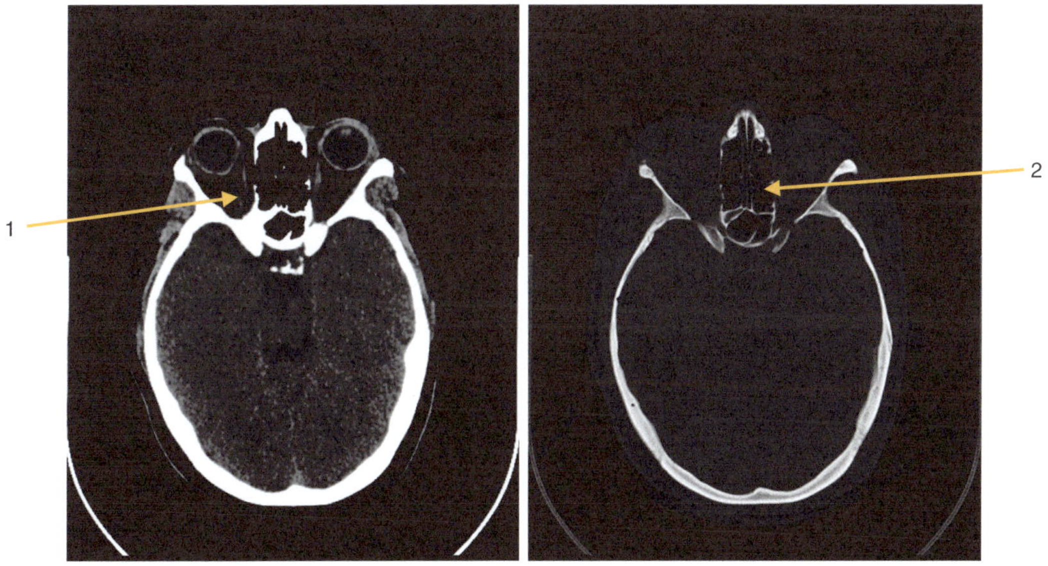

1. Optic nerve
2. Ethmoidal air cells

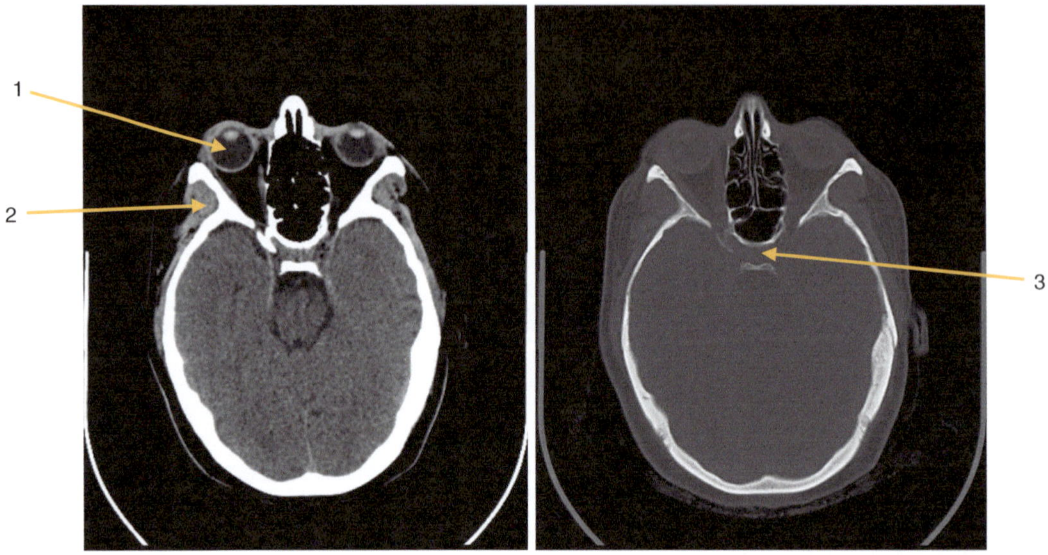

1. Eyeball
2. Temporalis muscle
3. Sella Turcica

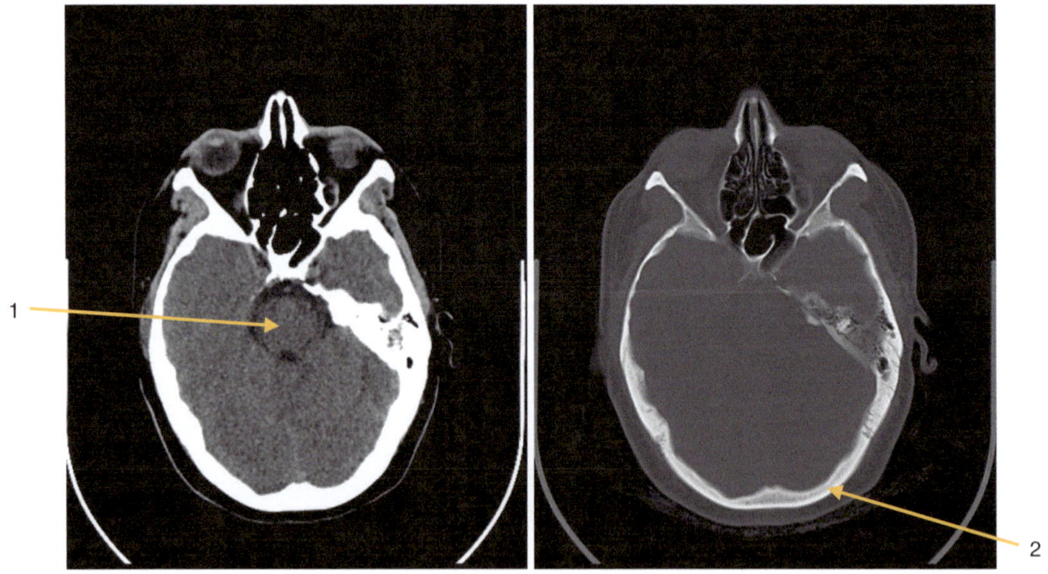

1. Pons
2. Occipital bone

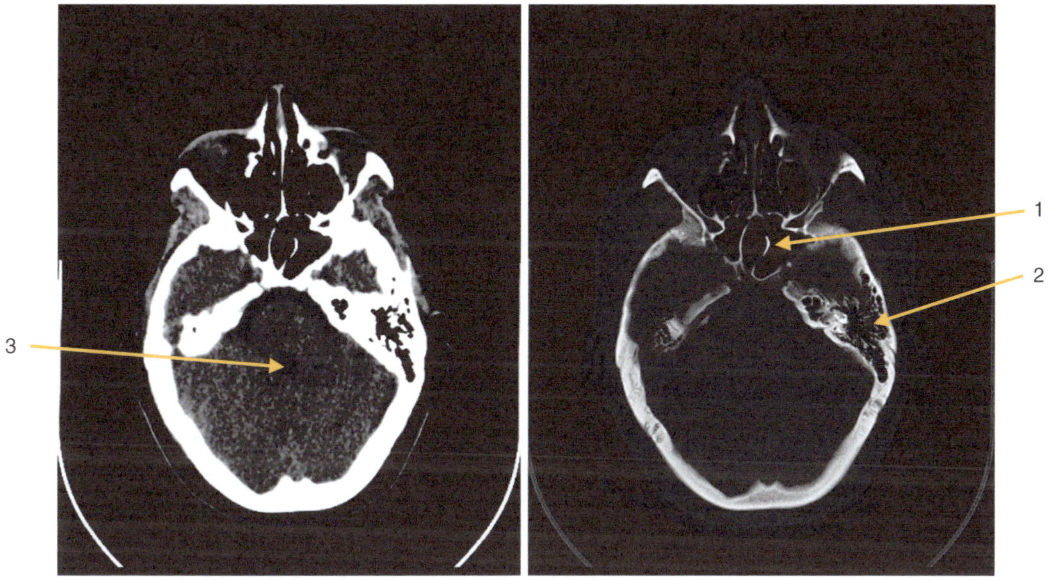

1. Sphenoid sinus and septa
2. Mastoid air cells
3. Fourth ventricle

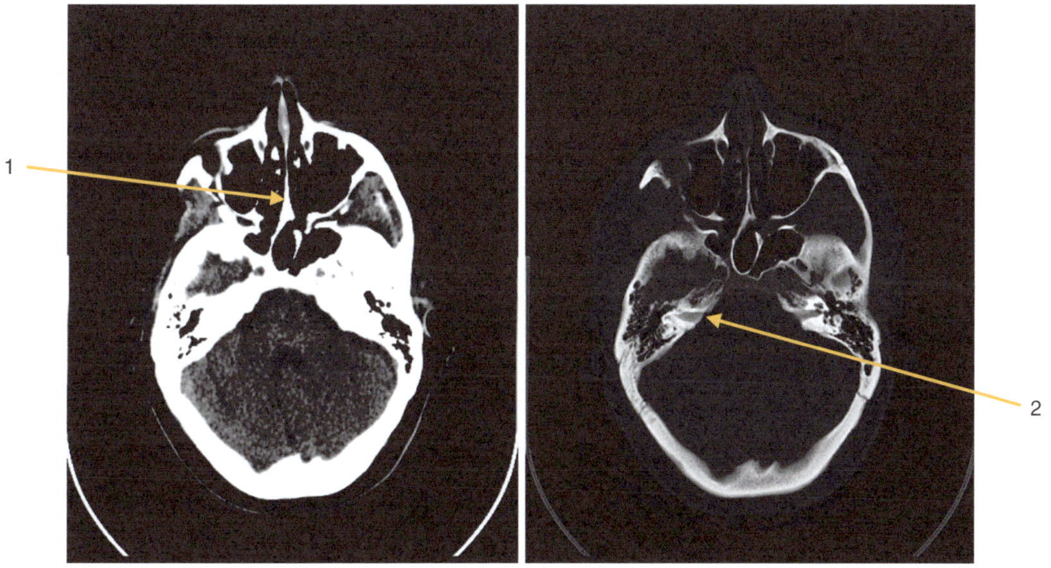

1. Nasal septum
2. Internal acoustic meatus

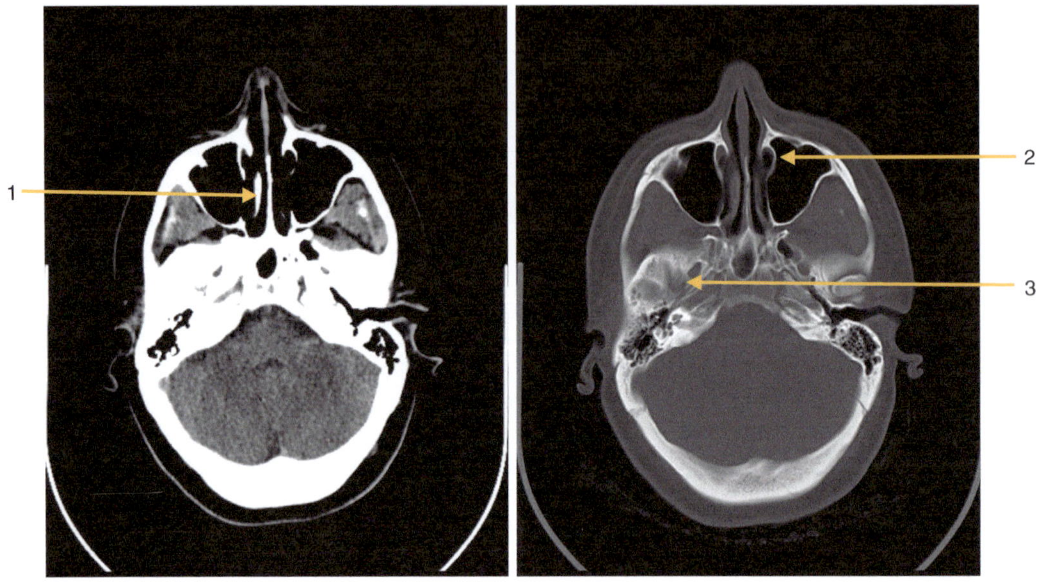

1. Middle nasal concha
2. Nasolacrimal duct
3. Temporal bone

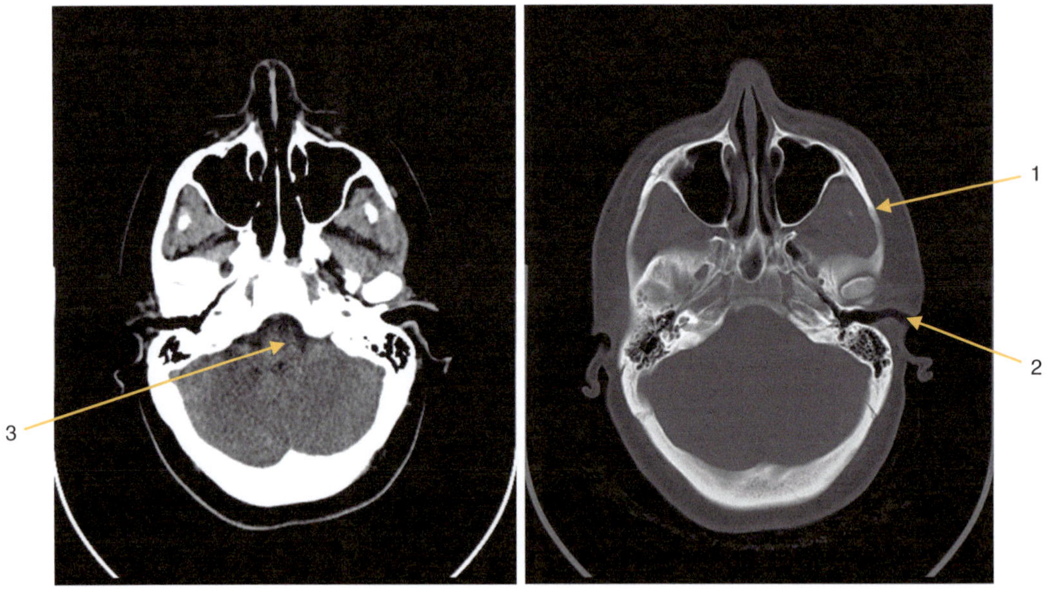

1. Zygomatic arch
2. External acoustic meatus
3. Medulla oblongata

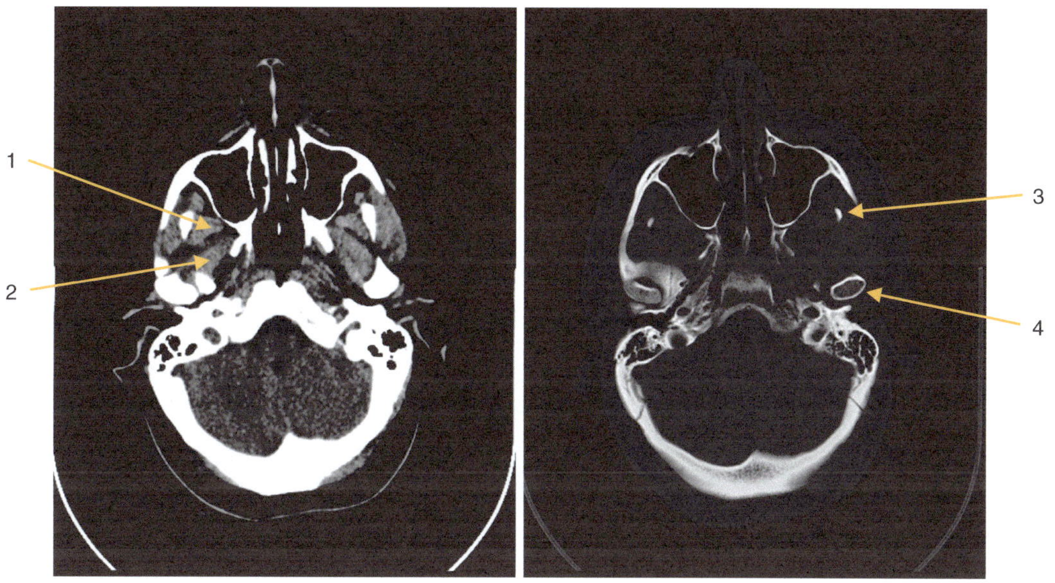

1. Lateral pterygoid muscle
2. Medial pterygoid muscle
3. Coronoid process
4. Condyle of Mandible

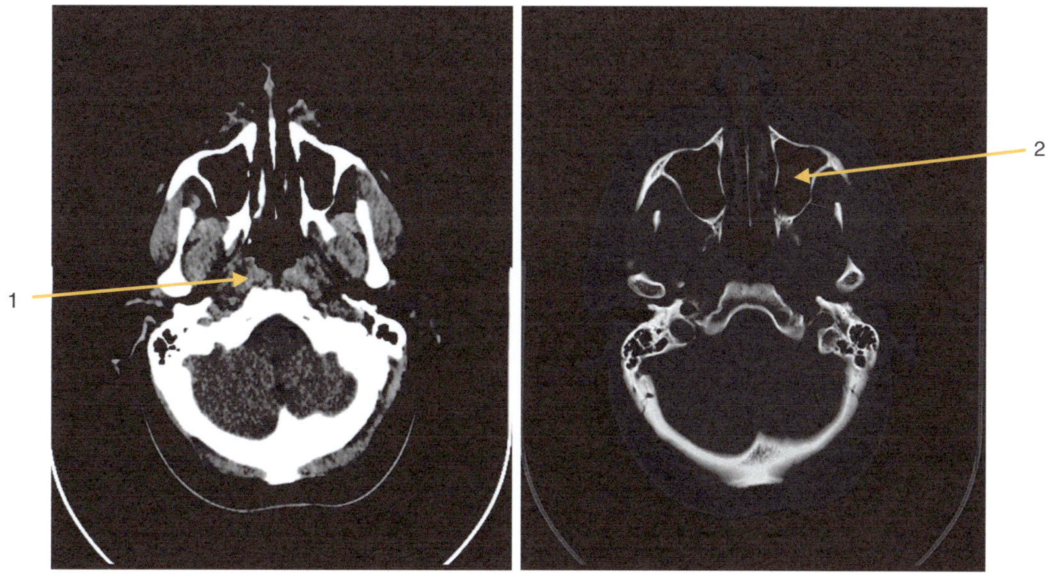

1. Longus capitis muscle
2. Maxillary sinus

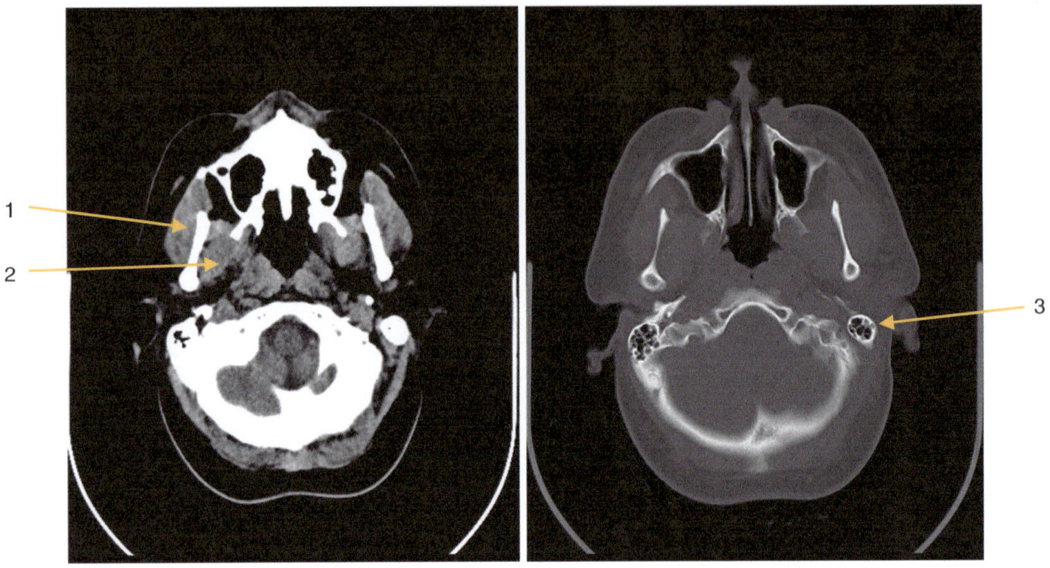

1. Masseter muscle
2. Medial pterygoid muscle
3. Mastoid process

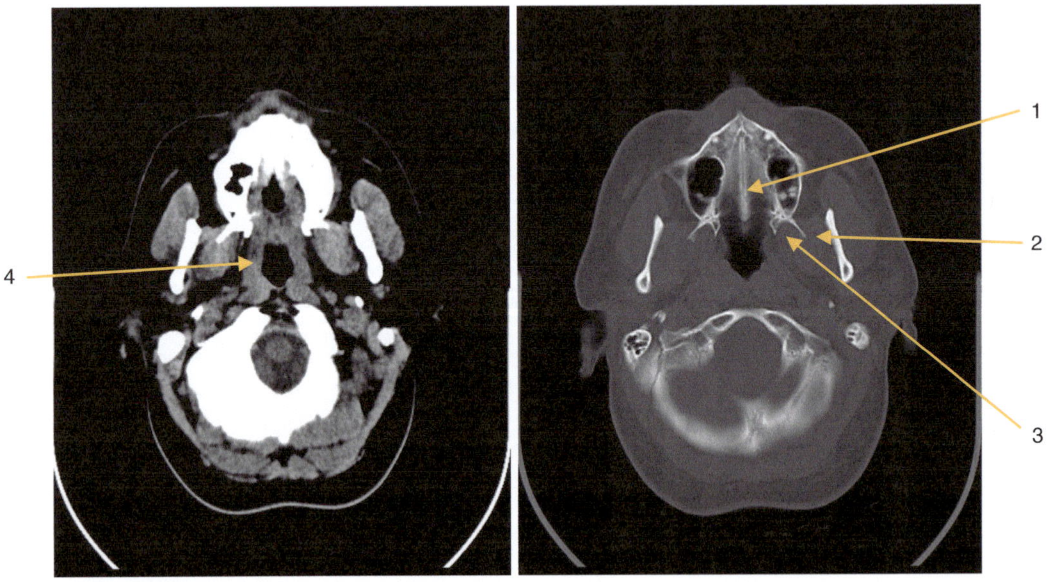

1. Hard palate with medial palatal suture (line)
2. Pterygoid process (lateral)
3. Pterygoid process (medial)
4. Levator veli palatini muscle

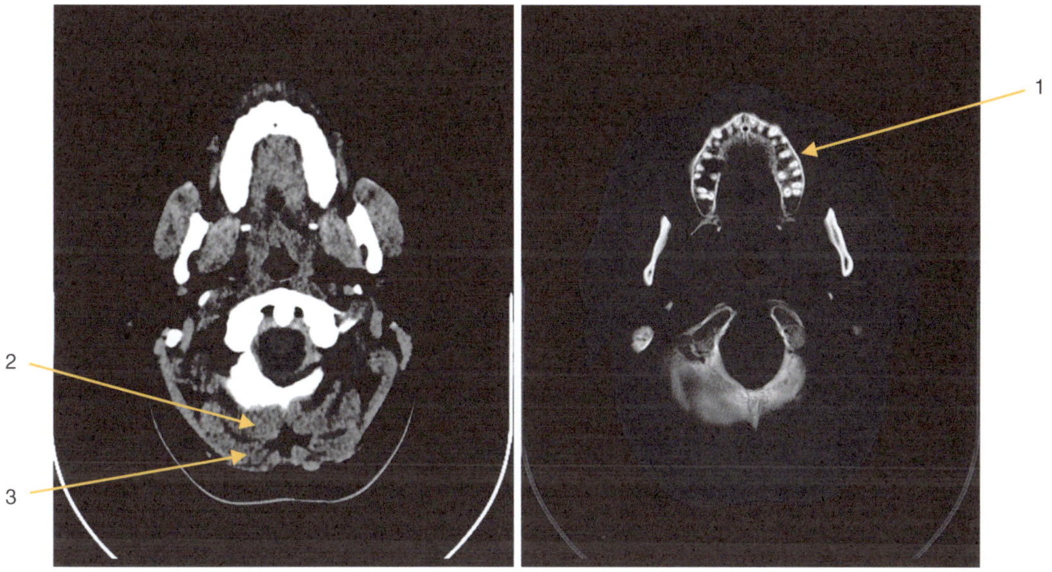

1. Maxilla with teeth apices
2. Rectus capitis posterior minor muscle
3. Semispinalis capitis muscle

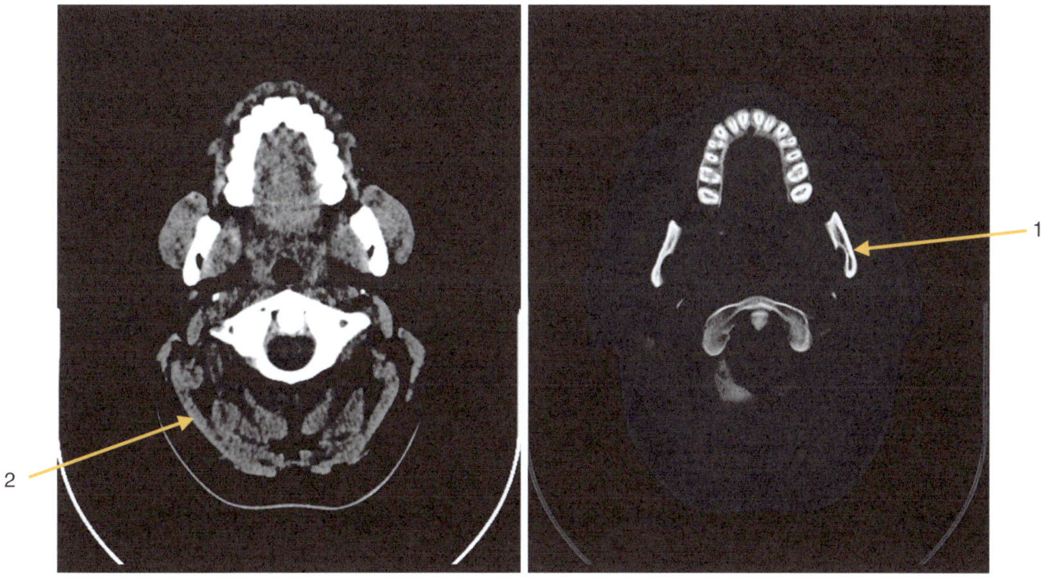

1. Ramus of mandible
2. Splenius capitis muscle

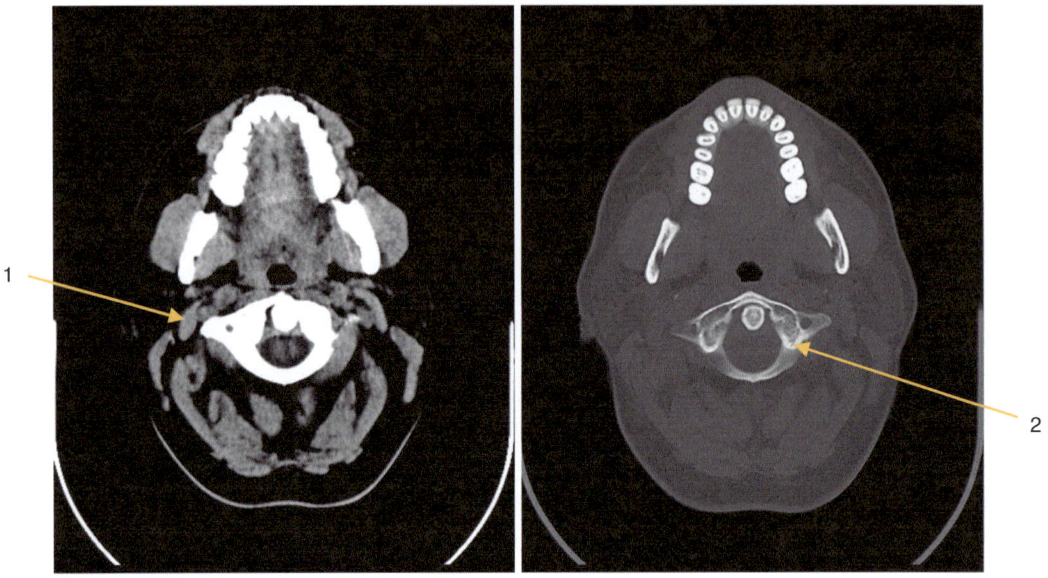

1. Digastric muscle
2. Atlas bone

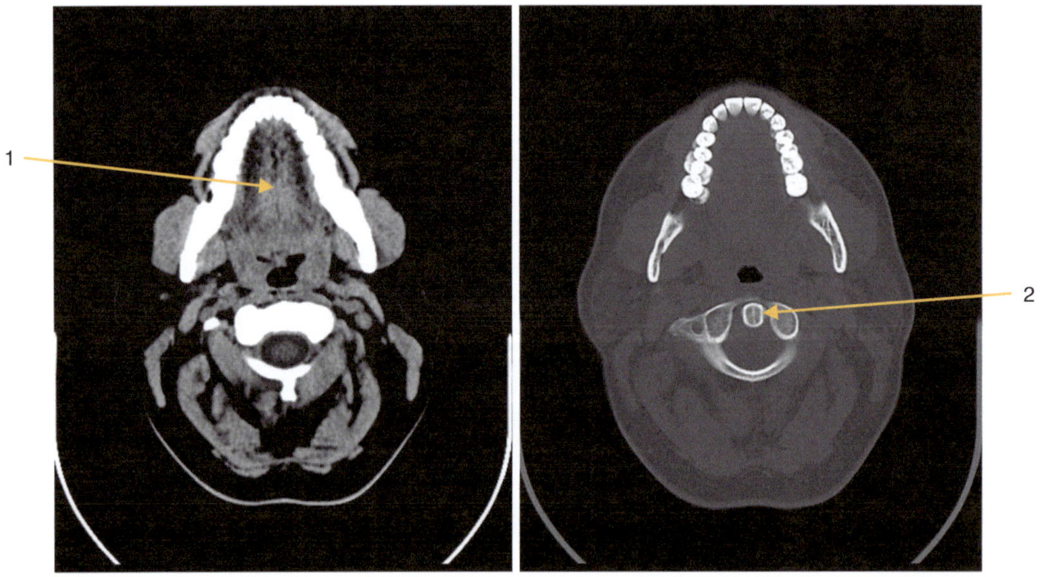

1. Tongue
2. Dens of axis

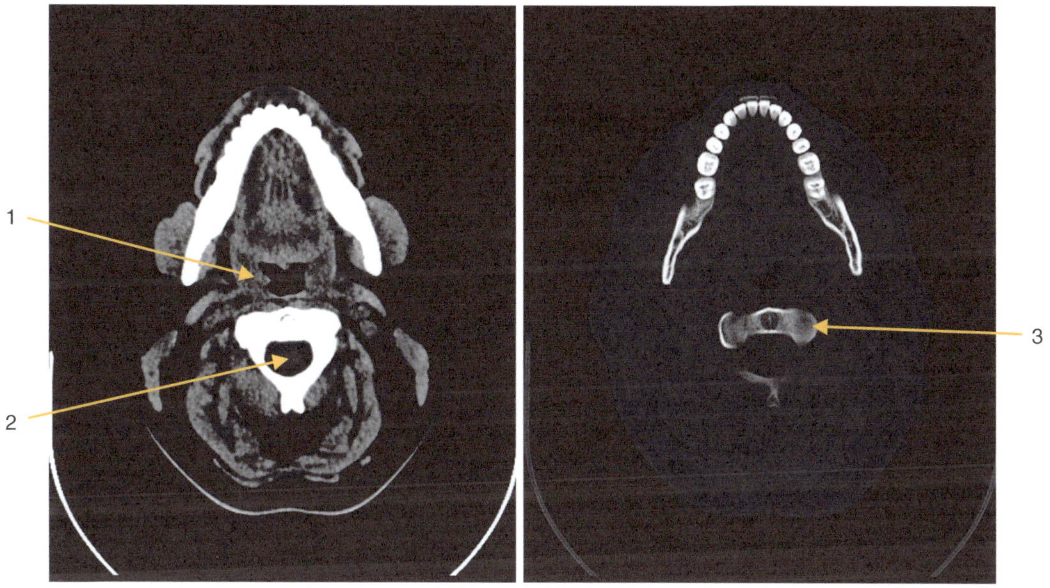

1. Palatine tonsil
2. Spinal cord
3. Axis bone

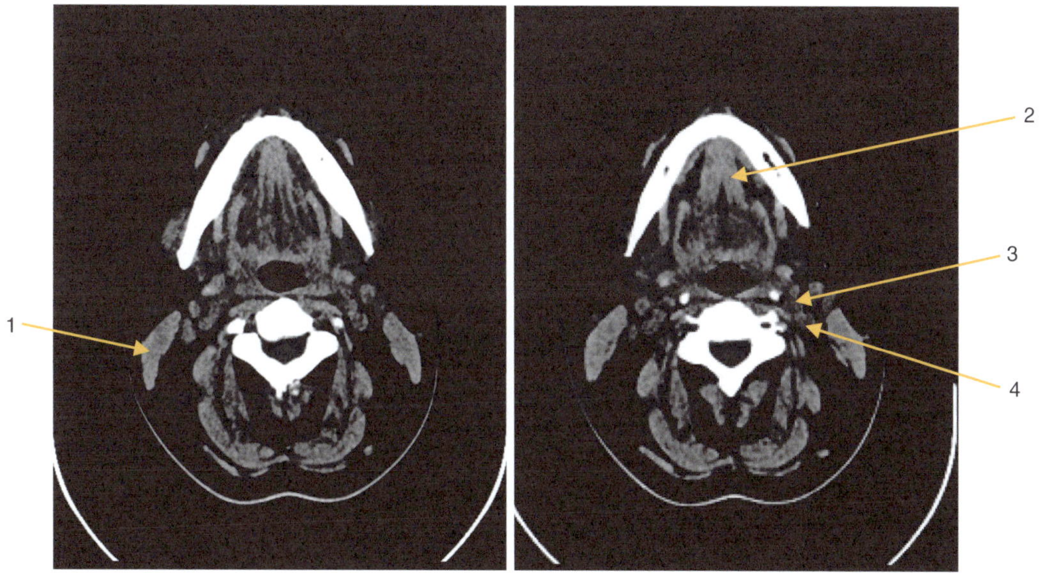

1. Sternocleidomastoid muscle
2. Genioglossus muscle
3. Common carotid artery
4. Internal jugular vein

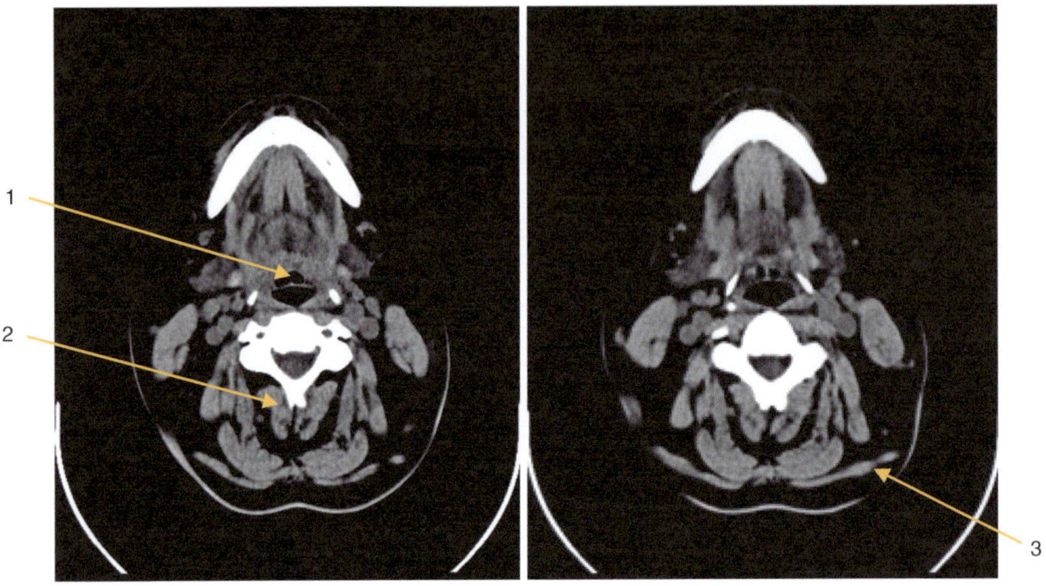

1. Oropharynx
2. Spinalis cervicis muscle
3. Trapezius muscle

9.3 Frontal/Coronal

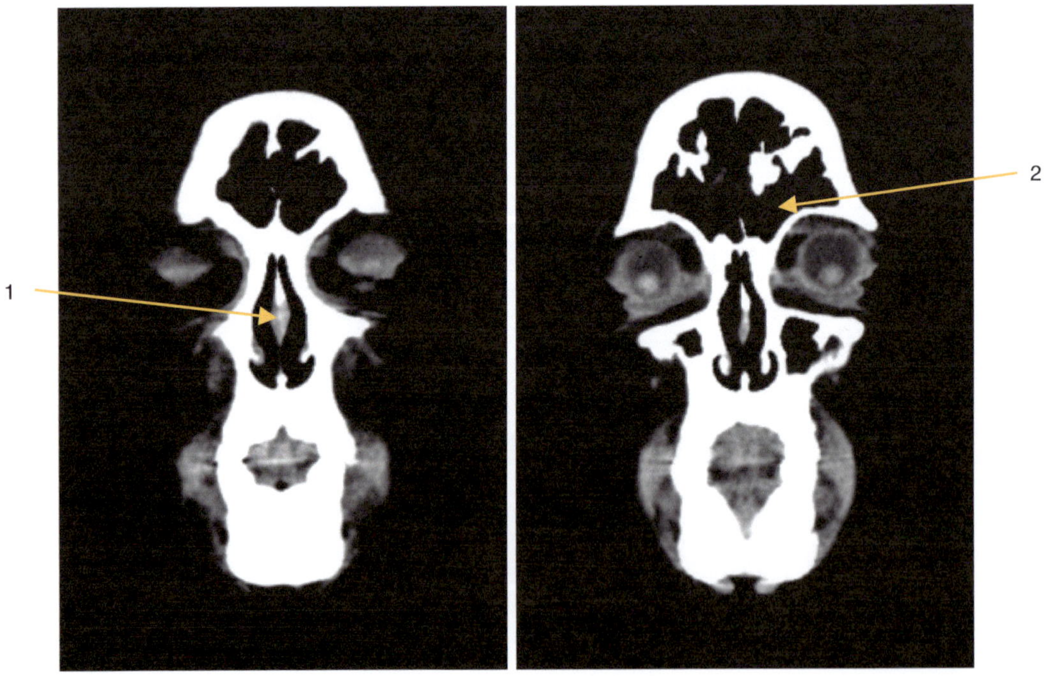

1. Nasal septum
2. Frontal sinus

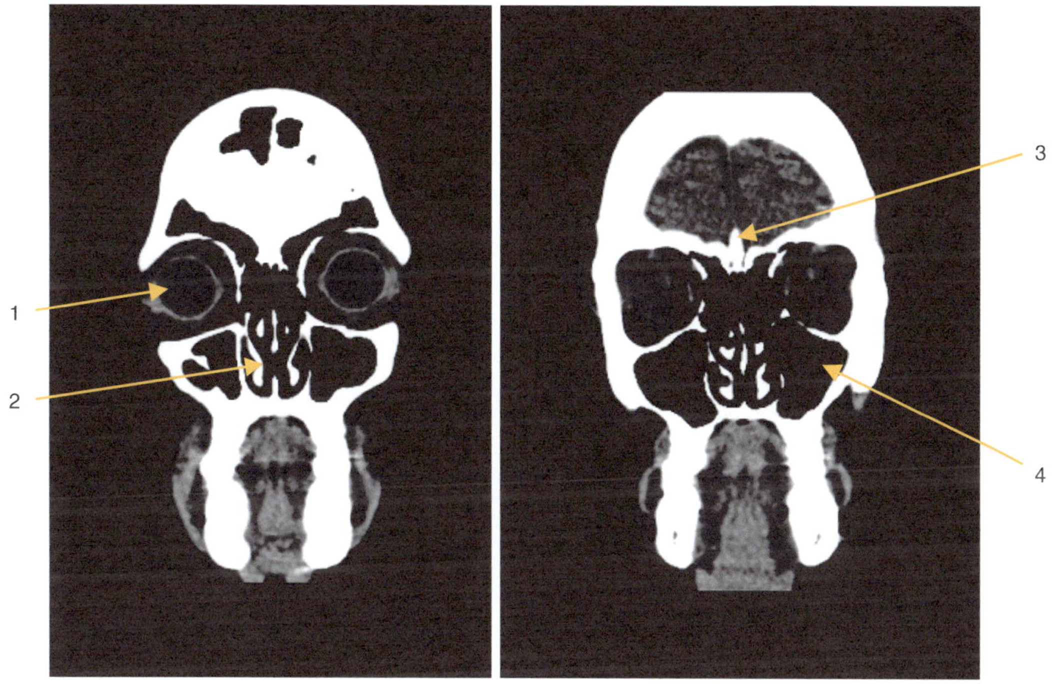

1. Eyeball
2. Nasal concha
3. Crista Galli
4. Maxillary sinus

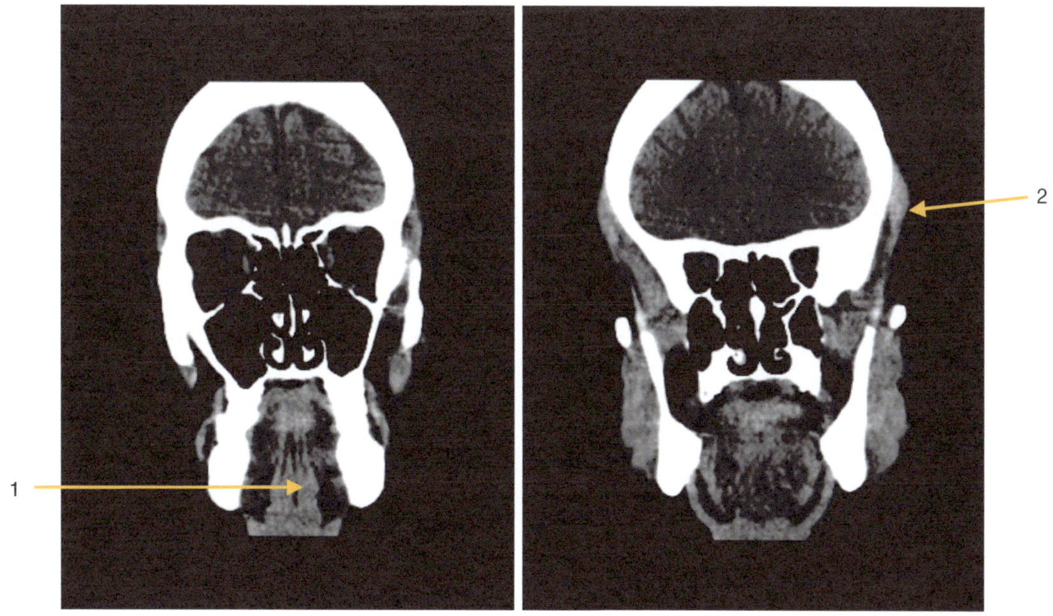

1. Genioglossus muscle
2. Temporalis muscle

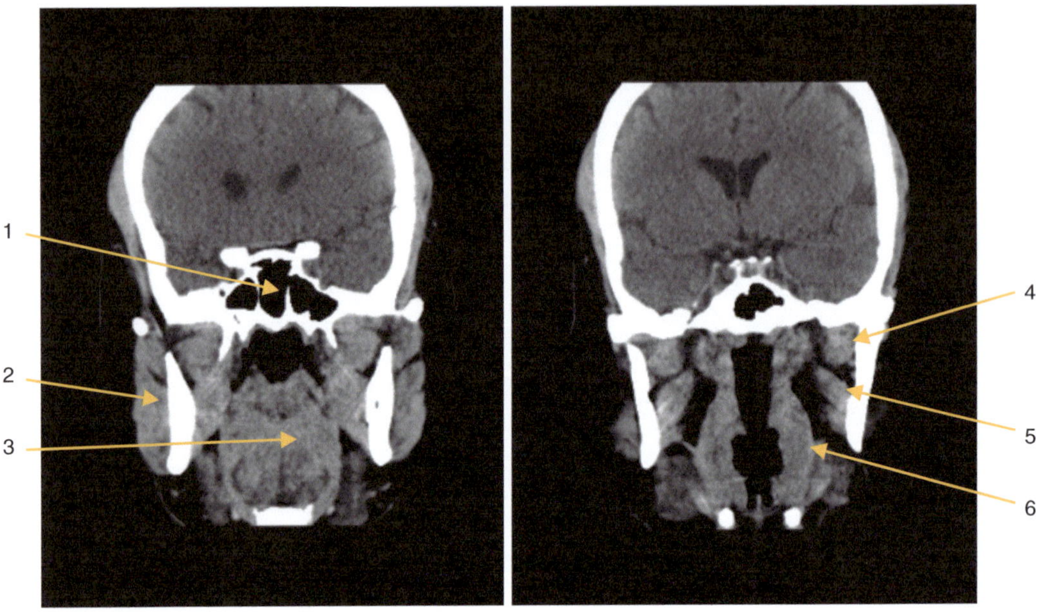

1. Sphenoid sinus
2. Masseter muscle
3. Tongue
4. Lateral pterygoid muscle
5. Medial pterygoid muscle
6. Superior constrictor muscle of pharynx

9.4 Sagittal

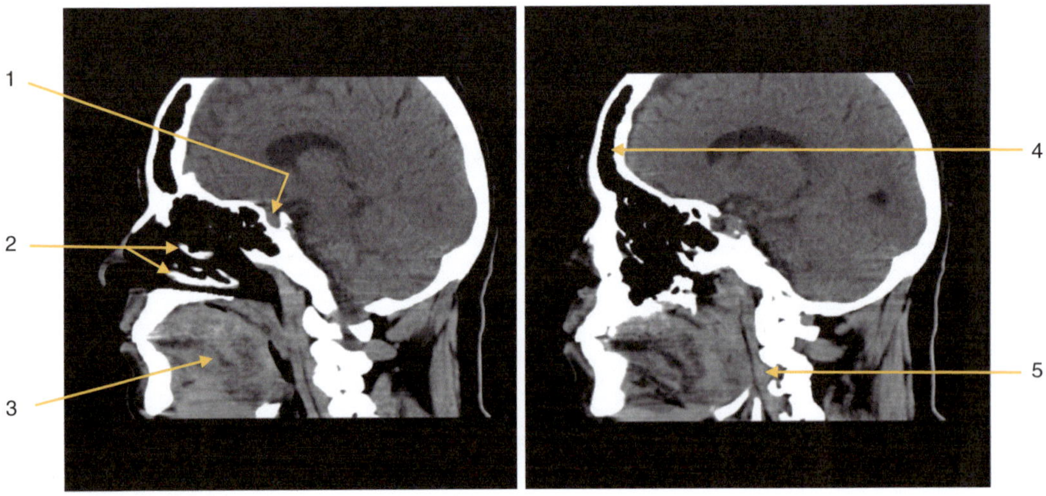

1. Pituitary gland
2. Middle and Inferior nasal concha
3. Tongue
4. Frontal Sinus
5. Longus capitis muscle

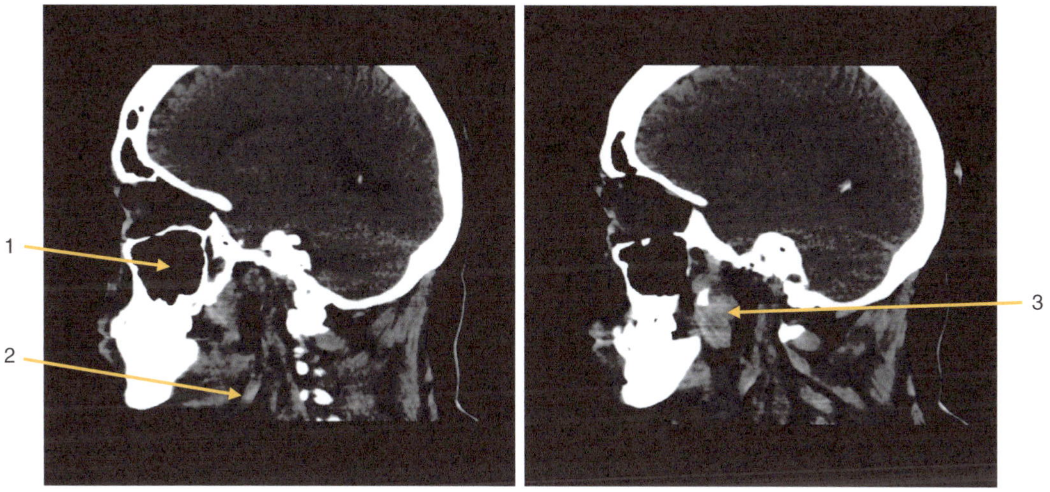

1. Maxillary sinus
2. Digastric muscle
3. Medial pterygoid muscle

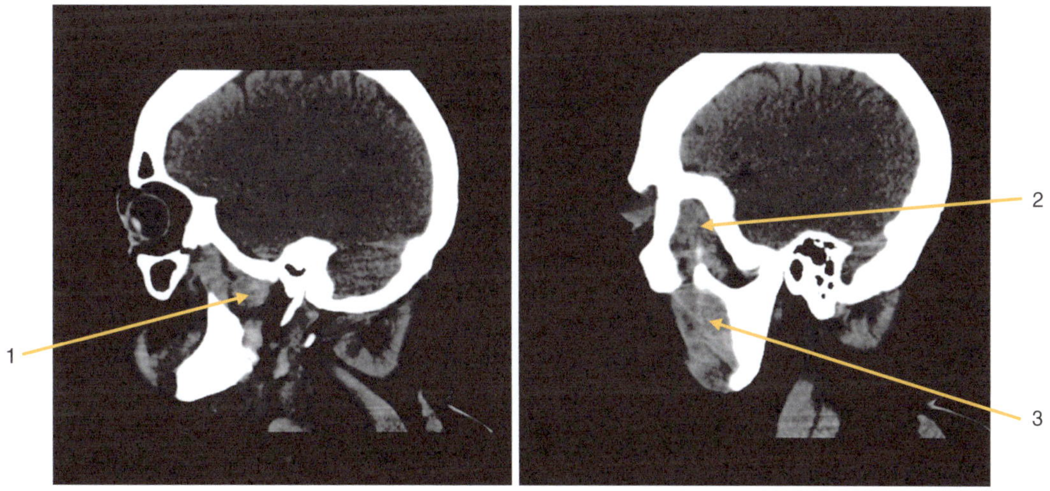

1. Lateral pterygoid muscle
2. Temporal muscle
3. Buccinator muscle

9.5 3D Imaging

Simple plain X-rays are 2D images of the area we are interested in.

They play a vital role in the diagnosis and treatment planning of the patient's condition. Though 2D images are more widely used and are still the method of choice in many cases, they only depict a 2D projection of the anatomy of interest. The addition of 3D tools, renders accessing the third dimention of the image such as the precise anatomical shape, and provides a very useful tool to the observer. The 3D imaginf is very useful to orientate the doctor in space and the three dimentions of the lesion in total. The addition of the third dimention can be useful to the dentist in cases of measuring symmetries etc and provides valuable information that could be useful to set the patients treatment plan, in more complex lesions and surgical treatment planning.

In the section that follows, 3D imaging of the osseous skull is presented and the major anatomical features of the osseous structured are identified in the sections.

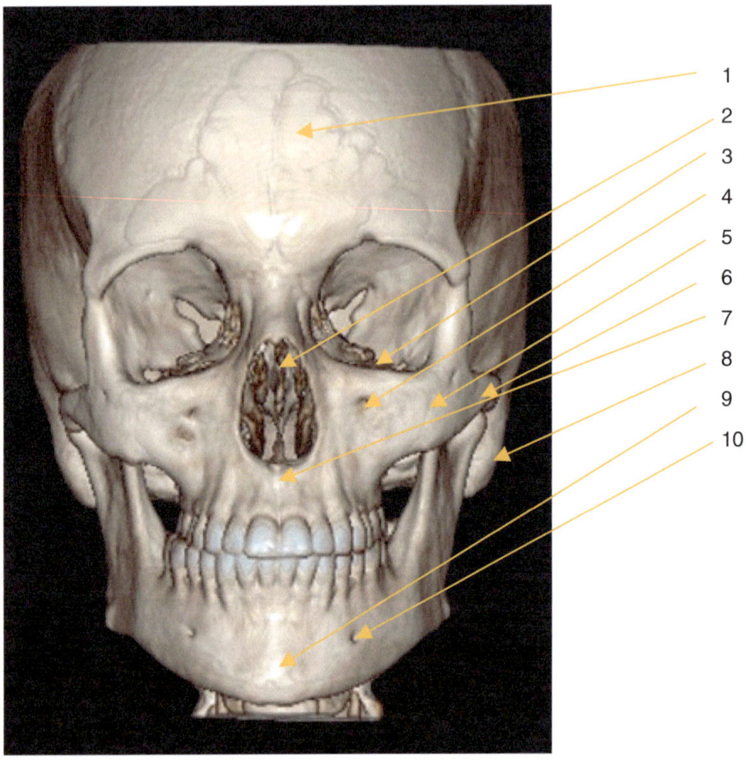

1. Frontal bone and sinus outline
2. Nasal cavity with nasal conchae
3. Orbital process of the maxilla
4. Infraorbital foramen
5. Zygomatic process of maxilla
6. Zygomatic arch
7. Anterior nasal spine
8. Mastoid process
9. Genial Tubercle
10. Mental foramen

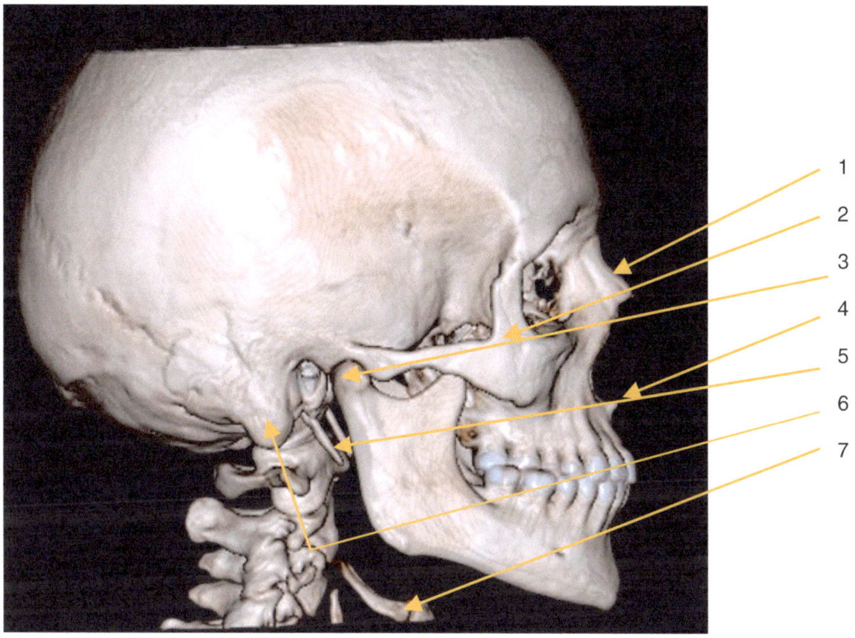

1. Nasal bone
2. Zygomatic bone
3. Condyle
4. Anterior nasal spine
5. Styloid ptocess
6. Mastoid process
7. Hyoid bone

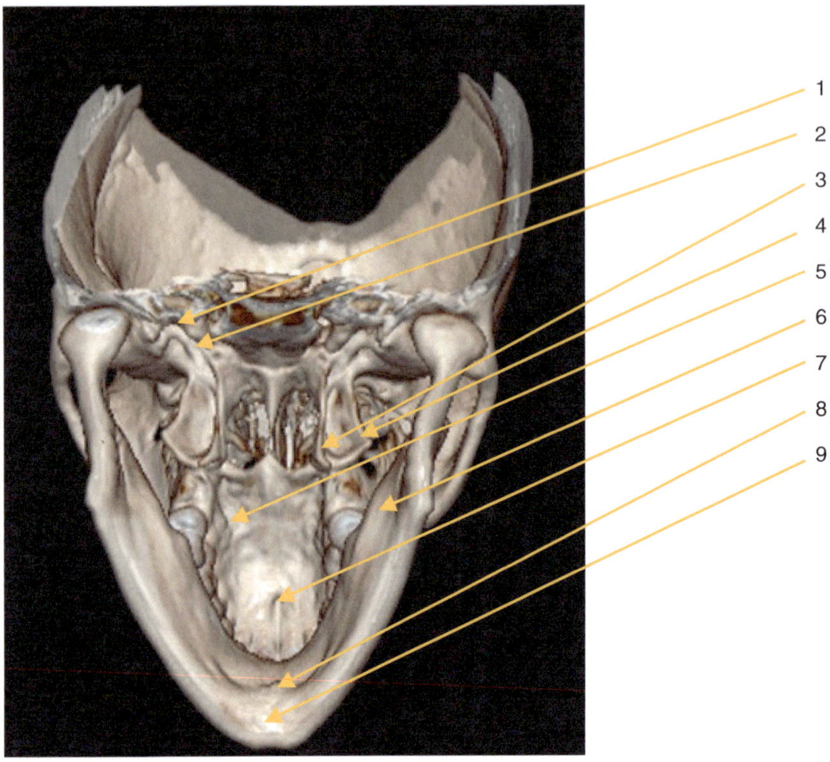

1. Foramen ovale
2. Pterygoid tubercle
3. Pterygoid hamulus
4. Lateral pterygoid plate
5. Palatine grooves
6. Mylohyoid groove
7. Incisive canal
8. Lingual foramen
9. Mental spine

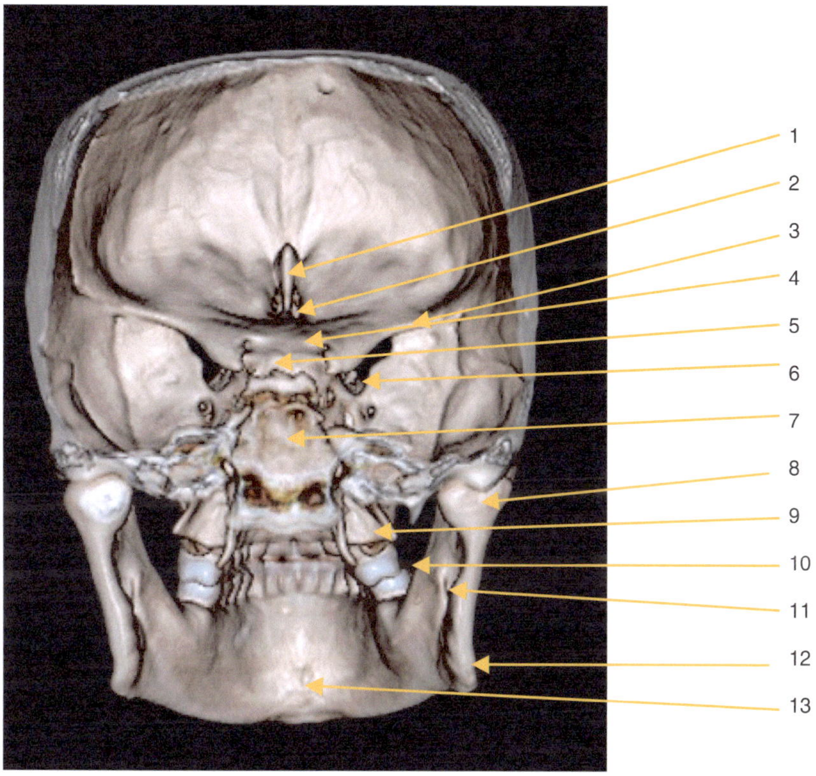

1. Crista galli
2. Ethmoid air cells
3. Lesser wing
4. Anterior Clinoid process
5. Sella Turcica
6. Lacrimal groove
7. Dorsum Sellae
8. Condyle of mandible
9. Pterygoid process
10. Internal oblique ridge
11. Mandibular foramen
12. Angle of mandible
13. Mental spine

9.6 Additional Planes of Section

The following images are sequences of various images in all planes of imaging with specifications to the exact location (smaller images) to help the dentist identify the exact slice position.

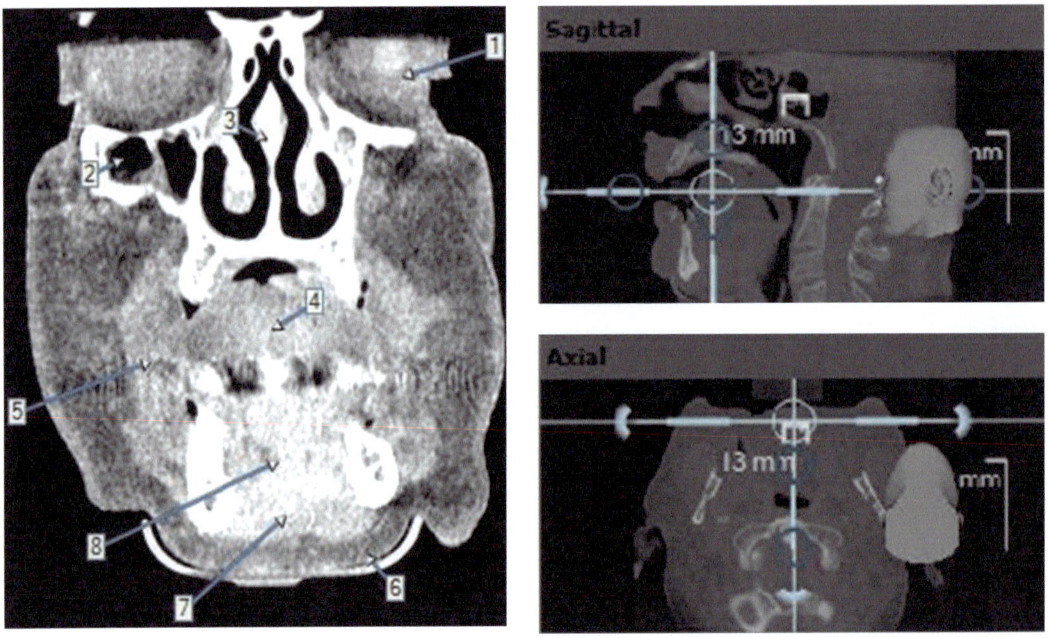

Coronal section figure 1:

1. Orbit
2. Maxillary sinus
3. Nasal septum
4. Tongue
5. Masseter muscle
6. Mylohyoid muscle
7. Geniohyoid muscle
8. Genioglossus muscle

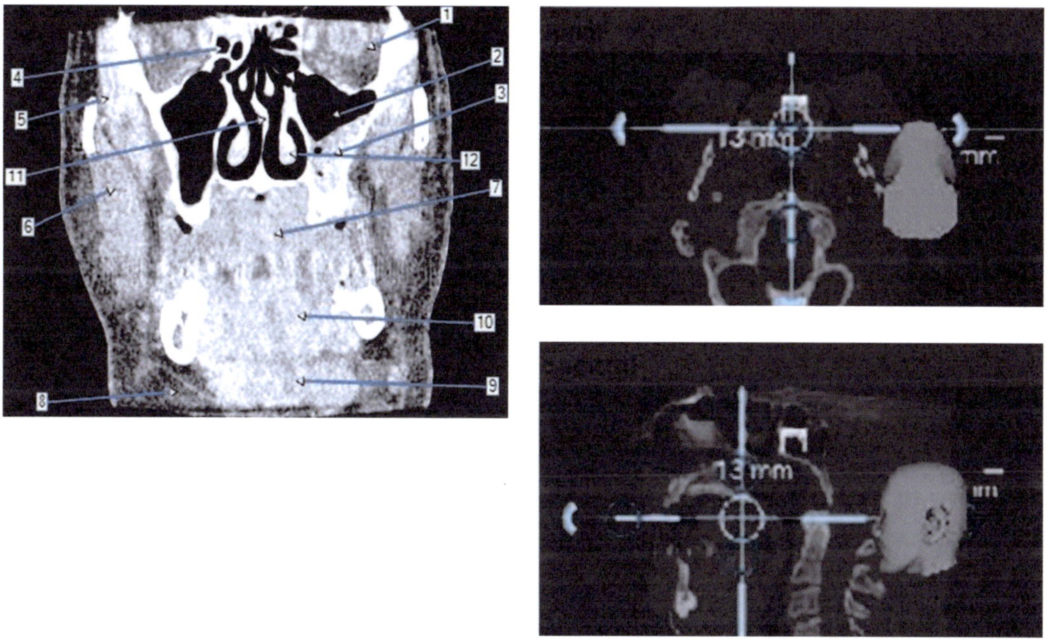

Coronal section figure 2:

1. Orbit
2. Maxillary sinus
3. Maxillary sinus mucosal hypertrophy
4. Ethmoid sinus
5. Temporal muscle
6. Masseter muscle
7. Tongue
8. Mylohyoid muscle
9. Geniohyoid muscle
10. Genioglossus muscle
11. Nasal septum
12. Concha nasalis inferior

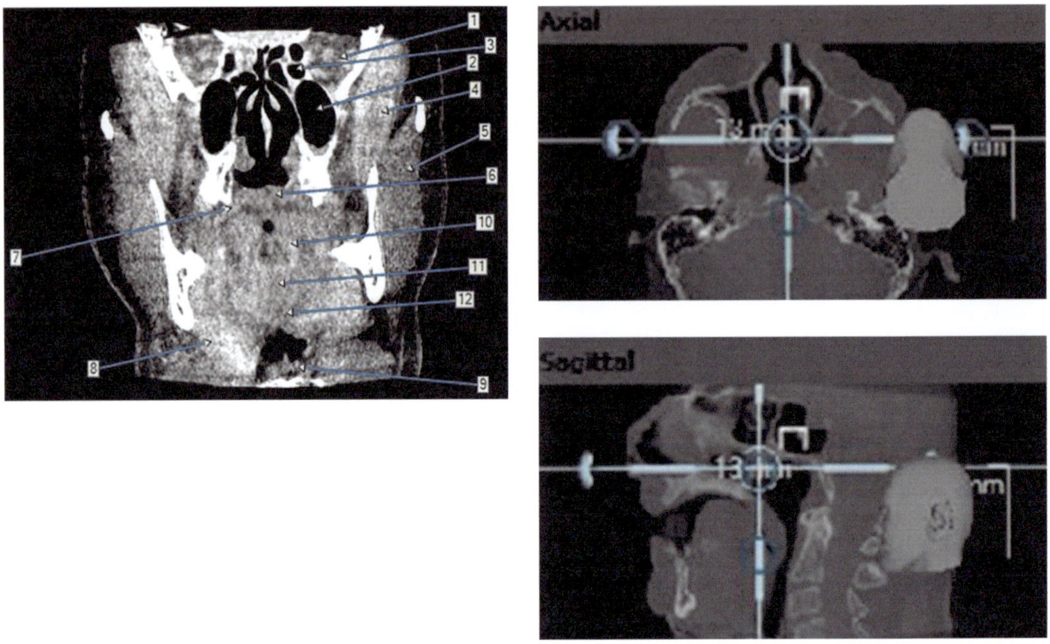

Coronal section figure 3:

1. Orbit
2. Maxillary sinus
3. Ethmoid sinus
4. Temporal muscle
5. Masseter muscle
6. Soft Palate
7. Styloglossus muscle
8. Submandibular gland
9. Epiglottis
10. Tongue
11. Genioglossus muscle
12. Geniohyoid muscle

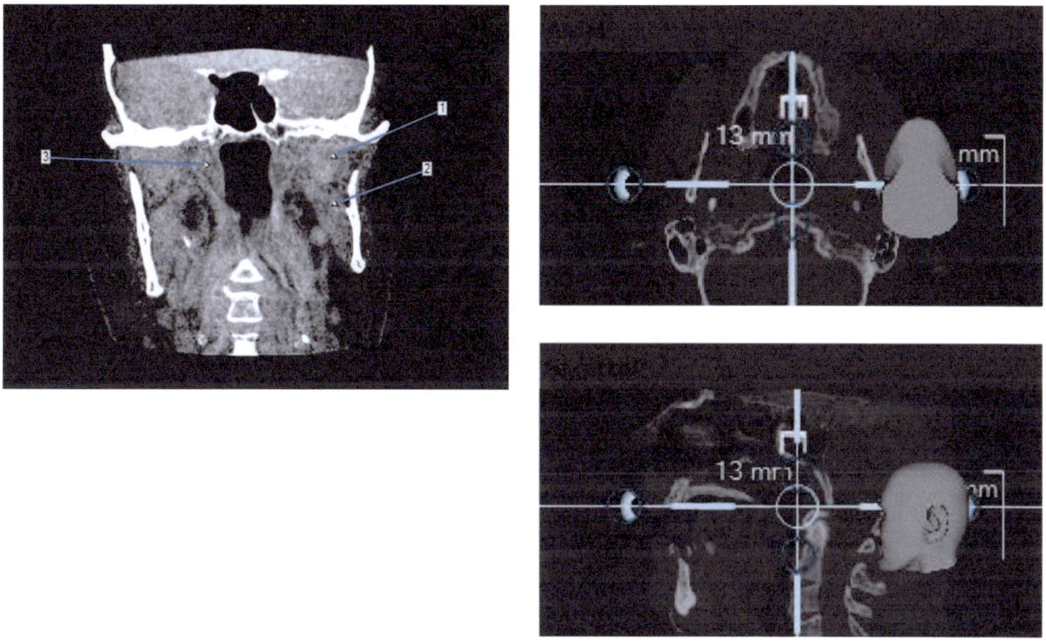

Coronal section figure 4:

1. Lateral pterygoid muscle
2. Medial pterygoid muscle
3. Levator veli palatini muscle

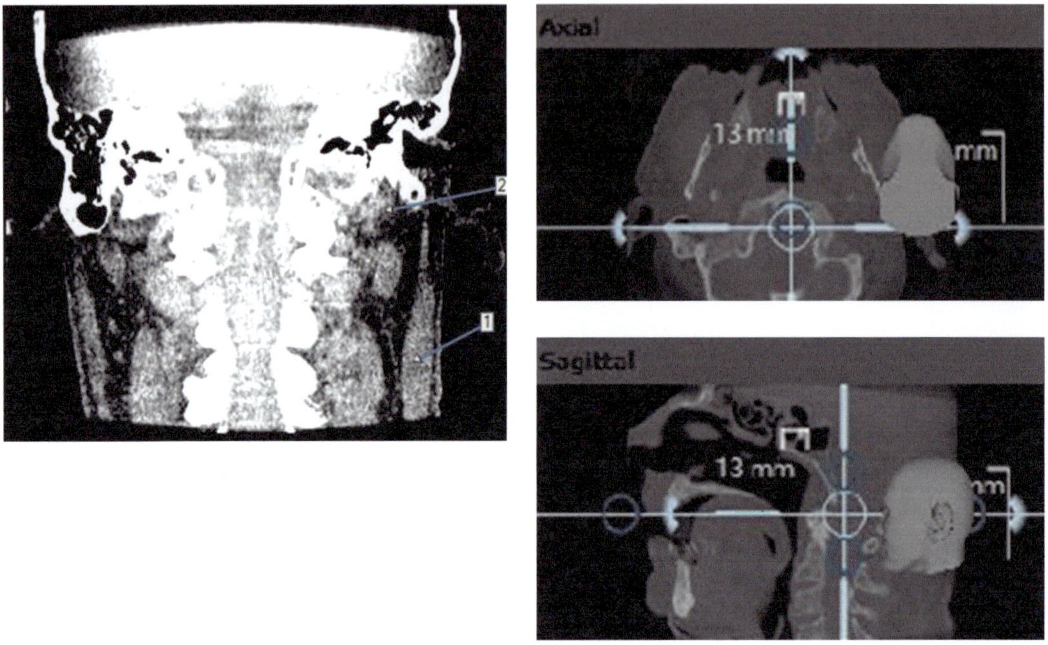

Coronal section figure 5:

1. Sternocleidomastoideus muscle
2. Digastric muscle (posterior belly)

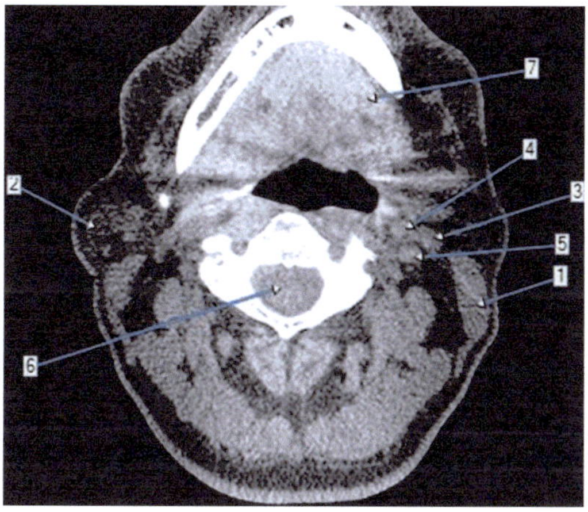

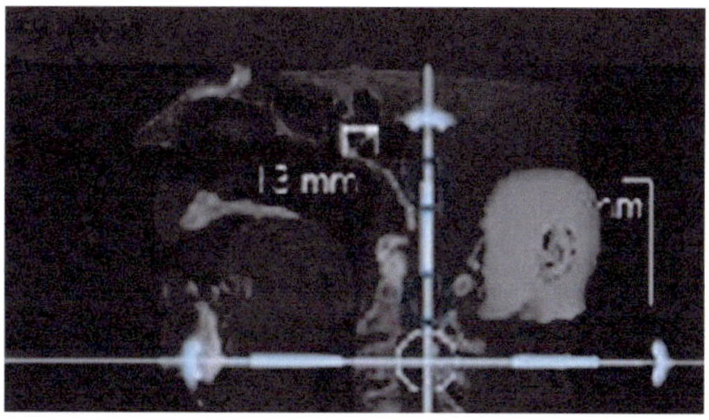

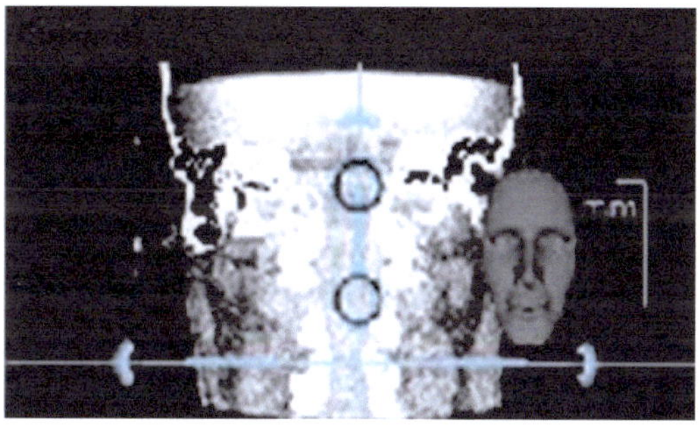

Axial section figure 1:

1. Sternocleidomastoid muscle
2. Submandibular gland
3. İnternal jugular vein
4. External carotid artery
5. İnternal carotid artery
6. Spinal cord
7. Mylohyoid muscle

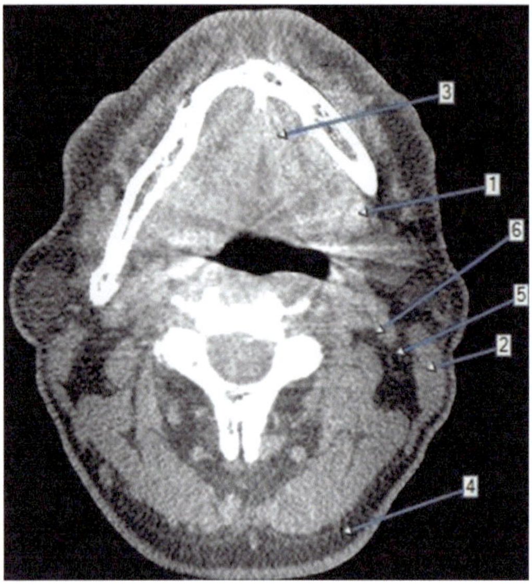

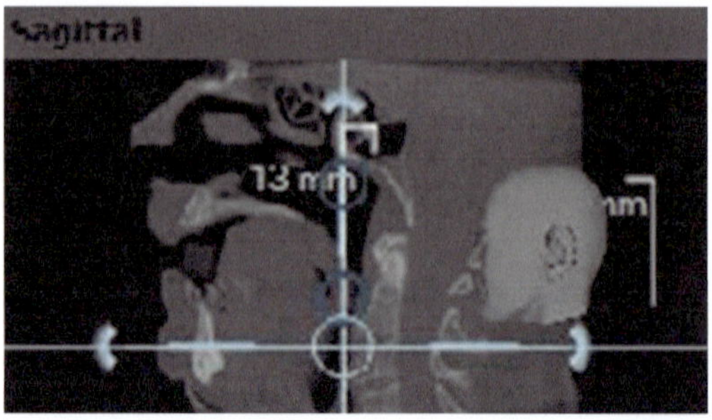

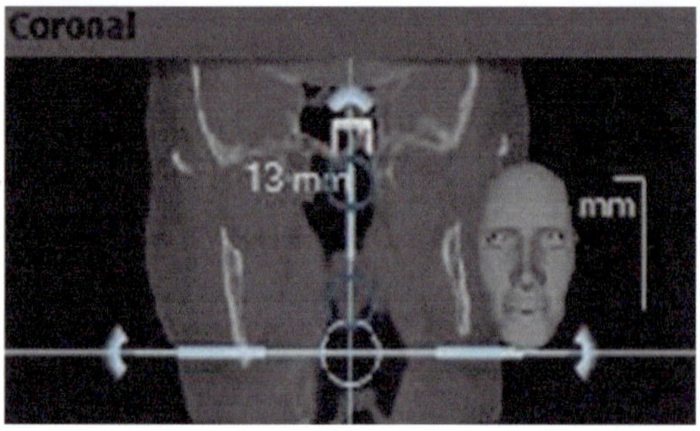

Axial section figure 2:

1. Submandibular gland
2. Sternocleidomastoid muscle
3. Mylohyoid muscle
4. Trapezius muscle
5. İnternal jugular vein
6. Common carotid artery

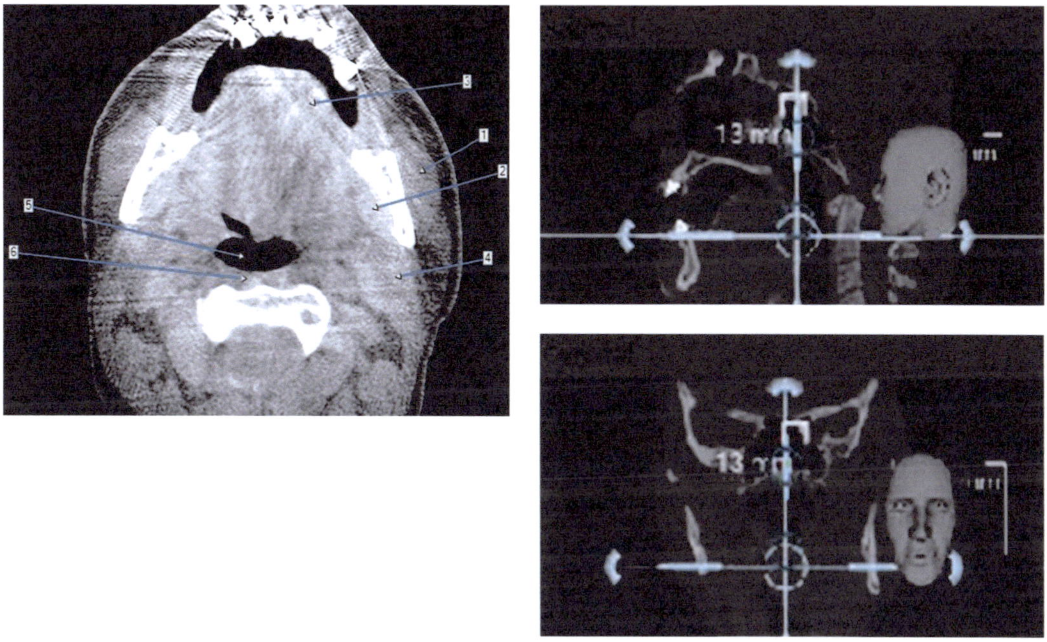

Axial section figure 3:

1. Masseter muscle
2. Submandibular gland
3. Tongue
4. Sternocleidomastoid muscle
5. Pharynx
6. Retropharynngeal space

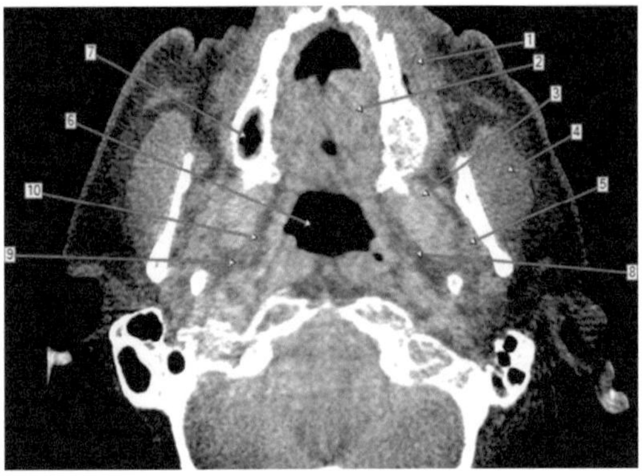

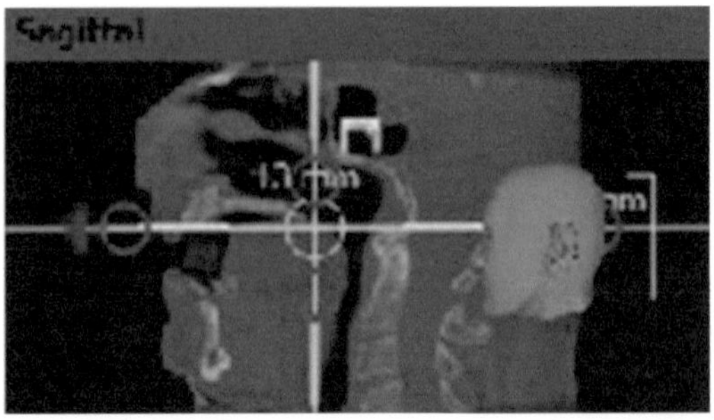

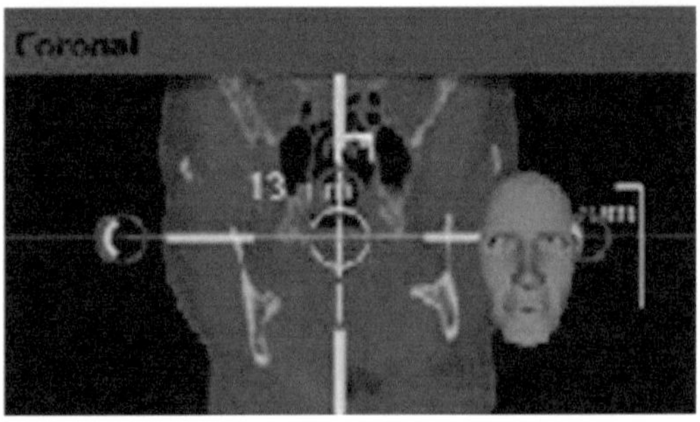

Axial section figure 4:

1. Buccinator muscle
2. Tongue
3. Medial pterygoid muscle
4. Masseter muscle
5. Parotid gland
6. Pharynx
7. Maxillary sinus
8. İnternal jugular vein
9. İnternal carotid artery
10. External carotid artery

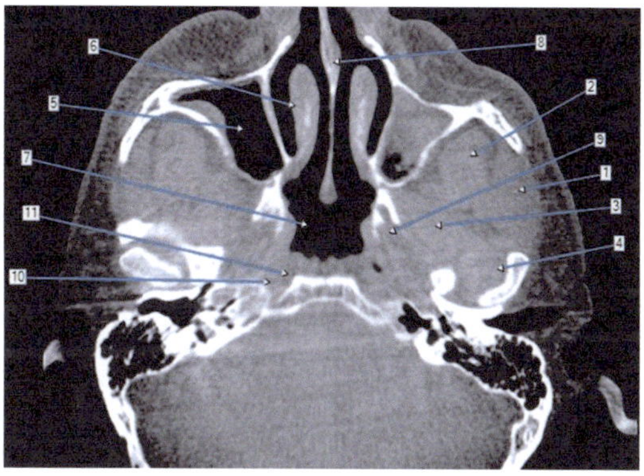

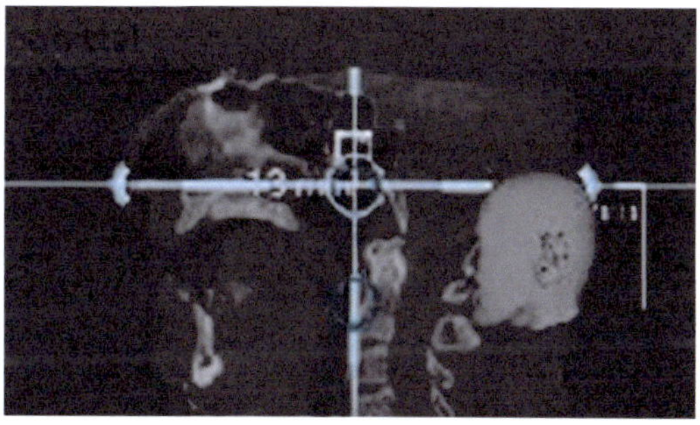

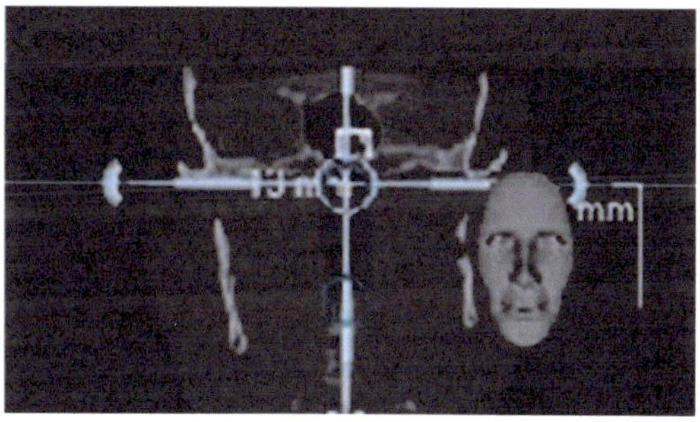

Axial section figure 5:

1. Masseter muscle
2. Lateral pterygoid muscle
3. Medial pterygoid muscle
4. Parotid gland
5. Maxillary sinus
6. İnferior nasal concha
7. Nasal pharynx
8. Nasal septum
9. Levator veli palatine muscle
10. İnternal jugular vein
11. İnternal carotid artery

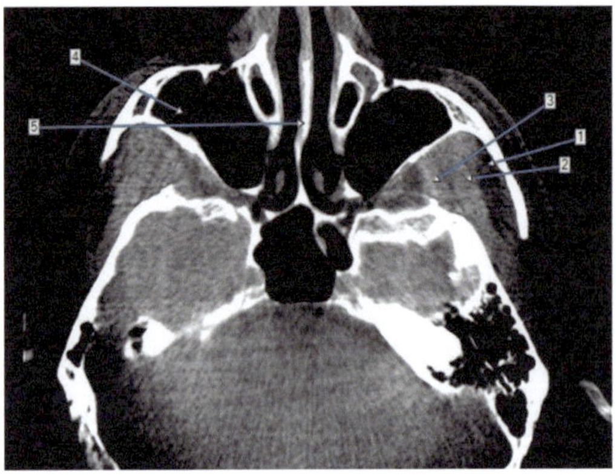

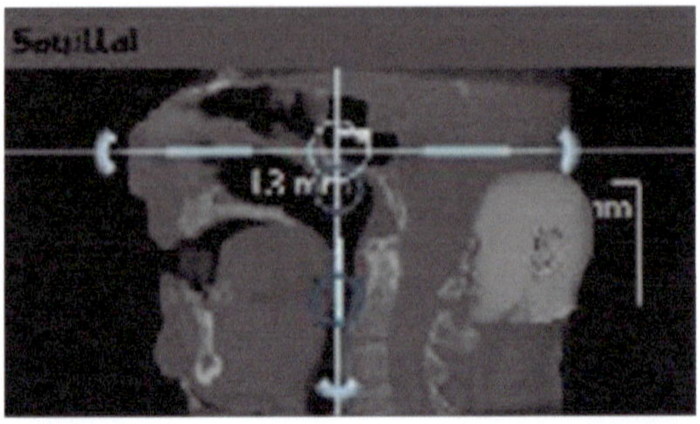

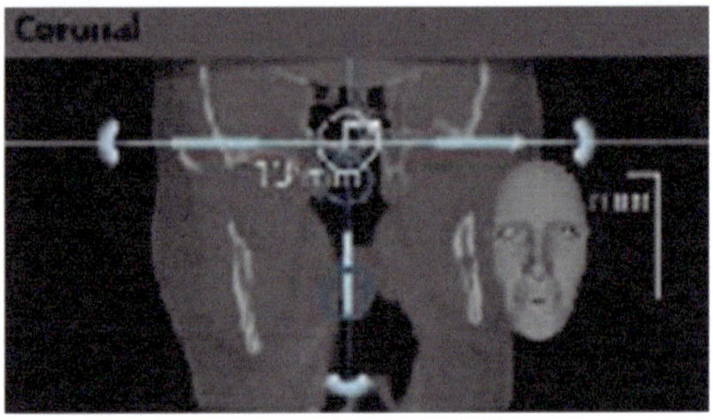

Axial section figure 6:

1. Masseter muscle
2. Temporalis muscle
3. Lateral pterygoid muscle
4. Maxillary sinus
5. Nasal septum

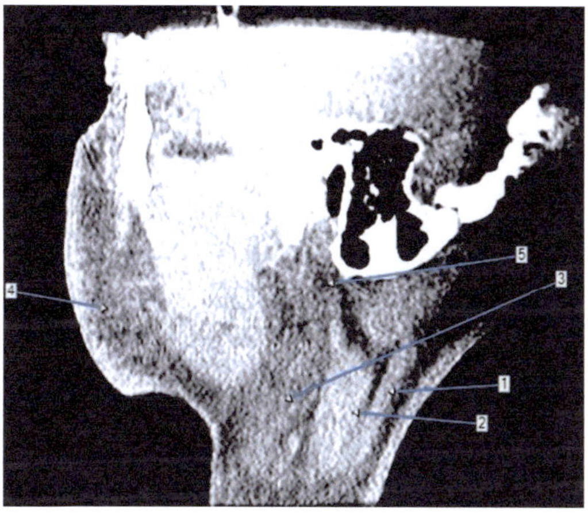

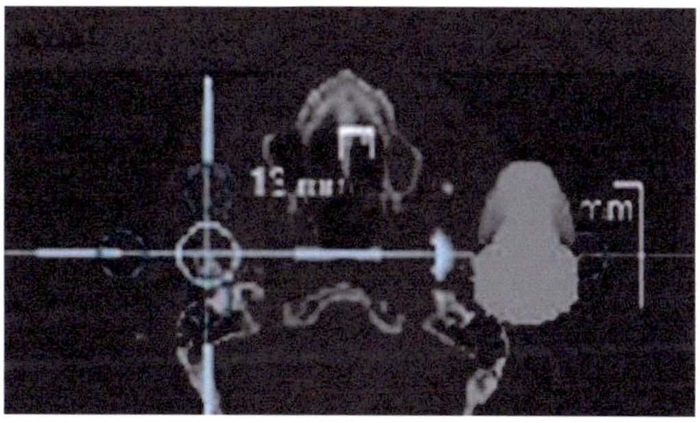

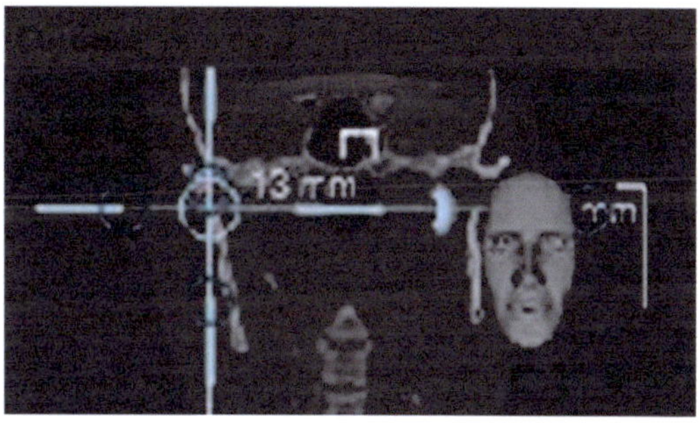

Sagittal section figure 1:

1. Trapezius muscle
2. Levator scapula muscle
3. Sternocleidomastoid muscle
4. Masseter muscle
5. Maxillary artery

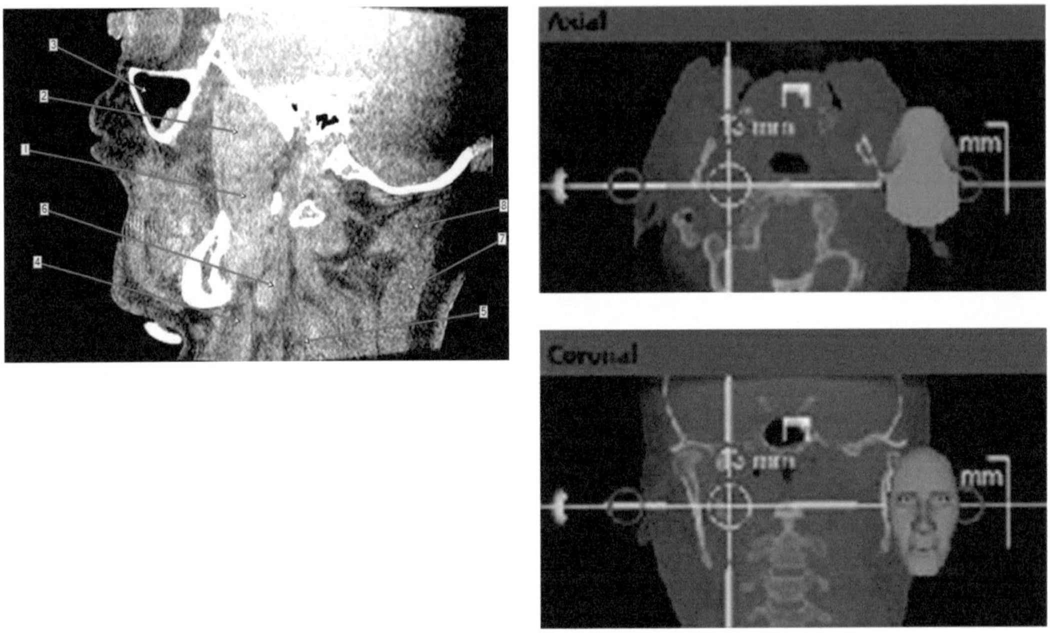

Sagittal section figure 2:

1. Medial pterygoid muscle
2. Lateral pterygoid muscle
3. Maxillary sinus
4. Sternocleidomastoid muscle
5. Scalenus anterior muscle
6. Submandibular gland
7. Trapezius muscle
8. Obliquus capitis superior muscle

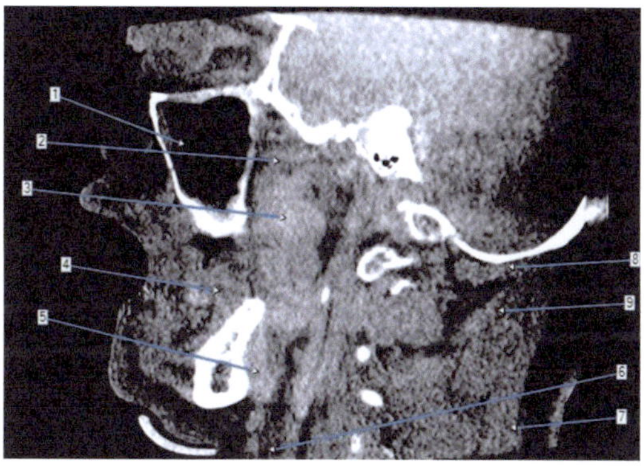

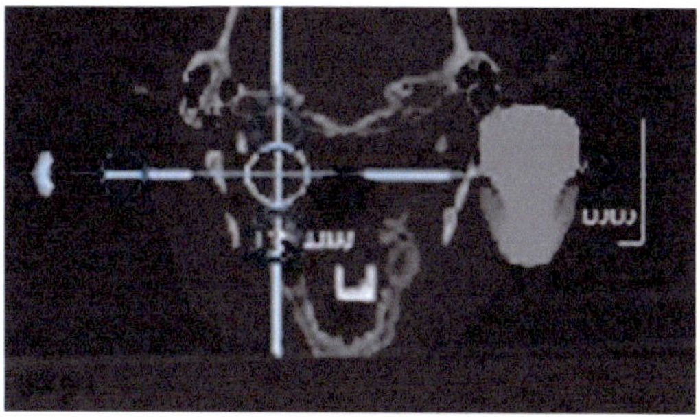

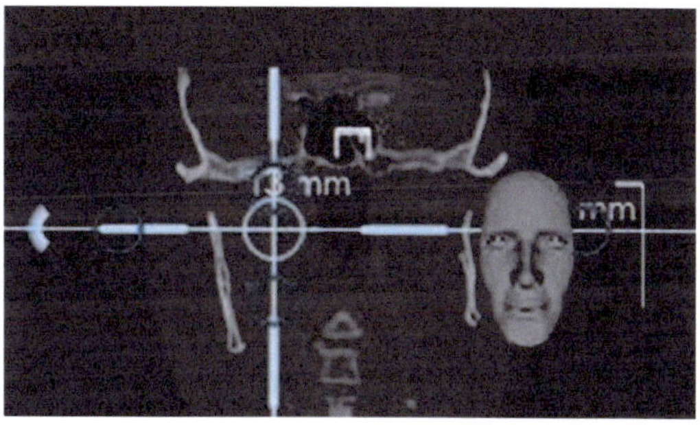

Sagittal section figure 3:

1. Maxillary sinus
2. Lateral pterygoid muscle
3. Medial pterygoid muscle
4. Tongue
5. Parotid gland
6. Sternocleidomastoid muscle
7. Trapezius muscle
8. Rectus capitis posterior major muscle
9. Obliquus capitis inferior muscle

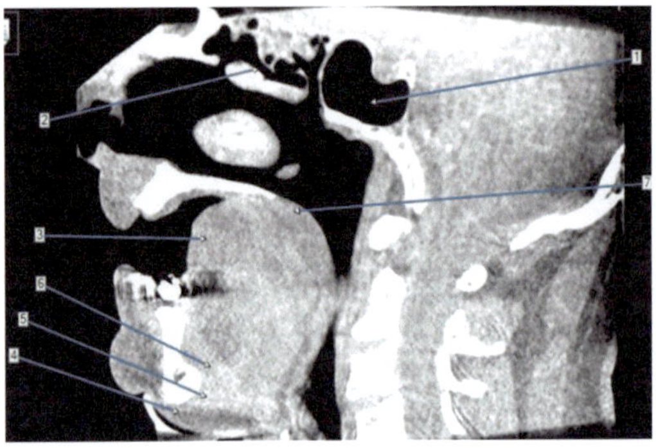

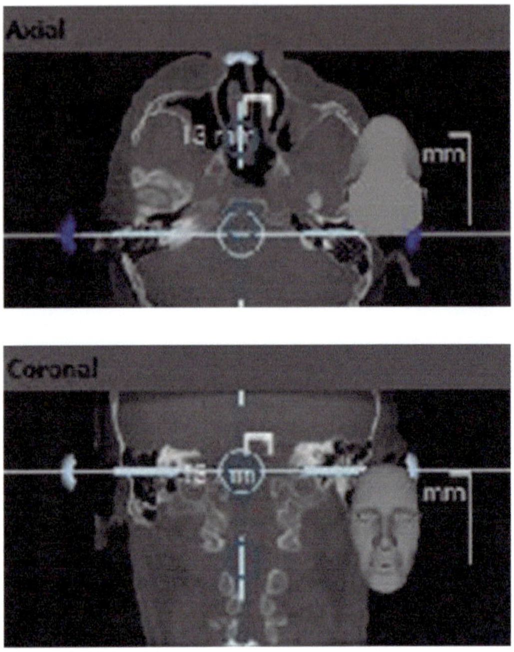

Sagittal section figure 4:

1. Sphenoid sinus
2. Ethmoid sinus
3. Tongue
4. Mylohyoid muscle
5. Geniohyoid muscle
6. Genioglossus muscle
7. Soft palate

Further Reading

Abrahams JJ, Rock R, Hayt MW. Embryology and anatomy of the jaw and dentition. In: Som PM, Curtin HD, editors. Head and neck imaging. 4th ed. St. Louis, MO: Mosby; 2003. p. 889–906.

American Dental Association. Dental radiographic examinations: recommendations for patient selection and limiting radiation exposure. ADA Council on Scientific Affairs, US Dept of Health and Human Services, Public Health Service, Food and Drug Administration; 2012.

American Dental Association Council on Scientific Affairs. The use of dental radiographs: update and recommendations. J Am Dent Assoc. 2006;137:1304–12.

Smoker WRK. The oral cavity. In: Som PM, Curtin HD, editors. Head and neck imaging. 4th ed. St. Louis, MO: Mosby; 2003. p. 1377–464.

Som PM, Shugar JMA, Brandwein MS. Sinonasal cavities: anatomy and physiology. In: Som PM, Curtin HD, editors. Head and neck imaging. 4th ed. St. Louis, MO: Mosby; 2003a. p. 87–147.

Som PM, Smoker WRK, Balboni A, Reidenberg JS, Hudgins PA, Weissman JL, Laitman J. Embryology and anatomy of the neck. In: Som PM, Curtin HD, editors. Head and neck imaging. 4th ed. St. Louis, MO: Mosby; 2003b. p. 1757–827.

10 Dentomaxillofacial Ultrasonography: Basic Principles and Radiographic Anatomy

Antigoni Delantoni and Apostolos Sarafopoulos

10.1 Introduction

Ultrasound is a common radiographic exam in patients with clinical findings and symptoms from the neck, buccal area, and oropharynx.

Adequate evaluation of a pathological structure should be based primarily on the recognition of normal anatomical structures. This presupposes the appropriate equipment, the familiarity of the operator, and the understanding of the examination techniques.

In the following sections we will describe the methods and the way of handling the ultrasound unit in order to achieve the optimal display of the anatomical structures of the soft tissues of the face and neck area in individuals—volunteers with normal non-pathological findings.

The authors state that the chapter does not contain any information or images or other third party material that is not copyrighted by the authors.

A. Delantoni (✉)
Department of Dentoalveolar Surgery, Implant Surgery and Radiology, Faculty of Dentistry, Aristotle University of Thessaloniki,
Thessaloniki, Greece
e-mail: andelant@dent.auth.gr

A. Sarafopoulos
AHEPA General Hospital, Thessaloniki, Greece

10.2 Equipment and Method

Ultrasound imaging of the structures of the face, upper neck, and the floor of the oral cavity is achieved using high-frequency transdermal transducers and a linear probe. Appropriate frequencies for an adequate scan range from approximately 6–15 MHz.

The choice of the appropriate frequency of ultrasound is individualized depending on the body types of the examinee and depends mainly on the thickness of the tissues that will absorb the sound, i.e., the skin, subcutaneous fat, muscle layers and the target organ. Low frequencies allow tissue imaging at greater depths compared to high frequencies, but lag far behind in sharpness and resolution. Therefore in people with increased thickness of soft particles we prefer the lowest frequencies 6–9 MHz. In contrast to patients with thin soft tissue, higher frequencies of 10–15 MHz are usually sufficient to examine deep tissues and produce higher resolution images.

It is of high significance and most helpful to the examiner, that the ultrasound equipment used in the maxillofacial area, should include color and spectral Doppler. With Color Doppler the examiner can control the perfusion of the tissues and the direction of blood flow while with Spectral Doppler the examiner can record the flow velocities in units of cm/s. The detection of a chromatic signal in the lumen of the arteries

A. Delantoni, K. Orhan (eds.), *Atlas of Dentomaxillofacial Anatomical Imaging*,
https://doi.org/10.1007/978-3-030-96840-3_10

and veins helps initially to distinguish the vascular branches from the secretory ducts of the salivary glands. In some tissues, such as the lymph nodes, the emergence of a characteristic pattern of perfusion allows them to be easily separated and located in the anatomical compartments of the neck, between the muscle groups and within the fatty layers [1].

The power Doppler method is a complementary test that detects weaker flows and measures the amount of vascularization with high resolution and higher resolution images compared to the Color Doppler. It cannot, however, determine the direction of flow and therefore separate the arterial from the venous network (Fig. 10.1).

In recent years, strain and shear wave elastography techniqyes have been added to the most advanced ultrasonographic equipment. They capture on a special color map and measure with Kpa units the rigidity of the tissues. This is obtained with the use of mechanical oscillation of the soft molecules at the device of the transducer in the first case and the electric emission, horizontal waves from the transducer in the second case.

Differences in tissue elasticity can confirm and to some extent determine the examiner's findings regarding the composition of the depicted anatomical structures such as muscle, cartilage, fat, and solid organs (Fig. 10.2).

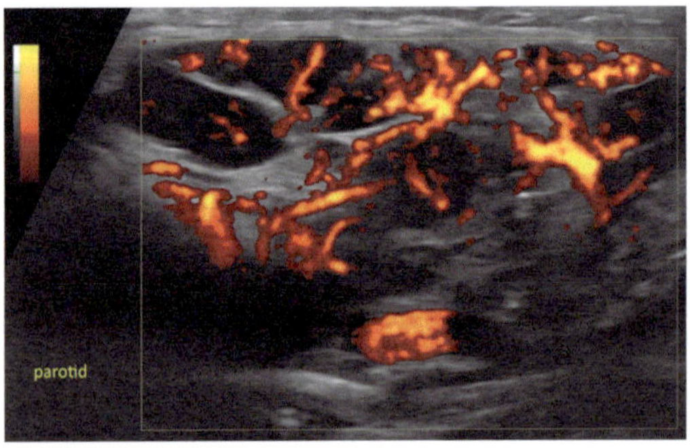

Fig. 10.1 The power Doppler method reveals in detail the increased perfusion of the parotid gland in a patient with chronic Sjogren's syndrome. Disorganization of the gland texture with reduced echogenicity, parenchyma reduction, and fibrous septa

10.3 Bone Structures

The visceral skull consists of the bones of the nasal cavity and the bones of the face. The second category includes the maxilla, zygomatic bones, and mandible [1–3].

The two maxillas are the main part of the facial skeleton. They form a triangular pyramid shape bone with three walls: anterior, posterior, and upper.

The maxilla as a bone has a body and four protuberances, the frontal, the buccal, the palatal, and the alveolar. The two alveolar ones join at the midline and form the alveolar arch or hard palate. They are areas of sonographic interest because they are directly related to the pathology of the oral cavity and teeth (Fig. 10.3).

The lower jaw or mandible is the largest bone in the face. It consists of the (A) body and the two (B) branches.

(A) The mandibular body shows in the midline the genial tuberocity and on the upper surface the alveoli of the mandibular teeth. On the inner surface of the body one can observe the sublingual and submandibular fossae for the homonymous salivary glands.
(B) The two rami of the mandible are merged with the body and form the two mandibular angles. The upper surface of the ramus ends in the coronary process towards the front and in the condylar process towards the back. The temporomandibular joint is created by the condylar process and the articular eminence of the temporal bone. A cartilaginous disc is located between the two articular surfaces, the anterior surface of which is concave in front due to the projection of the articular tubercle and convex to the back due to the temporal lobe.

The hyoid bone lies in the midline of the upper cervical region and serves mainly to support the tongue. It is U-shaped with the convex part facing forward and shows a middle degree, the body,

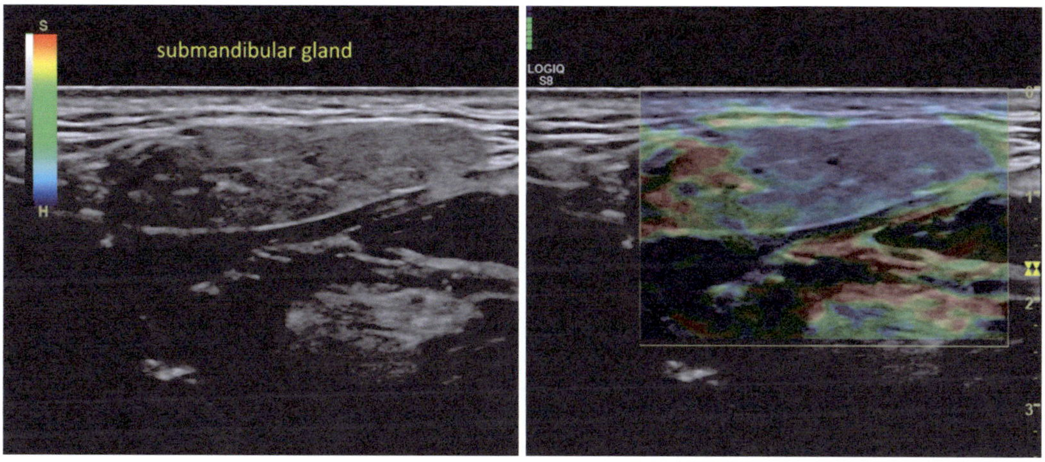

Fig. 10.2 Strain elastography of the submandibular salivary gland. The red areas correspond to soft tissues, while the dark blue ones to the hard ones. The normal submandibular gland (light blue color) shows increased stiffness compared to the surrounding tissues. In the elderly, the gland becomes harder due to fibrosis and parenchyma atrophy

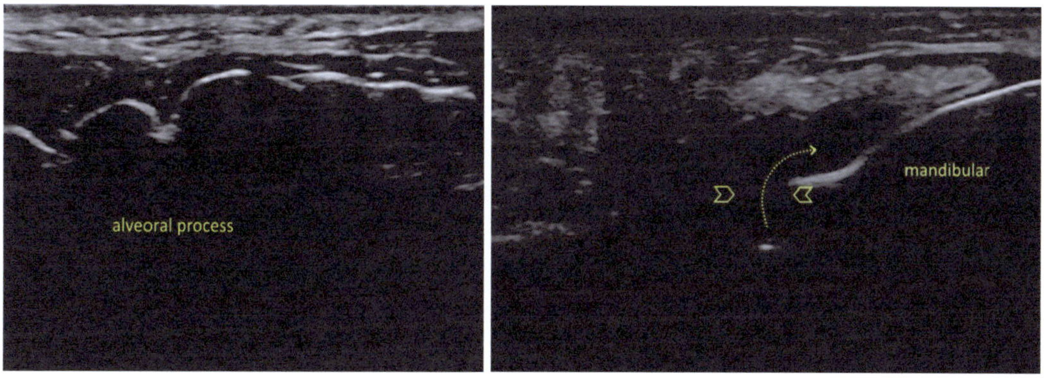

Fig. 10.3 Arched shaped morphology of the alveolar process in the normal maxilla. Osteomyelitis of the lower jaw with ultrasonographic disruption of the bone capsule (arrowheads) and diffusion of the inflammatory contents into the soft tissues of the area (arrow)

and two pairs of protuberances, the major and minor horns (Fig. 10.4).

10.3.1 Head Muscles

They are subdivided into (A) mimics and (B) masseter group of muscles [3–6].

(A) The mimic muscles that are located within the subcutaneous tissue, are small in size and are not surrounded by fascia. They adhere to the skin and are extremely sensitive to facial nerve impulses. With their contractions they change the facial expressions depending on the psychological state and the emotional changes of the person.

They are summarized to the muscles of the skull, mouth, nose, eyelids, and outer ear.

The buccal fat layer is located between the anterior edge of the massager and the buccinator muscle. The buccinator is a thin base of the buccal country, has a quadrangular shape and occupies the space between the upper and lower jaw. The duct of the parotid gland, pierces the buccinator muscle at the height of the second molar of the upper jaw.

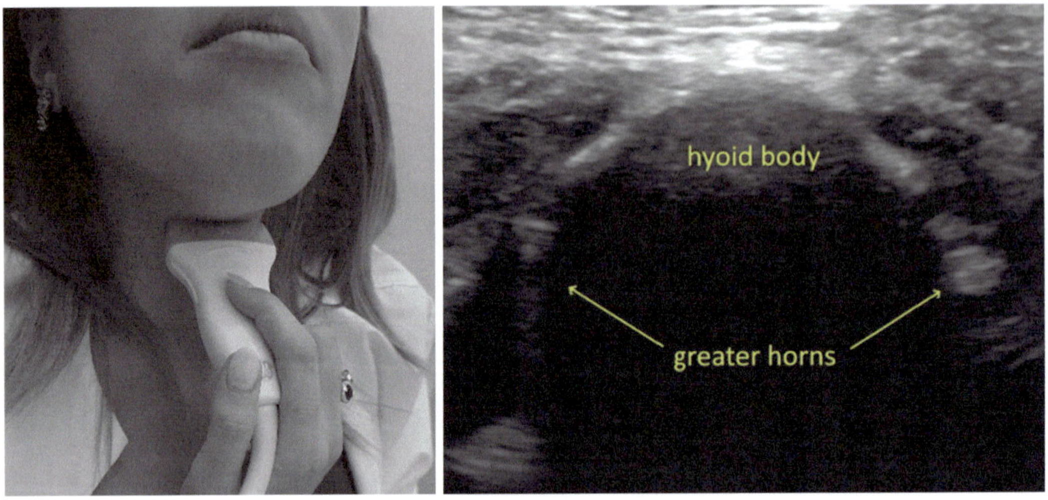

Fig. 10.4 The transducer is placed transversely at the boundaries between the floor of the oral cavity and the upper neck area. The hyoid bone is depicted as a curvilinear, hyperechoic formation

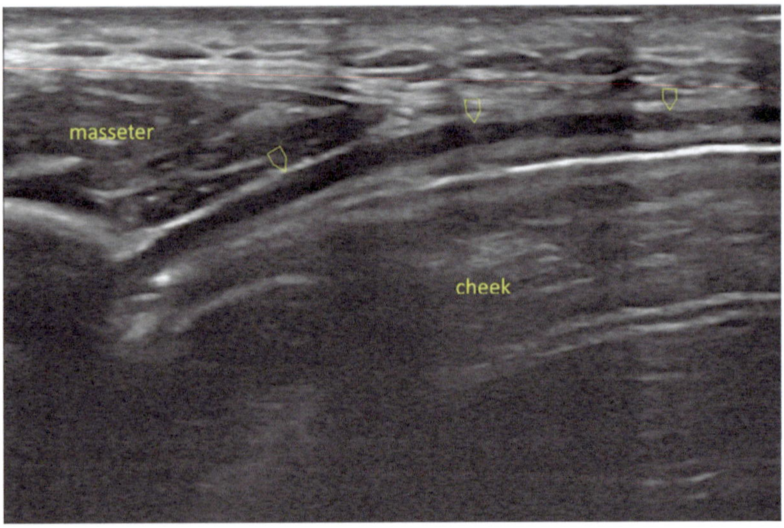

Fig. 10.5 Buccinator muscle (arrow heads) has the morphology of a thin hypoechoic zone and is readily visualized with the patient puffing (blowing and extending) his cheeks

The buccinator muscle helps in swallowing movements and air exhaling. Due to the close anatomical relationship with the oral cavity it is important to include it in our ultrasound examination (Fig. 10.5).

(B) The masseter muscles are four on each side: masseter, temporalis, median, and lateral pterygoid.

These are very strong muscles that rest on the lower jaw and control the chewing movements. They are innervated by the third branch of the trigeminal nerve.

The masseters show superficial and deep area. It arises from the cheek and ends in the masticatory area of the mandibular ramus. The outer surface of the muscle intersects with the parotid duct (Fig. 10.6).

The temporalis muscle is large and different from the masticatory muscles. It exits from the temporal fossa and the temporal bone and ends at the coronoid process of the mandible (Fig. 10.7).

The lateral pterygoid muscle appears with two sections the upper and lower. The

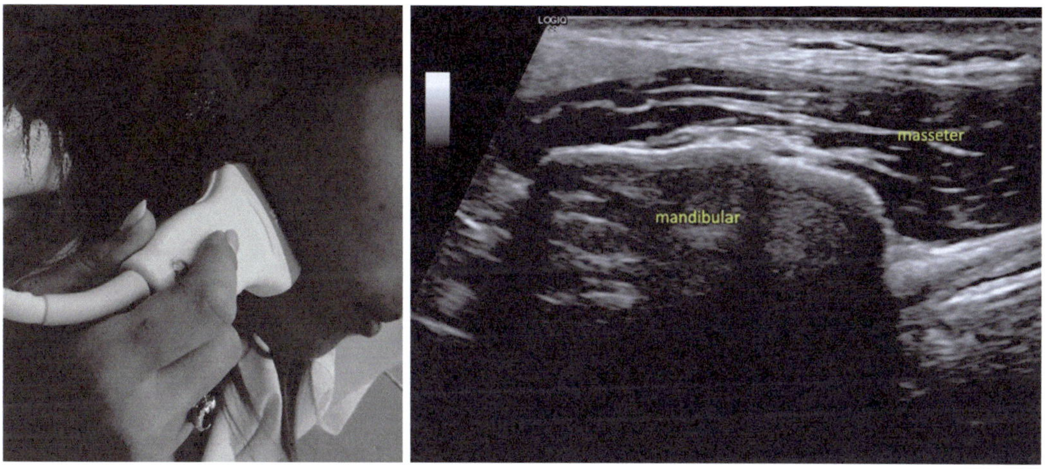

Fig. 10.6 Cross section of the masseter muscle at the corner of the lower jaw. Scanning the area starts at the height of the coronoid process of the mandible and continues downward

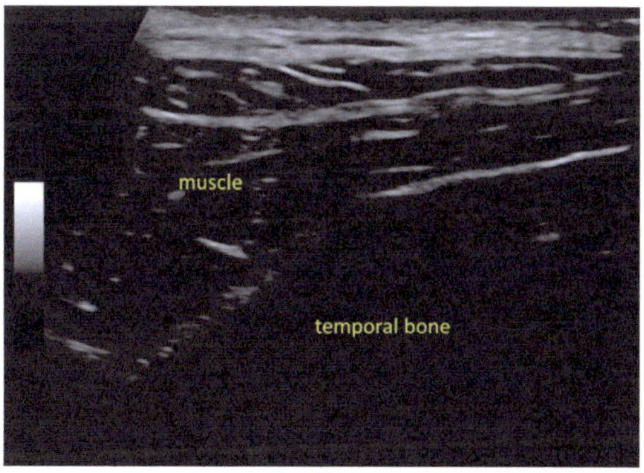

Fig. 10.7 Elongated cross section of the temporalis muscle above the zygomatic arch. The longitudinal, transverse, and vertical groups of muscle fibers are highlighted with proper positioning of the transducer and are depicted as linear or spotted/dotted sound reflections

upper surface rises from the infratemporal fossa. The lower section is larger and arises from the outer part of the pterygoid process of the sphenoid bone. The two sections proceed sagitally in the submandibular fossa, with a common tendon and lead to the pterygoid hamulus of the maxilla and the termporomandibular joint disc (Fig. 10.8).

10.4 Muscles of the Neck

One can readily distinguish the (a)anterior, (b) laterals, and (c) posterior or prevertebral.

The muscles that can be identified by ultrasonography are the mandibular digastor, geniohyoid muscle, sternocleidomastoid muscle, and the platysma (Fig. 10.9).

The digastric muscle belongs to the anterolateral group of cervical muscles located above the hyoid bone. It shows two bellies the anterior and posterior which are connected by an intermediate tendon. The posterior section rises from the mastoid process of the temporal bone and passes to the interstitial tendon that pierces the stylohyoid muscle and connects to the body of the hyoid. The anterior belly starts from the medial tendon and rests in the digastric fossa of the mandible at the inner surface of the mandibular angle [2–7].

The maxillohyoid belongs to the group of anterior cervical muscles located above the hyoid bone. It is triangular in shape and joins with its insertion of a central suture with the opposite muscle, forming a kind of septum between the oral cavity and the cervix. It protrudes from the inner oblique line of the lower jaw and lodges in the body of the hyoid bone.

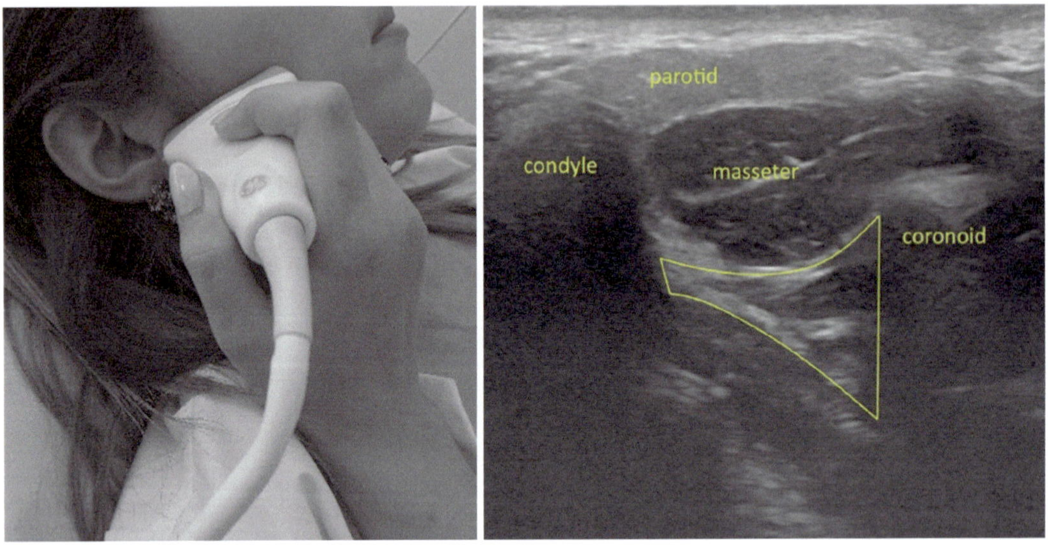

Fig. 10.8 The lateral pterygoid muscle (yellow frame) is shown in the cross-sections as a triangular formation interposed between the acoustic shadow of the coronoid process and the mandibular condyle

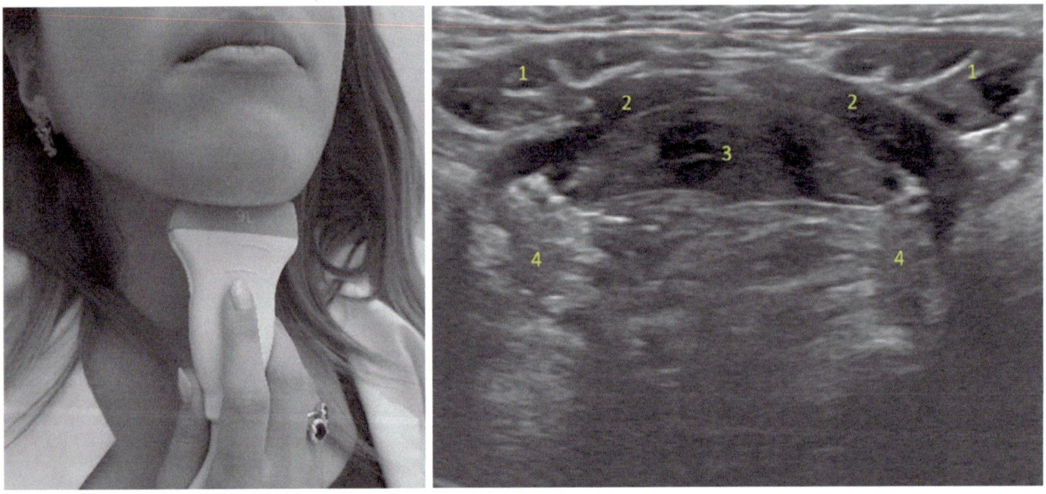

Fig. 10.9 Cross section by placing the transducer in the anterior part of the floor of the oral cavity (1) Digastric muscle, (2) Mylohyoid muscle, (3) geniohyoid muscle, (4) Sublingual salivary gland

Genoihyoid muscle lies above the previously mentioned muscle. It arises from the genial tubercle of the mandible and ends at the body of the hyoid bone.

The sternocleidomastoid muscle is responsible for the movements of the head. In abnormal contraction or shortening it causes differences in the skull shape. It is visible upon palpation in clinical examination. It consists of two sections, the sternal and the clavicular. They course obliquely upwards and outwards, they join in a common belly, which eventually rests on the mastoid process of the temporal bone (Fig. 10.10). Deep in the muscle is the angioneural bundle of the cervix and from its posterior rim emerge the dermal branches of the cervical plexus and the vagus nerve.

The platysma muscle is located in the subcutaneous fascia of the cervix, has a quadrilateral shape and a thin membrane morphologically. It

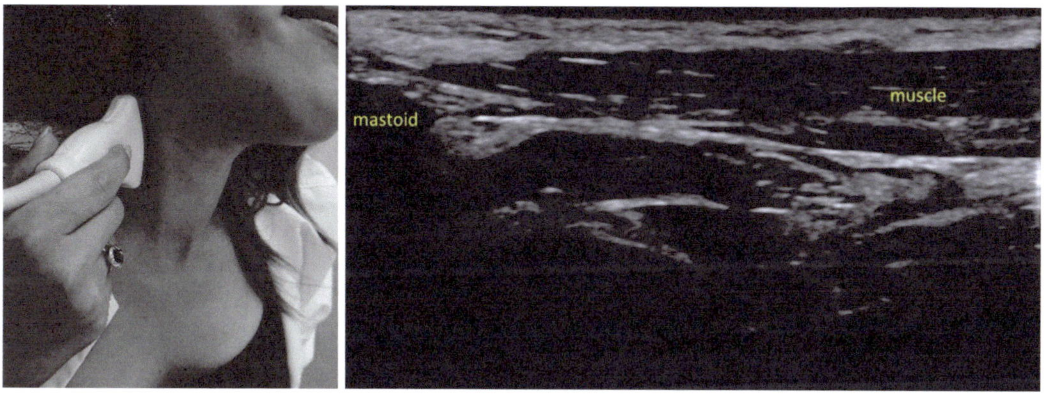

Fig. 10.10 Depiction of the linear morphology of the sternocleidomastoid muscle with superficial location

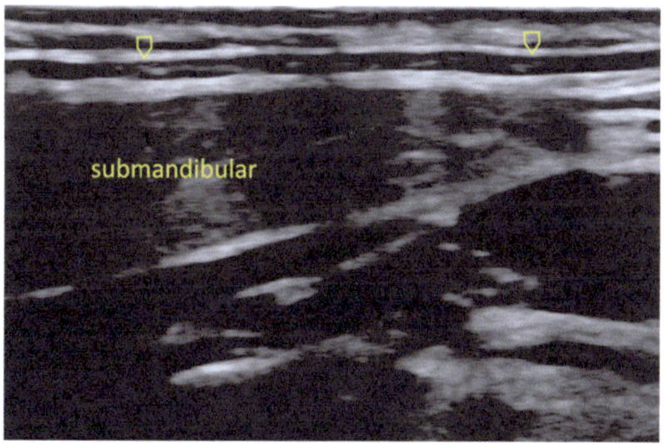

Fig. 10.11 The muscular platysma is relatively indistinguishable. It has the form of a hypoechoic wall on the anterior surface of the neck, below the subcutaneous fat (arrowheads)

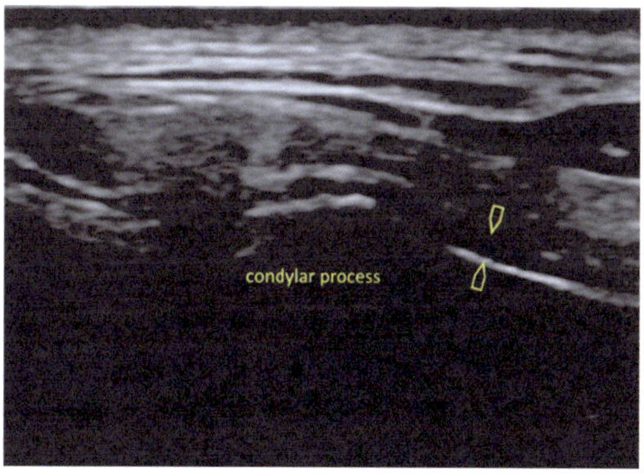

Fig. 10.12 Horizontal section. The normal synovial sac is depicted as a thin, subechoic edge at the neck of the mandibular condyle (arrowheads). In situations of increased amount of fluid the follicle swells and acquires the shape of a biconvex lens

protrudes from the upper part of the chest and penetrates the lower rim of the lower jaw and the skin of the lower lip of the face (Fig. 10.11).

10.4.1 Temporomandibular Joint

The temporomandibular joint is formed by the mandibular condyle and the articular eminence of the temporal bone. With the insertion of the articular disc, it is divided into two smaller structures, the upper and lower compartments or sections. In the non pathological temporomandibular joint the distance between the tubercle and the temporomandibular joint ranges from 1.5 mm to 2.5 mm and is even.

The articular capsule is extremely loose, allowing the lower jaw to move freely in all directions during chewing and speaking (Fig. 10.12). The most important ligaments that strengthen the joint are the outer lateral that surrounds the pocket from the outer surface and the inner mesial one, that covers the pocket from the inner surface.

The articular disc or meniscus is not static, but moves normally within the joint. When the mouth is closed, the mandibular condyle rests firmly on the posterior border of the disc. At the beginning of the contraction, it is displaced forward by the action of the lower part of the outer pterygoid muscle, moving at the same time the anterior lip of the disc on the articular ridge of the temporal bone (Fig. 10.13).

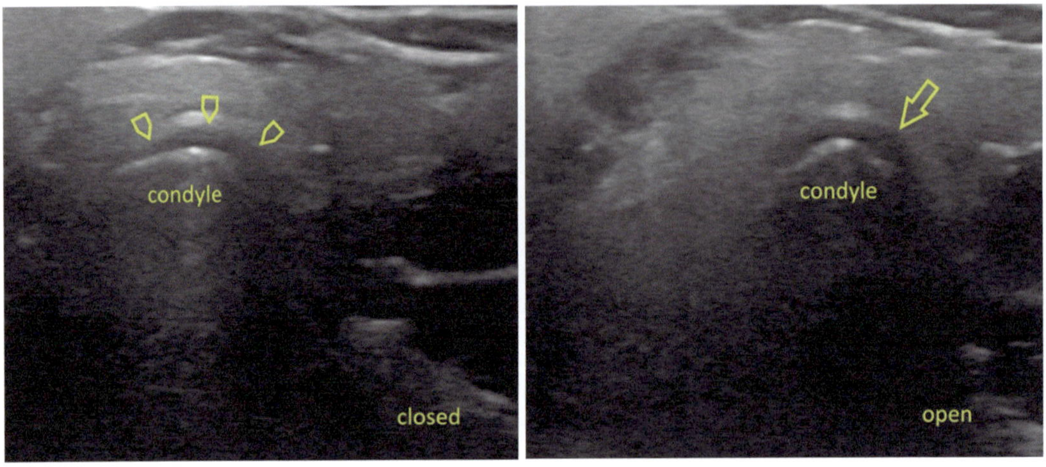

Fig. 10.13 Transverse sections of the disc in the preauricular region. With the mouth closed, the articular disc is recognized as a lunar formation of low echogenicity that touches the condyle of the lower jaw (arrowheads). With the mouth open there is a slight change in the position and thickness of the disc, more visible in the anterior section (arrow)

10.4.2 Tongue

The tongue is a muscular organ surrounded by mucosa and is used for speech, taste, chewing, and swallowing. It has a conical shape and shows three anatomical borders, the top, the body, and the root. Between the body and the root of the tongue there is a V-shaped groove, the apex of which corresponds to the blind foramen. This corresponds to the apex of a thin tube that extends down to another cervical level length and is the embryonic remnant of the thyroglossal canal.

Descriptively the tongue displays the upper and lower surface and the two lateral edges or borders or lips. On the lower surface there is a mucosal fold, the frenulum, which holds the tongue in the ground of the oral cavity. On either side of the base of the frenulum, the two sublingual salivary glands protrude, adjacent to the outlets of the submandibular gland and the major duct of the sublingual gland. From these tubercles rise the lunar folds of the mucosa, which have as a base the sublingual glands and on which the minor excretory pores flow.

The pharyngeal part of the dorsal surface of the tongue shows on the right and left side two appendages, the palatal tonsils that have as their base large lymph nodes and lymph follicles. Further down and backward, the lingual mucosa recovers on the anterior surface of the epiglottis forming elongated folds that enclose the lingual epiglottis.

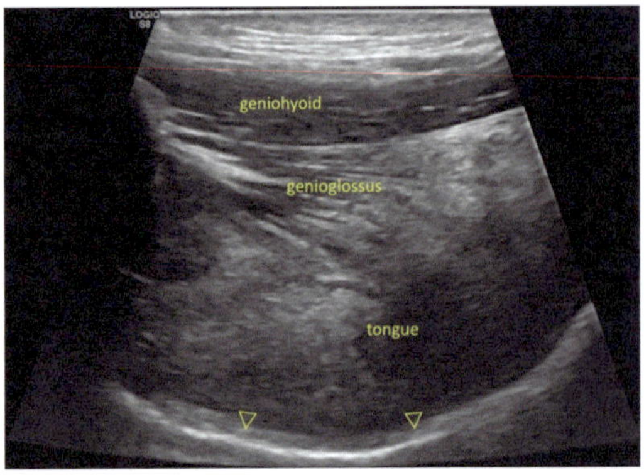

Fig. 10.14 Elongated section of the tongue in submandibular view. It is a compact instrument with a relatively homogeneous texture and intermediate echogenicity, surrounded by hypoechoic mucosa of increased thickness on the upper surface (arrowheads). The penetration depth of the ultrasound for the examination of the whole tongue should be set at 70 mm, with appropriate adjustments of frequency and degree of contrast

The muscles of the tongue are divided into heterogeneous and indigenous. They are lined and all ribbed by the 12th cranial nerve branch (sublingual nerve). The genioglossus muscle belongs to the group of intrinsic muscles of the tongue and is easily accessible during the ultrasound examination (Fig. 10.14).

10.4.3 Lymph Nodes

Normal lymph nodes are small kidney-shaped structures ranging from 0.1 up to 2.5 cm in size. They are surrounded by a thick connective tissue capsule. The parenchyma of the lymph nodes is distinguished in the cortical, subcortical, and medullary sections. A small opening in the middle of the glands creates an area rich in fibrous and fatty tissue designated as a portal. The medullary section surrounds the gate and is separated from the cortical section by insertion of the transitional zone of the subcortex. The blood supplying artery enters through the gate and the corresponding vein and the lymph nodes exit through it [10].

The lymph nodes are innervated by autonomic nervous system fibers and their innervation include in sections, the capsule, the inner diaphragms, and the smooth muscle of the blood vessels [8, 9].

They drain into the following groups.

Based on older and more recent literature data cervical lymph nodes are classified at least in six different anatomical levels (level I-VI) with different varying subclassifications aiming aid to the classification of pathology, surgical planning and better programming of the treatment head and neck cancer [10].

The major lymph node groups are classified according to their drainage and the major divisions are:

- Facial: skin and mucosa of the eyelids, the nose, the buccal area the temporal and subtemporal region and rinopharynx.
- Parotid: Skin of the temporal and frontal region. The maxilla, the buccal area, the external acoustic meatus and ear drum, the eyelids, and section of the nose (Fig. 10.15).
- Retroauricular: side section of the hairy part of the skin, the skin at the external acoustic meatus region and the external ear.
- Submental: Posterior section of the hairy part of the head.

Lymph nodes of the neck also drain the soft tissues of the region and the organs. In the upper section of the neck, the most important groups are as follows.

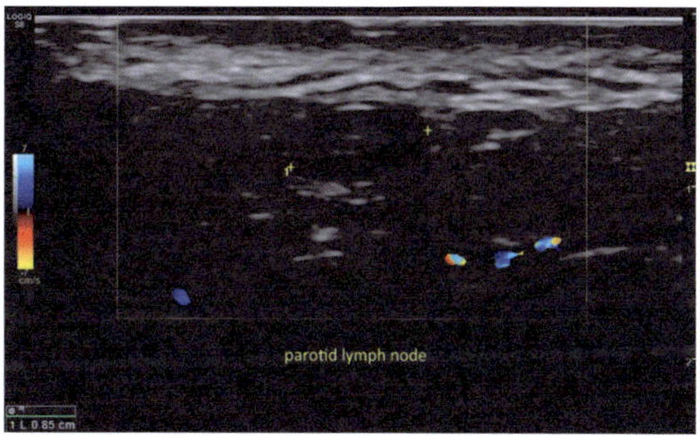

Fig. 10.15 Benign lymph node with donut morphology and elongated diameter <1 cm in the parenchyma of the parotid gland. In the parenchyma of the lymph nodes, the cortex is distinguished as a peripheral zone of low echogenicity and the hyperechoic marrow that is surrounded by the cortex and is located centrally

- Submental: Lower lip, tongue tip, gums, and anterior teeth (Fig. 10.16).
- Submandibular: Upper and lower lip, intraoral mucosa, tongue, mandible gums, and teeth (Fig. 10.17).
- Jugulodigastric: Lingual and pharyngeal tonsils, hard palate, sections of the tongue (Fig. 10.18).
- Deep cervical: Larynx, trachea, thyroid gland, parathyroid glands, and upper esophagus.
- Supraclavicular: Anterior thoracic wall, armpit region, shoulder, and upper limb.
- Superficial cervical lymph nodes on the surface of the sternocleidomastoid muscle, they drain the skin, and the superficial tissues.

10.4.4 Salivary Glands

The salivary glands produce the saliva that is necessary for the digestion of food in the oral cavity. They are divided into main and auxiliary. They consist of many small lobes, between which is inserted a thin connective tissue that forms the substrate of the pores. Individual lobes consist of glandular cells that erupt into the interstitial pores. The interstitial pores converge and form the large excretory pores that secrete saliva into the oral cavity.

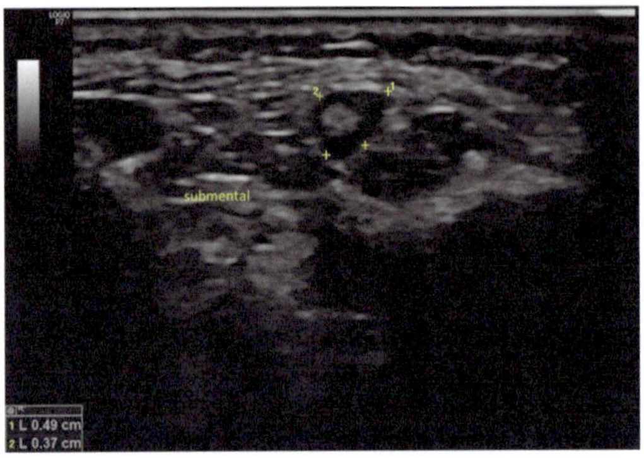

Fig. 10.16 Submental lymph nodes are smaller in size and often round in shape

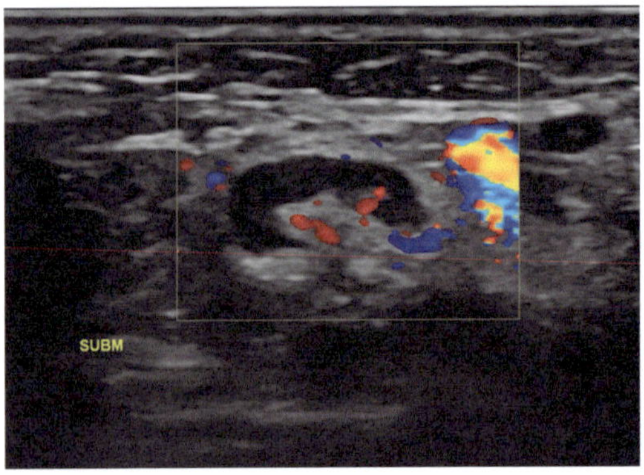

Fig. 10.17 Submandibular lymph node with color Doppler. In normal and reactive lymph nodes, the nutrient artery and the accompanying vein are depicted with small branches that are limited to the area of the hyperechoic portal and not beyond it

From the ultrasonographic point of view, the main salivary glands are:

(a) parotid,
(b) submandibular, and.
(c) sublingual gland.

and they should all be included in our imaging control.

10.4.5 The Parotid

(a) The parotid gland is the largest salivary gland weighing about 25 g. It is located in the retromandibular area and has the shape of a three-sided pyramid, with the top (or deep lobe) facing inwards into the pharynx and the base (or superficial lobe) facing outwards on the skin. In 20% of patients, an extra small lobe that often rests on the masseter muscle may coexist. The upper surface of the parotid gland comes in contact with the temporomandibular joint and the external auditory canal. The base of the parotid gland is covered by the skin and the muscular platysma (Fig. 10.19). The external carotid artery, the posterior facial vein, and the facial nerve pass through the parotid gland, with the former being located deeper than the latter (Fig. 10.20).

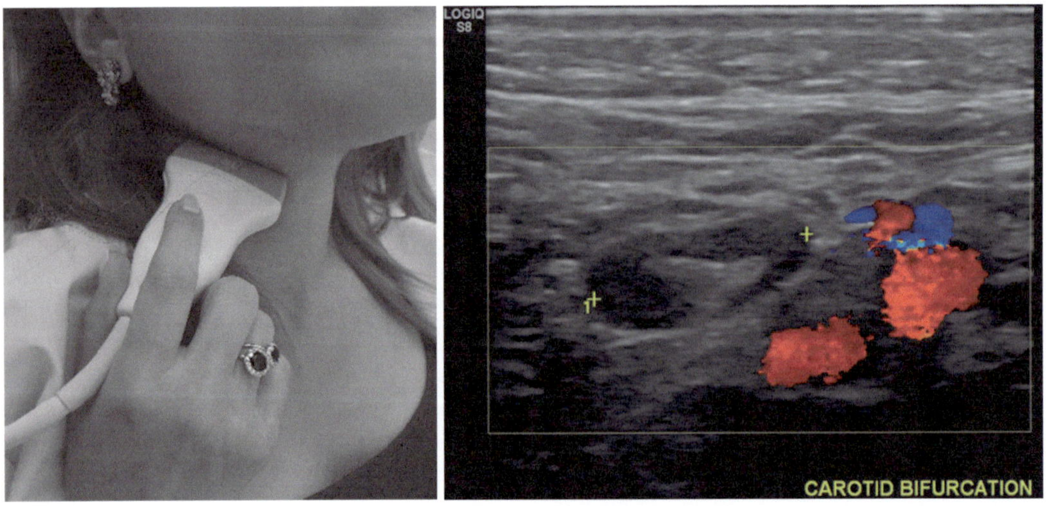

Fig. 10.18 Jugulodigastric lymph node above the carotid bifurcation. Characteristic location at the junction of the internal jugular vein with the posterior belly of the digastric muscle. Benign lymph nodes are bordered smoothly and move freely on ultrasound and palpation

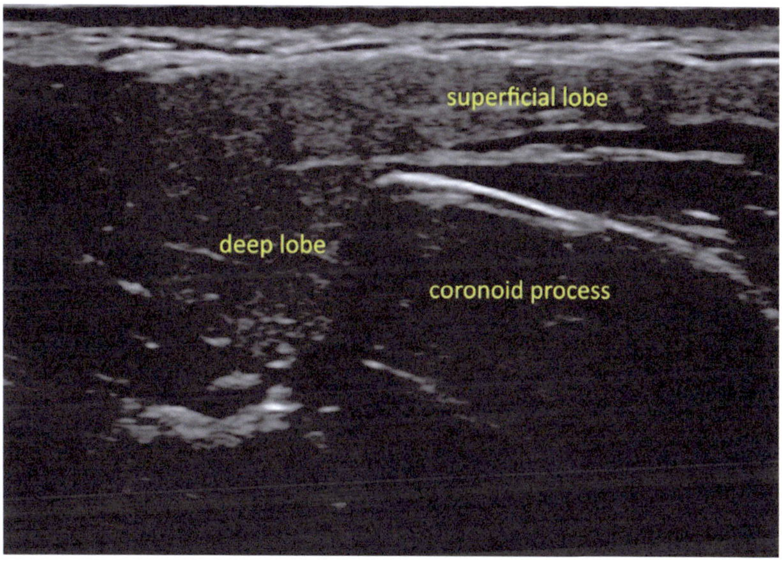

Fig. 10.19 Cross section of the parotid gland at the height of the coronoid process. The gland is homogeneous, with increased echogenicity and smooth margin

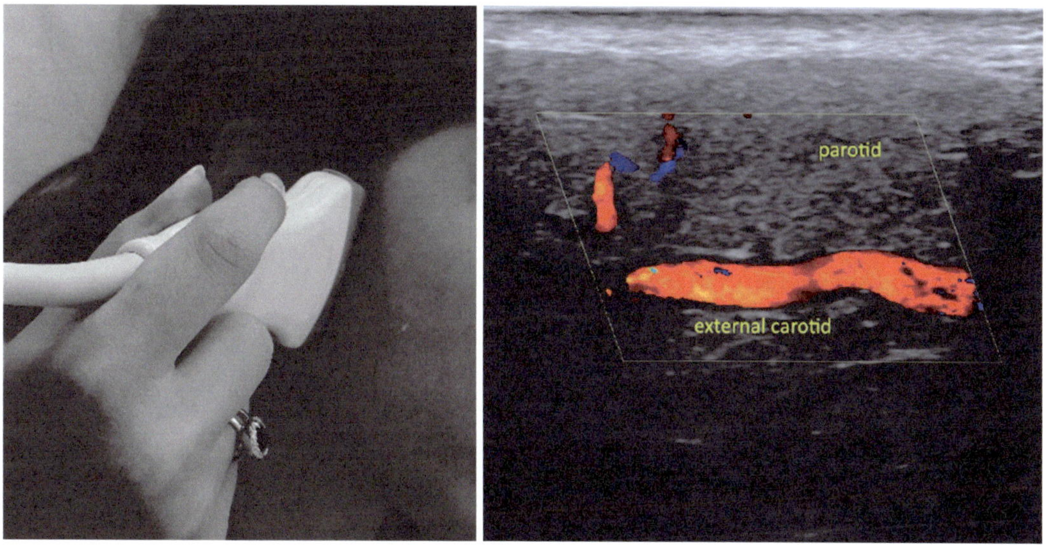

Fig. 10.20 Presence of a color signal in the intraparotid part of the external carotid artery during Doppler control. Each parotid should be evaluated for both transverse and sagittal scans

The Stensen secretory duct emerges from the upper part of the anterior rim of the base and travels forward onto the masseter muscle. After that, it pierces the buccinator muscle and the mucosa of the cheek, erupting into the pore opposite the second upper molar. Except in the case of dilation, it is not visible on the ultrasound examination (Fig. 10.21).

(b) The submandibular gland is the second largest salivary gland after the parotid gland. The superior exterior surface of the submandibular gland comes in relation to the homonymous cavity of the mandible. The lower-outer surface is covered by the skin, the muscular plate and the cervical fascia. The posterior end of the gland exhibits a groove through which the external maxillary artery travels and is separated from the parotid by the insertion of a fibrous band. The anterior part comes in direct contact with the anterior belly of the digastric muscle (Fig. 10.22).

Wharton's submandibular excretory pore starts from the middle of the inner surface of the submandibular gland and after passing between the maxillohyoid muscle and the sublingual salivary gland, it eventually flows to the top of the sublingual mucosa. As in the case of the parotid gland, the normal submandibular canal and endoparenchymal branches are subtle and usually do not show upon normal ultrasonographic examination (Figs. 10.23 and 10.24).

(c) The sublingual gland is the smallest of the salivary glands, is located below the sublingual fold, and comes in direct contact with the sublingual groove of the lower jaw. It has a flattened form, a major pore flowing into the sublingual mucosa, and many minor pores flowing into the free edge of the sublingual fold (Fig. 10.25).

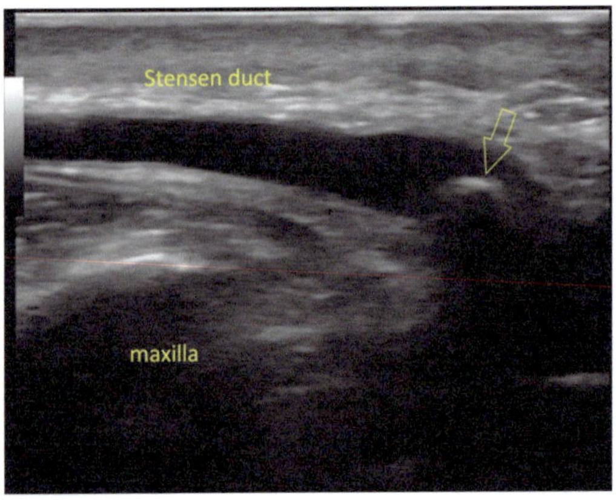

Fig. 10.21 Enlarged parotid duct with anechoic content due to obstruction of its final section by a calcified stone (arrow)

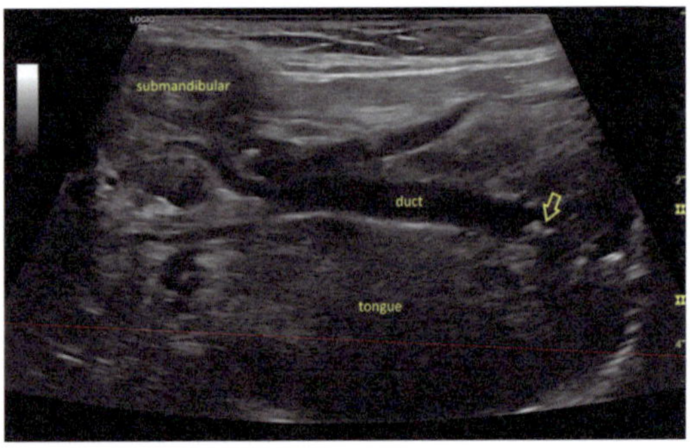

Fig. 10.23 Presence of a stone (arrow) in the sublingual area that causes stretching of the Wharton pore

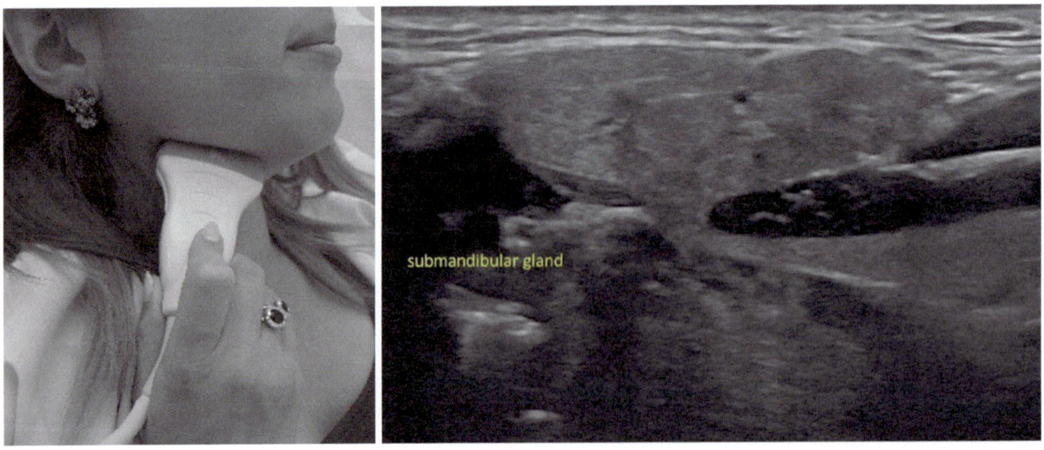

Fig. 10.22 The parenchyma of the submandibular gland is of medium echogenicity, with a relatively homogeneous texture and with a clear border

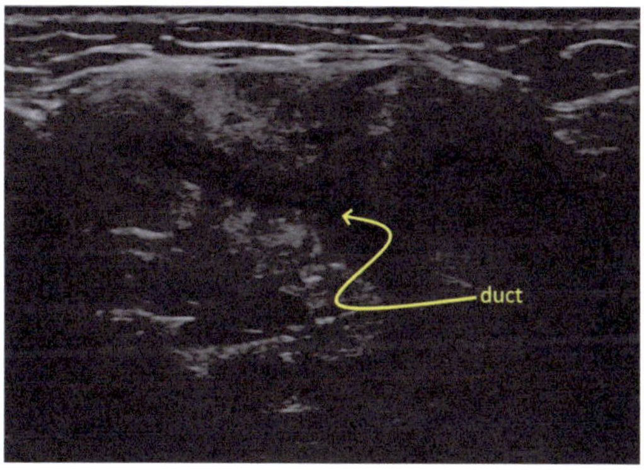

Fig. 10.24 Dilatation of the intermediate pores branches (arrow) in the case of sialadenitis

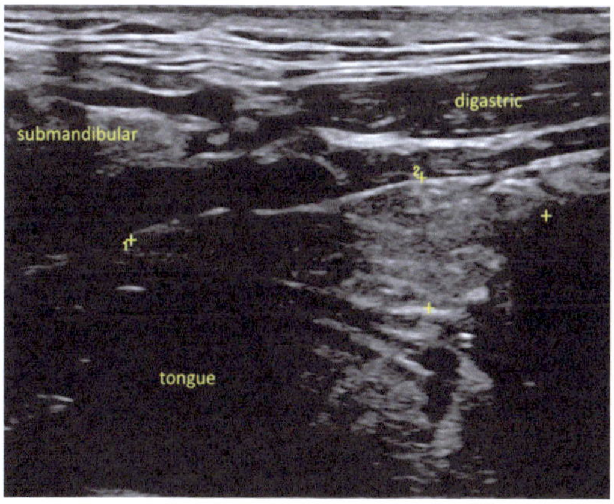

Fig. 10.25 Elongated transverse section of the sublingual gland by placing the transducer in front of the submandibular gland and parallel to the body of the mandible. Spindle morphology of the sublingual gland, in contact with the base of the tongue is observed

References

1. Standring S, editor. Gray's anatomy. 41st ed. London: Elsevier; 2016.
2. Moore KL, Dalley AF, Argus AMR. Clinically oriented anatomy. 7th ed. Philadelphia: Lippincott Williams & Wilkins; 2006.
3. Orhan K. Ultrasonography in maxillofacial diagnosis. Berlin: Springer; 2021.
4. Naqvi J, Yap KH, Ahmad G, Ghosh J. Transcranial Doppler ultrasound: a review of the physical principles and major applications in critical care. Int J Vasc Med. 2013;2013:629378.
5. Rasulo FA, De Peri E, Lavinio A. Transcranial Doppler ultrasonography in intensive care. Eur J Anaesthesiol Suppl. 2008;42:167–73.
6. Feigl G, Hammer GP, Litz R, Kachlik D. The inter carotid or alar fascia, other cervical fascias, and their adjacent spaces—a plea for clarification of cervical fascia and spaces terminology. J Anat. 2020;237:197.
7. Guidera AK, Dawes PJ, Fong A, Stringer MD. Head and neck fascia and compartments: no space for spaces. Head Neck. 2014;36:1058–68.
8. Kulzer MH, Branstetter BF 4th. Chapter 1 neck anatomy, imaging-based level nodal classification and impact of primary tumor site on patterns of nodal metastasis. Semin Ultrasound CT MR. 2017;38:454–65.
9. Som PM, Curtin HD, Mancuso AA. Imaging-based nodal classifcation for evaluation of neck metastatic adenopathy. AJR Am J Roentgenol. 2000;174:837–44.
10. Delantoni A, Sarafopoulos A. Sonographic anatomy and pathology: cervical lymph nodes in ultrasonography in dentomaxillofacial diagnostics. p. 77–87.

Basics of Magnetic Resonance Imaging (MRI)

11

Ingrid Rozylo-Kalinowska

11.1 Principles of Magnetic Resonance Imaging (MRI)

Magnetic resonance imaging (MRI) is a more and more frequently applied imaging technique in medical diagnostics. The name of the examination is derived from the physical phenomenon of magnetic resonance which is the foundation of image acquisition.

MRI is the imaging technique based on interactions of electromagnetic waves with protons in nuclei exposed to external magnetic field. Protons, that are elements of the atomic nuclei are characterized by positive charge, spinning movement around their axes and behaving as tiny magnets. Their movement is asynchronous and directions of spin movements chaotically distributed. The most commonly imaged proton is hydrogen as this element is prevalent in human organism, both in organic and inorganic compounds, water being the most widespread compound containing hydrogen [1–6].

An MRI scanner (Fig. 11.1) consists of several elements including:

- magnet with a bore creating external magnetic field—permanent (with lower induction of magnetic field) or, much more commonly, superconducting magnet (characterized by higher values of induction of magnetic field) cooled down by liquid helium;
- gradient coils—modifying external magnetic field;
- radio frequency transmitters—emitting and receiving signal;
- matrix—registering signals;
- patient table;
- computer system—controlling MRI unit;
- technical console—for programming of examination protocol and control throughout the examination;
- if contrast-enhanced examinations are required, also equipment for administration of contrast agent is used [1, 2, 4, 6, 7].

Patient is first placed in strong magnetic field, with induction up to 3 T, and in some conditions, especially experimental, up to 7 T. Action of external magnetic field forces synchronization of proton spins along the axis of induction of the field—majority of directions of their magnetic fields are placed in a parallel way to the direction of the magnetic field (B_0) and the rest antiparallel to it. Their net magnetization vector (being a sum up of all vectors of individual spinning protons) is aligned along the long axis of patient's body and longitudinal magnetic moment is created (Fig. 11.2). The number of parallel aligned protons increases together with increase in induc-

I. Rozylo-Kalinowska (✉)
Department of Dental and Maxillofacial Radiodiagnostics, Medical University of Lublin, Lublin, Poland
e-mail: rozylo.kalinowska@umlub.pl

A. Delantoni, K. Orhan (eds.), *Atlas of Dentomaxillofacial Anatomical Imaging*,
https://doi.org/10.1007/978-3-030-96840-3_11

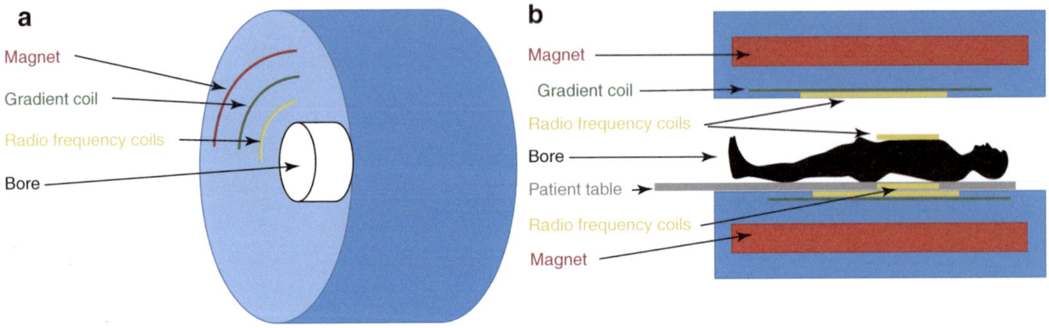

Fig. 11.1 (**a**, **b**) Schematic drawing of MRI scanner

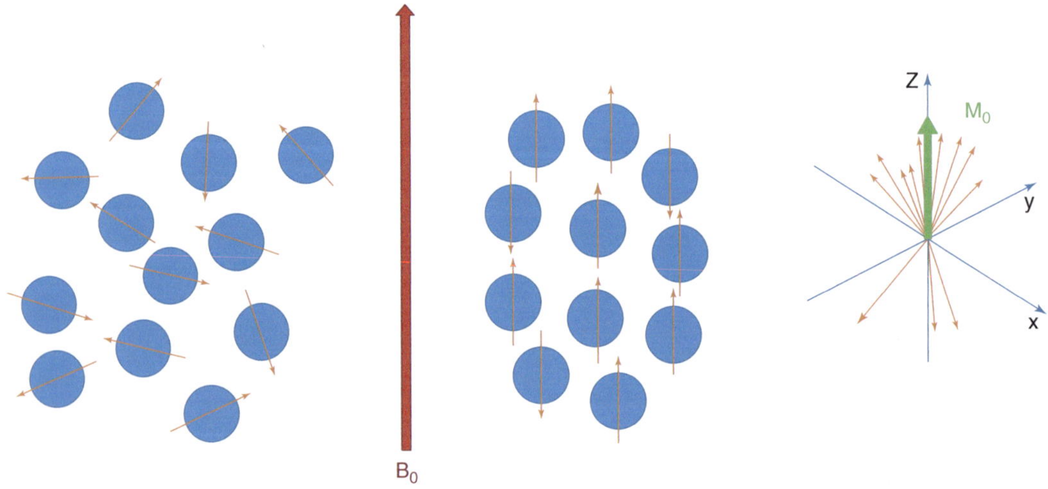

Fig. 11.2 Synchronization of proton spins in external magnetic field (B_0) with resulting longitudinal net magnetization vector

tion of magnetic field. However, the alignment is not purely parallel or anti-parallel as in external magnetic field also precession occurs. Precession is oscillation of protons around the lines of the magnetic field at a rate which is known as the Larmor frequency. The latter depends on the type of nucleus and on the induction of the magnetic field [1–5, 7].

The next stage of the MRI procedure is the emission of electromagnetic wave pulses with radio frequency (RF) by body coil transmitter at 90° to the direction of the magnetic field. The frequency of radio waves is chosen in such a way that it matches that of spinning protons of hydrogen. At the same time excitation of protons (resonance) is induced and absorption of pulses occurs which results in decrease of the longitudinal magnetic moment and appearance of the transverse magnetic moment (Fig. 11.3). The latter is capable of inducing electrical current in receiver coil. The duration of RF pulses is measured in microseconds and they have to be repeated multiple times. When the pulses cease, the protons relax, i.e. return to the original status and longitudinal magnetic moment is regained, while transverse magnetic moment is lost. The essence of imaging is registration of previously absorbed energy by receiver coil in the form of signal (the so-called echo). Registration includes disappearance of transverse vector of magnetization and reappearance of longitudinal vector of magnetization. As relaxation times of protons located in various tissues differ, the obtained

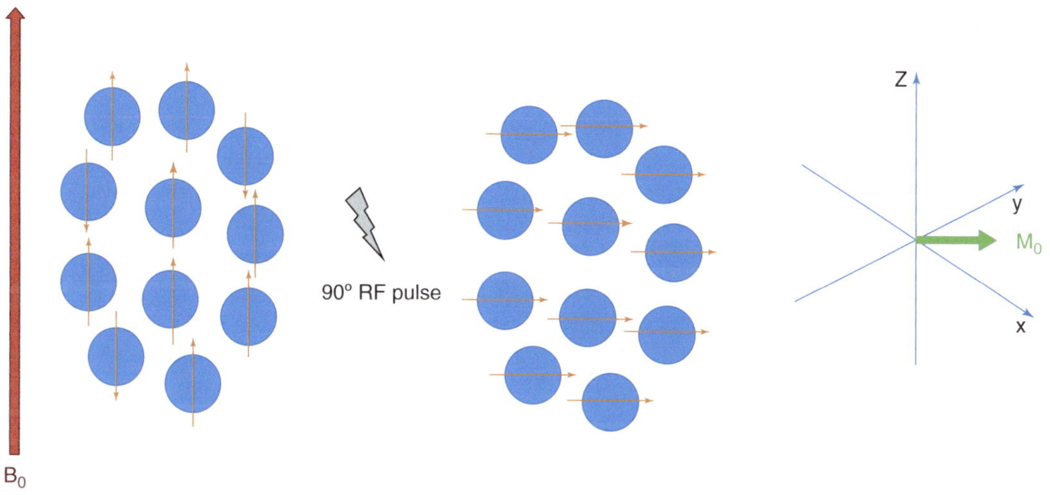

Fig. 11.3 Appearance of transverse net magnetization vector following a 90° radiofrequency (RF) pulse

images are not alike thus tissue differentiation is possible [1–5, 7–9].

The main images applied in MRI include:

- T1-weighted images based on registration of longitudinal relaxation times (TR below 500 ms, TE below 30 ms);
- T2-weighted images based on registration of transverse relaxation times (TR over 1500 ms, TE over 90 ms);
- PD-weighted images based on distribution of protons (TR over 1500 ms, TE below 30 ms).

For example, fluids have a long T1 so it takes a long time to re-establish their longitudinal magnetic moment. As a result their signal is weak (hypointense) in T1-weighted images. On the contrary, fluids have a long T2 which means that they dephase slowly and give a strong (hyperintense) signal [1–4, 7–9].

Gradients are used to enable excitation of a selected slice and not of the whole body, and protons outside the slice are not affected by the RF pulses. Gradient coils are capable of changing magnetic field magnitude and spatial encoding which is setting of specific frequency of precession along the axis of gradient. There are three sets of gradient coils corresponding to basic planes (*X*, *Y*, *Z*) and this way spatial localization is achieved in MRI. Amplitude of slice selection and bandwidth determine slice thickness, and bandwidth is the amount of frequencies that can be transmitted or received in a certain timeslot. Two gradients are differentiated—frequency-encoding gradient and phase-encoding gradient. Data from all gradients are recorded in an array called k-space which is being filled with data during acquisition. Horizontal axis of k-space contains information about frequency and vertical one is responsible for collecting data on phase [1–3, 7–9].

Essential parameters in designing an MRI scan are the times between RF pulses—repetition time (TR) and time to echo (TE). TR is time between application of two pulses and is responsible for T1 contrast. Shorter time between pulses means that protons are not able to fully recover longitudinal magnetization moment. TE is the time between application of 90° pulses and MR signal sampling. Longer TE is related to stronger T2 weighting, and on the contrary, shorter TE results in low T2 weighting [1–3, 7–9].

Based on the TR and TE different MRI acquisition techniques are available, the main division including spin echo techniques (SE), inversion recovery (IR) and gradient echo techniques (GE). In spin-echo techniques after 90° pulses, 180° pulses are used in order to reduce inhomogeneity of magnetic field. Gradient echo techniques are based on application of gradient coils instead of

180° RF pulses for producing an echo. In these techniques RF with various pulses between 10° and 90°, called flip angles, are used in order to induce appearance of transverse magnetization. In general acquisition of gradient sequences is shorter than of spin-echo techniques, and two categories of gradient sequences are differentiated—gradient spoiled (in other words, incoherent gradient echo) and coherent (refocused transverse magnetization). In inversion recovery sequences apart from TE and TR also time of inversion (TI) is relevant. This pulse is produced between 180° and 90° pulses and duration of TI influences T1-weighting of image [1, 2, 7–10].

Many sequences are already elaborated, and may differ in names according to manufacturer, and new sequences are being developed (Fig. 11.4) [1, 7–10].

Examples of SE sequences are:

- Fast sequences such as Fast Spin Echo (FSE) and Turbo Spin Echo (TSE) based on RARE (Rapid Acquisition Relaxation-Enhanced) sequence;
- Half-Fourier Acquisition Single-Short Turbo Spin Echo (HASTE)—allowing registration of all echoes necessary for image reconstruction after application of a single pulse;
- Spin-Echo Echo Planar Imaging SE-EPI [8, 10].

Inversion Recovery (IR) sequences contain e.g.:

- Fluid Attenuated Inversion Recovery sequence (FLAIR)—for suppression of image of free fluid with long TI.
- FatSat—fat saturated techniques for elimination of intense signal of fat tissue with short TI (e.g. Frequency Selective Fat Saturation—FS—and Short-Tau Inversion recovery—STIR);
- Double Inversion Recovery (DIR) with simultaneous suppression with two inversion times [8].

Gradient sequences include:

- Steady-State Free Precession (SSFP),
- Fast Low-Angle Shot (FLASH),
- Gradient echo Echo Planar Imaging (GE–EPI) [8].

MRI is a very fast developing and versatile imaging technique. Different MRI modalities include among others [7, 11–15]:

- MR angiography—Time of Flight (TOF), Phase Contrast (PC), and true FISP (True Fast Imaging with Steady-state Precession) imaging to demonstrate blood vessels without contrast media administration;
- Perfusion-Weighted Imaging (PWI)—imaging of tissue perfusion to visualize and measure vascular supply to a tissue;
- Diffusion-Weighted Imaging (DWI) to demonstrate diffusion of molecules in examined tissues;
- Diffusion Tensor Imaging (DTI) and tractography—based on multidirectional measurements of movement of molecules allowing for mapping of nerve fibers;
- MRI spectroscopy, i.e. analysis of chemical composition of tissues under in vivo conditions due to specific chemical shift of resonance frequency of different substances applied mainly in brain tumor examinations;
- Blood Oxygen Level Dependent (BOLD) which is functional technique used in order to visualize brain centers activated by different stimuli such as visual or sonic based on registration of increased use of oxygen in activated neurons;
- real-time MRI to register movements in real time, e.g. heart and joints such as temporomandibular joint;
- use of MRI as navigation tool in minimally invasive surgical procedures;
- functional MRI sialography based on registration of changes in the area of salivary ducts before and after stimulation with citric acid;
- use of deep learning algorithms (Artificial Intelligence, AI) for image reconstruction, processing, and segmentation.

11.2 Contrast-Enhanced MRI

In MRI it is also sometimes necessary to administer contrast media, mostly intravenously, rarely intraorally or into joint space (e.g. temporomandibular joint space). Contrast agents used in MRI

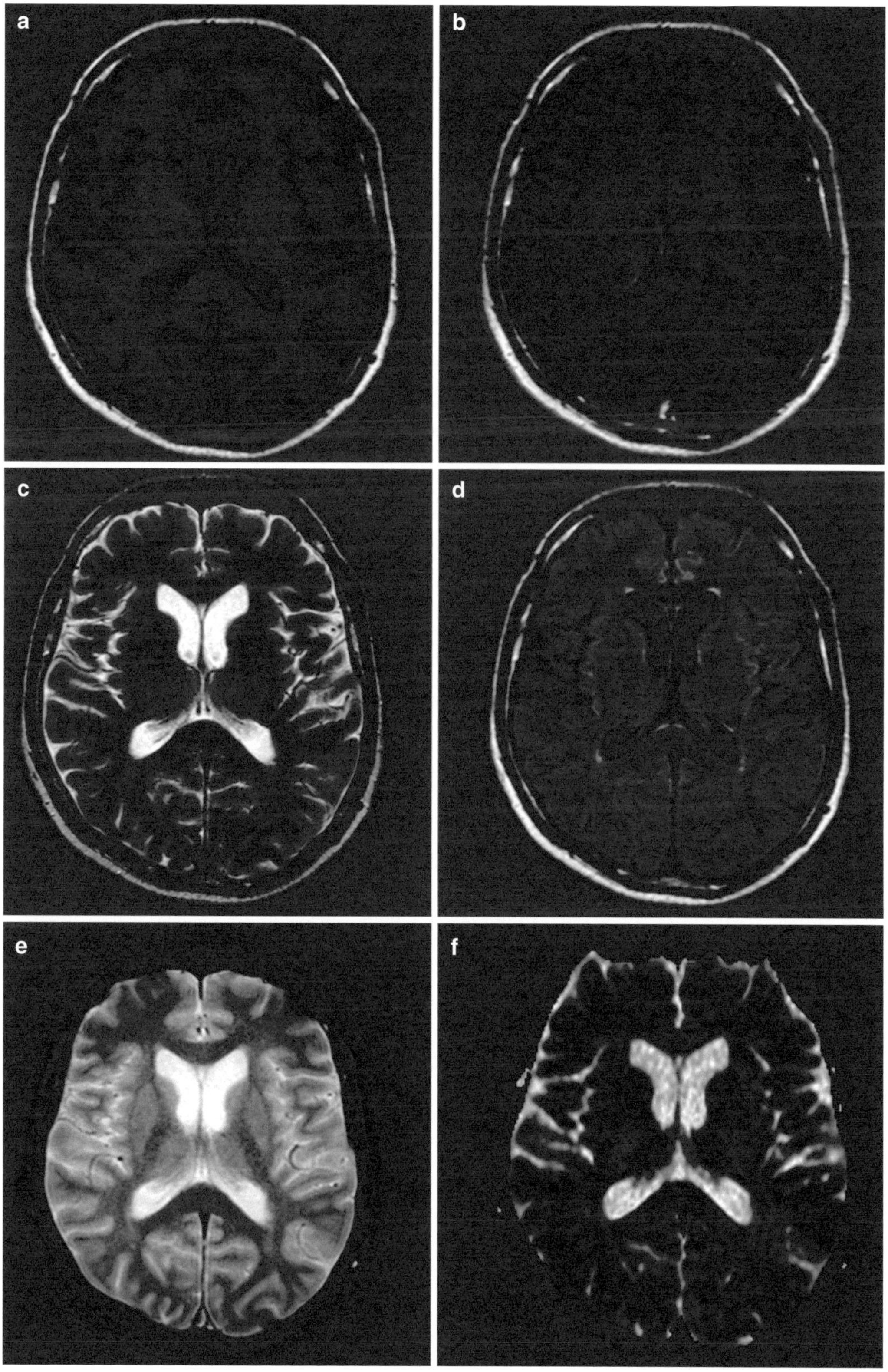

Fig. 11.4 Examples of images in MRI. (**a**) T1-weighted. (**b**) Contrast-enhanced T1-weighted. (**c**) T2-weighted. (**d**) FLAIR. (**e**) T* FLASH. (**f**) DWI

are paramagnetics, i.e. compounds that locally change intensity of proton signals. They cause significant shortening of T1and T2 relaxation times of areas filled with contrast media such as blood vessels and extracellular space. It is difficult to demonstrate shortening of T2 relaxation time (reduction of signal intensity), therefore contrast-enhancement is best visualized in T1-weighted sequences. The most often used contrast agents are water soluble gadolinium-based chelates, such as gadolinium-diethylenetriamine pentaacetic acid (Gd-DTPA) available under various commercial names [16].

Patient preparation for MRI scanning with contrast agents requires the presence of the patient's empty stomach (at least 5 h after last meal and at least 3 h after intake of fluids), however regularly taken medications must be administered [7].

Side effects of MRI are to a large extent and in most cases related to paramagnetic contrast media and do not occur in case of unenhanced MRI studies. Most of the side effects are mild (flushing, nausea, headache, vomiting) and allergy-like reactions occur (ranging from pruritus and urticaria to rarely encountered anaphylaxis), but still paramagnetic contrast media in MRI are considered safer than iodine-based contrast agents applied in imaging studies based on X-rays [17]. One of the serious side effects of MRI contrast agents is nephrogenic systemic fibrosis (NSF) affecting skin and internal organs in patients with renal failure. In order to decrease the risk of development of this debilitating and potentially fatal systemic disease in all patients referred for contrast-enhanced MRI it is necessary to obtain creatinine blood level in order to estimate glomerular filtration rate (GFR) and GFR of 30 is the threshold for administration of paramagnetic contrast agents [18]. Another recently reported effect of gadolinium-based contrast media is accumulation of minor amounts of gadolinium in bones and in brain, however, so far the long-term effect of these collections is unknown. Nevertheless, as a precaution some gadolinium-based contrast agents (with linear composition) are not administered intravenously anymore, while cyclic compounds are still in use.

11.3 Advantages and Disadvantages of MRI

Advantages of MRI examination include [1–5, 7]:

- no exposure to ionizing radiation and related risks;
- no negative effects of strong magnetic fields on human organisms in patients, including pregnant women and fetuses;
- very high resolution of imaging of soft tissues;
- direct acquisition of multiplanar images (axial, coronal, sagittal, their modifications such as parasagittal) without necessity of secondary reformatting of images;
- recent advances regarding shortening of acquisition times and enhanced image processing.

Disadvantages of MRI examination [1–5, 7, 19–21]:

- absolute and relative contraindications (see below);
- no signal from structures poor in hydrogen protons such as compact bone, cancellous bone trabecula, mineralized dental structures, calcifications, ossifications, however, new developments allow visualization of bone tissue, as well;
- necessity of maintaining motionless position during long sequences in order to avoid motion artefacts, this may not be feasible in neurological patients (nervous twitches and involuntary movements not controlled by medications) and may cause discomfort to pregnant females;
- necessity of administration of sedation or general anesthesia in new borns and small children due to lack of cooperation during scanning;

- unknown long-term effects of exposure of fetuses to noise during image acquisition;
- claustrophobia is a limitation in older generations of MRI scanners with more narrow bores;
- in some systems and some sequences—considerable noise generated by gradient coils, up to 120 dB, currently reduced in some newer MRI scanners;
- many types of image artifacts, e.g. generated by metallic elements (such as fixed prosthetic appliances, dental implants, fixed orthodontic appliances, some dental materials, surgical clips), aliasing, chemical shift, magnetic susceptibility, partial volume, shading, herringbone, zipper; artifacts in head and neck area can be reduced by use of other imaging planes, FSE and TSE techniques as well as avoiding gradient sequences.

11.4 Contraindications to MRI

Contraindications to MRI are derived from the presence of foreign bodies in patient organism—following trauma or as a consequence of therapeutic procedures such as prostheses, stimulators, other implanted devices. The source of risk to patient may be displacement of a ferromagnetic object in tissues leading to their damage or in case of larger objects not easily displaced within the body—overheating resulting in tissue burns. Usually before MRI scan starts, patient fills in a questionnaire containing questions related to potential contraindications including presence of foreign bodies.

Absolute contraindications concern patients with:

- implanted cardiac pacemakers of older design due to possible disruption of their work resulting in heart arrythmias that can be life-threatening; however, nowadays special MRI-safe stimulators are available with shielding of electric circuits and fitted with special electrodes that are resistant to external magnetic field as well as with special software mode activated during MRI examination. Another risk is imposed by obsolete fragments of old electrodes not completely removed during exchange of pacemaker as the fragments may overheat in magnetic field and cause uncontrolled ablation of a part of myocardium that can also lead to cardiac arrythmia;
- implanted ferromagnetic vascular clips and orthopedic prostheses;
- implanted neurostimulators such as cochlear implants of older type (not MRI-safe);
- implanted subcutaneous pumps for drug delivery such as insulin pump;
- some types of cardiac valves;
- metallic foreign bodies in the eyeball as a result of trauma or professional exposure—some authors indicate necessity of taking a radiograph of orbits before MRI scan in risk groups [7, 22, 23].

Relative contraindications include patients with:

- contraceptive intrauterine devices (those containing metallic elements may be displaced during scanning);
- stents in coronary and other blood vessels 8 weeks from stenting procedure;
- hemostatic clips 6 weeks from implantation;
- orthopedic implants 6 weeks from surgery.

Although metallic prostheses, dental implants, orthodontic appliances, and dental implants are not always ferromagnetic, they still cause artefacts that can considerably degrade quality of MRI images of the head and neck. Knowledge on composition of dental alloys and their ferromagnetic properties is necessary when qualifying for head and neck MRI to avoid artefacts and potential overheating of metallic appliances that may lead to premature termination of scanning. Strength of fixation of metallic elements of orthodontic appliances should be checked before MRI and all removable elements of these appliances such as wires should be removed [22, 24, 25].

References

1. Dale BM, Brown MA, Semelka RC. MRI basic principles and applications. Hoboken, NJ: Wiley; 2015.
2. Elmaoğlu M, Çelik A. MRI handbook. Berlin: Springer; 2012.
3. Gibby WA. Basic principles of magnetic resonance imaging. Neurosurg Clin N Am. 2005;16:1–64.
4. Grover VP, Tognarelli JM, Crossey MM, Cox IJ, Taylor-Robinson SD, McPhail MJ. Magnetic resonance imaging: principles and techniques. Lessons for clinicians. J Clin Exp Hepatol. 2015;5:246–55.
5. Mallaya S, Lam E. White and Pharoah's oral radiology. Principles and interpretation. 8th ed. London: Mosby.
6. Weishaupt D, Köchli VD, Marincek B. How does MRI work? 2nd ed. Berlin: Springer; 2006.
7. Rozylo-Kalinowska I, Rozylo TK. Współczesna radiologia stomatologiczna. 3rd ed. Lublin: Wydawnictwo Czelej; 2021.
8. Bitar R, Leung G, Perng R, Tadros S, Moody AR, Sarrazin J, McGregor C, Christakis M, Symons S, Nelson A, Roberts TP. MR pulse sequences: what every radiologist wants to know but is afraid to ask. Radiographics. 2006;26:513–37.
9. Calle D, Navarro T. Basic pulse sequences in magnetic resonance imaging. Methods Mol Biol. 2018;1718:21–37.
10. Jung BA, Weigel M. Spin echo magnetic resonance imaging. J Magn Reson Imaging. 2013;37:805–17.
11. Bammer R, Bammer R, Skare S, Newbould R, Liu C, Thijs V, Ropele S, Clayton DB, Krueger G. Foundations of advanced magnetic resonance imaging. NeuroRx. 2005;2:167–96.
12. Börnert P, Norris DG. A half-century of innovation in technology-preparing MRI for the 21st century. Br J Radiol. 2020;93:20200113.
13. Glover GH. Overview of functional magnetic resonance imaging. Neurosurg Clin N Am. 2011;22:133–9.
14. Insko EK, Carpenter JP. Magnetic resonance angiography. Semin Vasc Surg. 2004;17:83–101.
15. Yousaf T, Dervenoulas G, Politis M. Advances in MRI methodology. Int Rev Neurobiol. 2018;141:31–76.
16. Czeyda-Pommersheim F, Martin DR, Costello JR, Kalb B. Contrast agents for MR imaging. Magn Reson Imaging Clin N Am. 2017;25:705–11.
17. Li A, Wong CS, Wong MK, Lee CM, Au Yeung MC. Acute adverse reactions to magnetic resonance contrast media – gadolinium chelates. Br J Radiol. 2006;79:368–71.
18. Cowper SE, Rabach M, Girardi M. Clinical and histological findings in nephrogenic systemic fibrosis. Eur J Radiol. 2008;66:187–90.
19. Bulas D, Egloff A. Benefits and risks of MRI in pregnancy. Semin Perinatol. 2013;37:301–4.
20. Dewey M, Schink T, Dewey CF. Claustrophobia during magnetic resonance imaging: cohort study in over 55,000 patients. J Magn Reson Imaging. 2007;26:1322–7.
21. Yanasak NE, Kelly MJ. MR imaging artifacts and parallel imaging techniques with calibration scanning: a new twist on old problems. Radiographics. 2014;34:532–4822.
22. Rozylo-Kalinowska I, Orhan K, editors. Imaging of the temporomandibular joint. Berlin: Springer; 2019.
23. Soto DM. Current guidelines for MRI safety in patients with cardiovascular implantable electronic devices. Nursing. 2020;50:24–9.
24. Klinke T, Daboul A, Maron J, Gredes T, Puls R, Jaghsi A, Biffar R. Artifacts in magnetic resonance imaging and computed tomography caused by dental materials. PLoS One. 2012;7:e31766.
25. Rozylo-Kalinowska I, Walawska B, Prędko-Engel A, Jurkiewicz E, Urbanik A. Magnetic resonance imaging in orthodontic patients. Guidelines of the polish orthodontic society (PTO), the polish medical radiological society (PLTR), and the polish dental association (PTS). J Stoma. 2019;72:1–3.

12 MRI Anatomy

Ingrid Rozylo-Kalinowska

Magnetic resonance imaging (MRI) is diagnostic imaging technique providing high-resolution, detailed images of human body in an non-invasive manner and moreover, not exposing the patient to harmful ionizing radiation.

During an MRI examination patient is placed in a strong magnetic field which forces protons (hydrogen nuclei) within the scanned area to spin in a synchronous way with the formation of longitudinal net magnetization vector. Application of external radiofrequency wave causes change in directions of spins and occurrence of transverse magnetization vector. Once radiofrequency impulse ceases, protons return to the basic position and this process is called relaxation. As the relaxation times (measured in milliseconds) differ in various tissues hence registered images are also slightly different which enables visualization of tissues and organs.

MRI does not use ionizing radiation therefore is potentially non-harmful to human beings. Nevertheless, there are many contraindications for MRI scans that exist, which have to be taken into account when referring a patient for the study. Moreover, the examination is not free from artifacts and technical problems.

A detailed description of the methodology as well as contraindications is presented in the previous chapter.

Within the maxillofacial area MRI primarily serves as a means of imaging of soft tissues, especially tumors, cysts, and inflammatory processes. It is also currently the best method of imaging of soft tissues of temporomandibular joint thus is crucial to dentists, especially those dealing with prosthodontics and temporomandibular joint disorders.

The following is a series of magnetic resonance images of maxillofacial area with emphasis on the soft tissue imaging (Figs. 12.1, 12.2, and 12.3).

I. Rozylo-Kalinowska (✉)
Department of Dental and Maxillofacial Radiodiagnostics, Medical University of Lublin, Lublin, Poland
e-mail: rozylo.kalinowska@umlub.pl

A. Delantoni, K. Orhan (eds.), *Atlas of Dentomaxillofacial Anatomical Imaging*,
https://doi.org/10.1007/978-3-030-96840-3_12

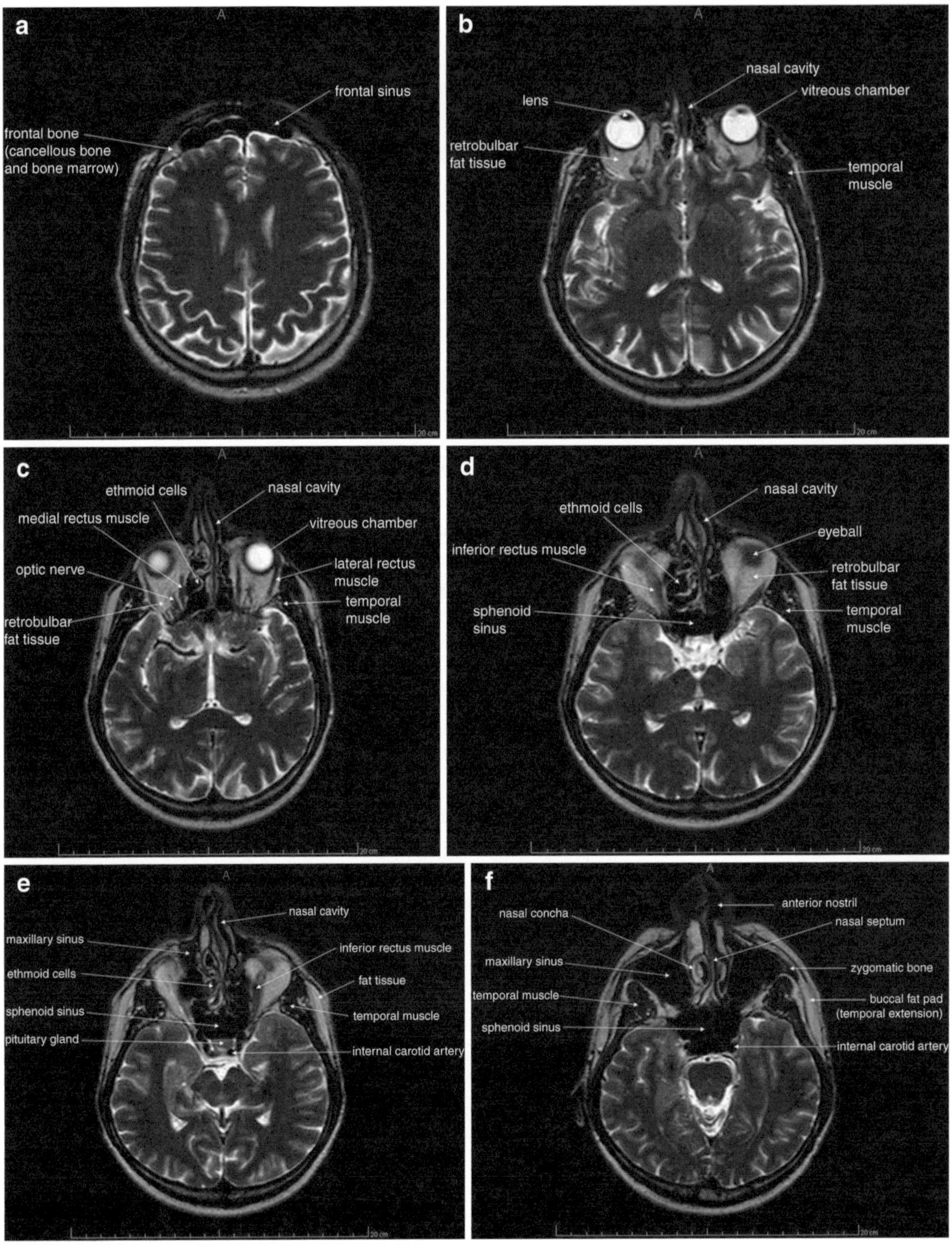

Fig. 12.1 MR anatomy in axial slices

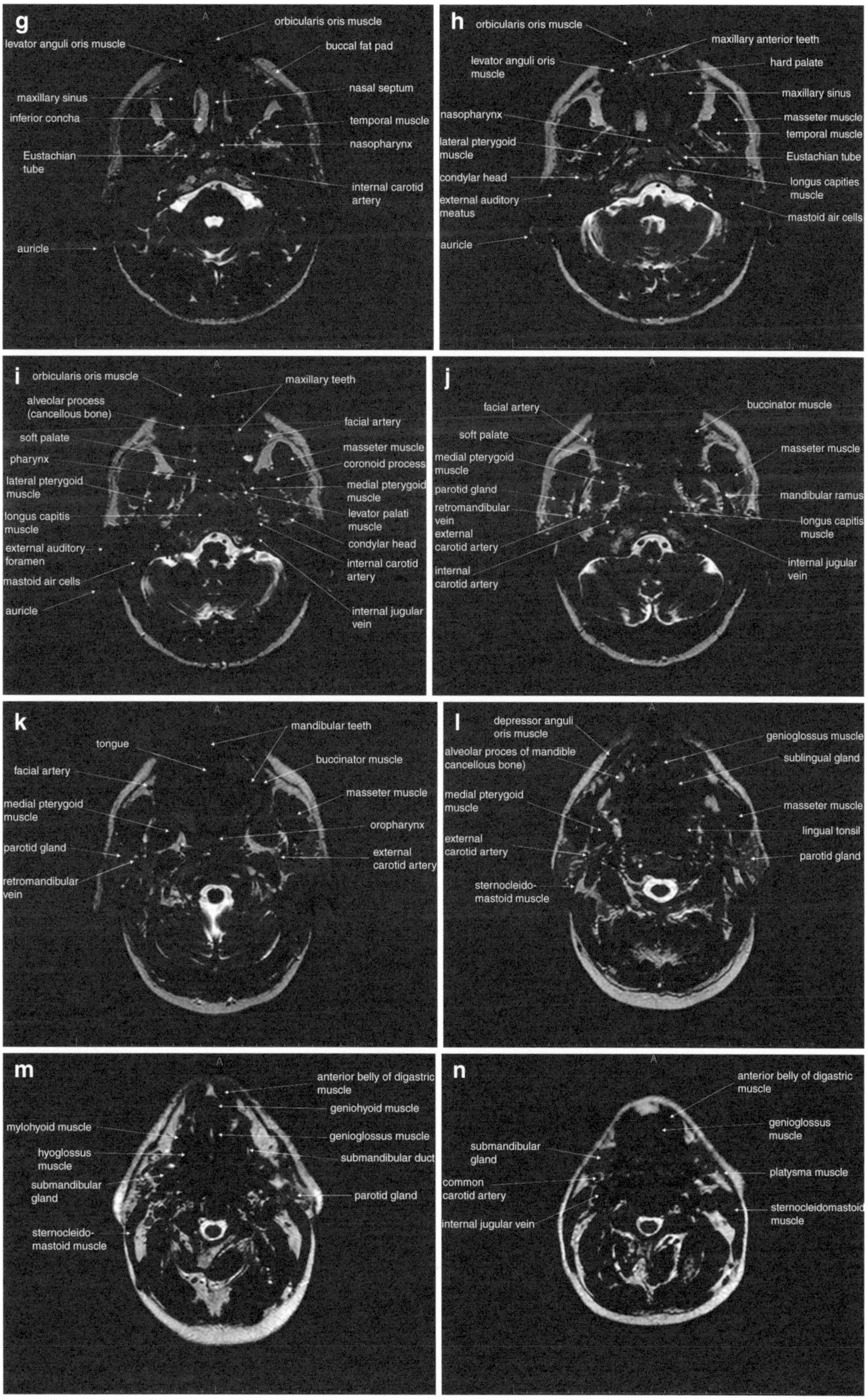

Fig. 12.1 (continued)

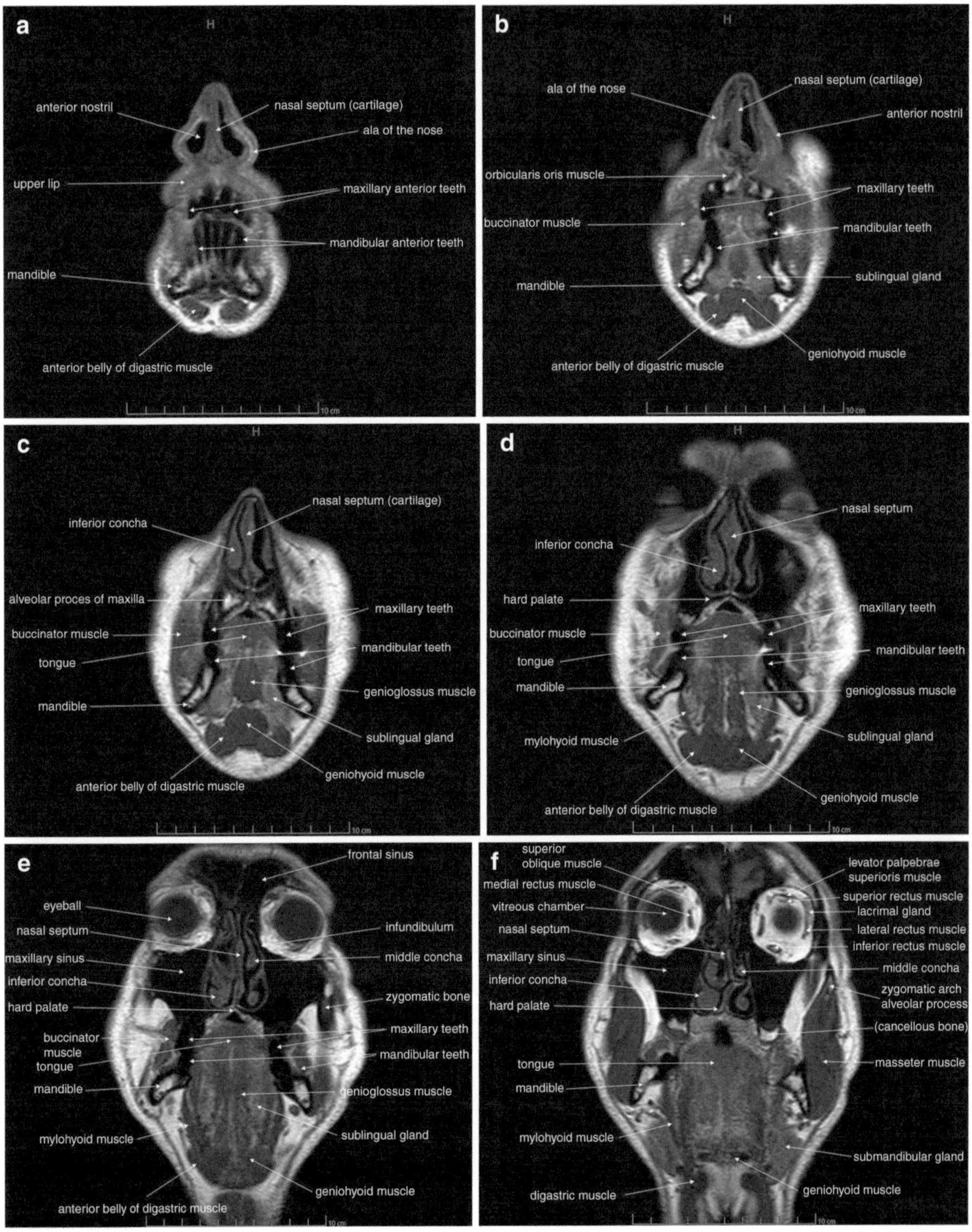

Fig. 12.2 MR anatomy in coronal slices

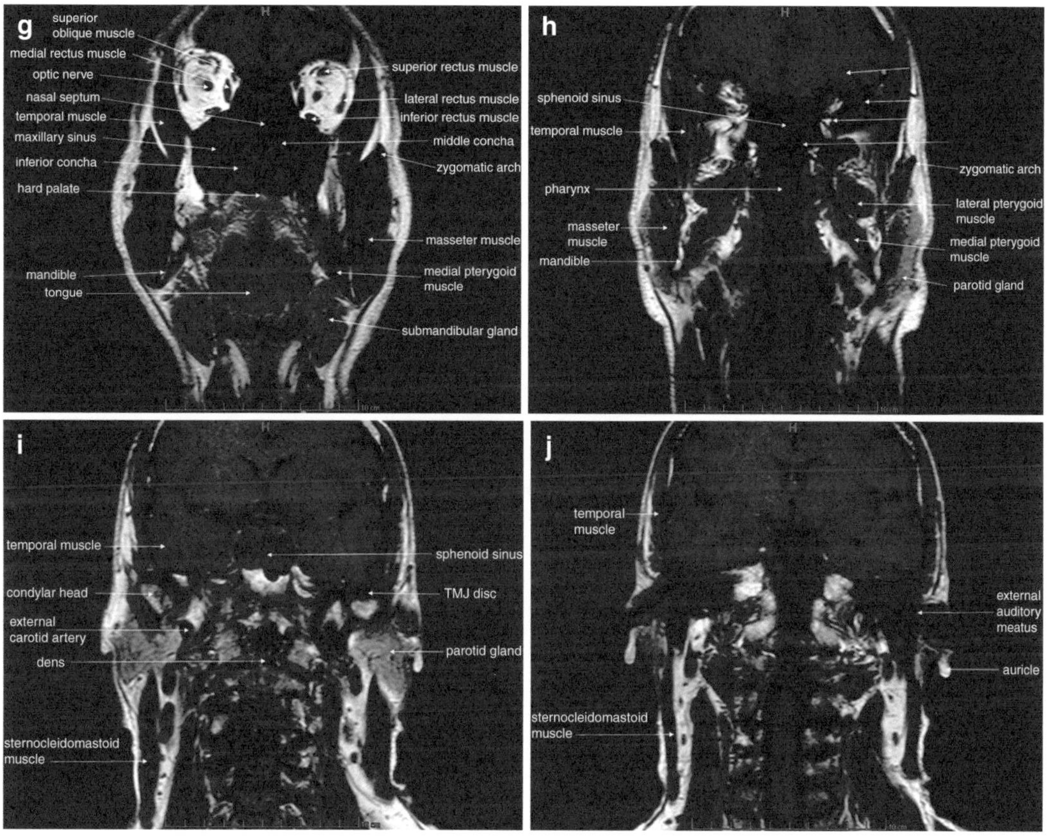

Fig. 12.2 (continued)

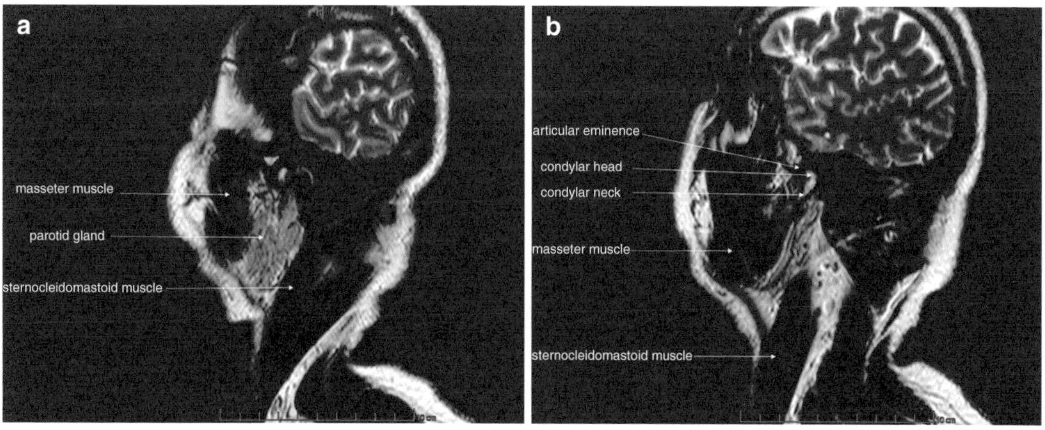

Fig. 12.3 MR anatomy in sagittal slices

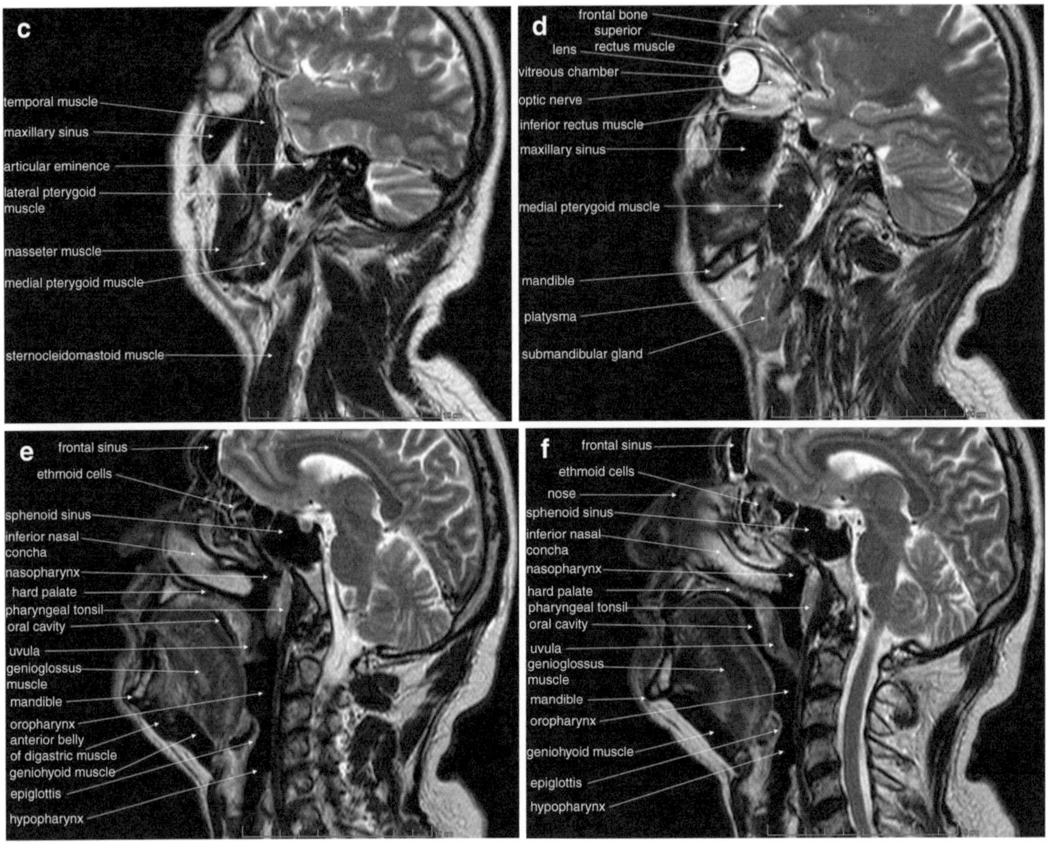

Fig. 12.3 (continued)

Further Reading

Braitinger S, Pahnke J. MR atlas of ENT anatomy. Diagnostic planning. Interpretation. Illustration of surgical approaches. Stuttgart: Schattauer; 1995.

Dale BM, Brown MA, Semelka RC. MRI basic principles and applications. Hoboken, NJ: Wiley; 2015.

Elmaoğlu M, Çelik A. MRI handbook. Berlin: Springer; 2012.

Mallaya S, Lam E, editors. White and Pharoah's oral radiology. Principles and interpretation. 8th ed. London: Mosby.

Moeller TB, Reif E. Pocket atlas of sectional anatomy. In: Computed tomography and magnetic resonance imaging. Head and neck, vol. 1. New York: Theime; 2007.

Rozylo-Kalinowska I, Rozylo TK. Współczesna radiologia stomatologiczna. 3rd ed. Lublin: Wydawnictwo Czelej; 2021.

13 Principles of Maxillofacial Angiography

Stefanos Finitsis

13.1 Materials

Angiography of the maxillofacial region consists of the selective catheterization of the internal maxillary artery to study its main trunk and branches. The injection of radiopaque contrast material achieves visualization of these vessels. Whether the interest of the study involves arteries or veins, a minimum of two orthogonal projections is mandatory. Continuous advancements of catheter material technology have made the catheterization of cervical cephalic vessels easier and more reliable. Several puncture techniques are available.

13.1.1 Puncture Techniques

13.1.1.1 Femoral Puncture

It is the most employed route for head and neck and cerebral angiography in general. Following local anesthesia, the common femoral artery is punctured directly under the inguinal ligament at the internal portion of the femoral head (Fig. 13.1).

This approach allows the operator to work at a distance from the X-ray tube and compress the punctured artery on stable osseous support after retrieving the catheterization material. Its primary disadvantage is that the common femoral artery is sometimes challenging to compress (for example, in obese patients), and the patient is required to stay in the hospital several hours before normal ambulation.

13.1.1.2 Brachial and Radial Puncture

Brachial puncture is rarely used and consists of the direct puncture of the brachial artery at the elbow level. It allows a more accessible axis of the arterial brachiocephalic trunk on the right and the subclavian artery and its branches on the left side. This approach has the advantage of an eas-

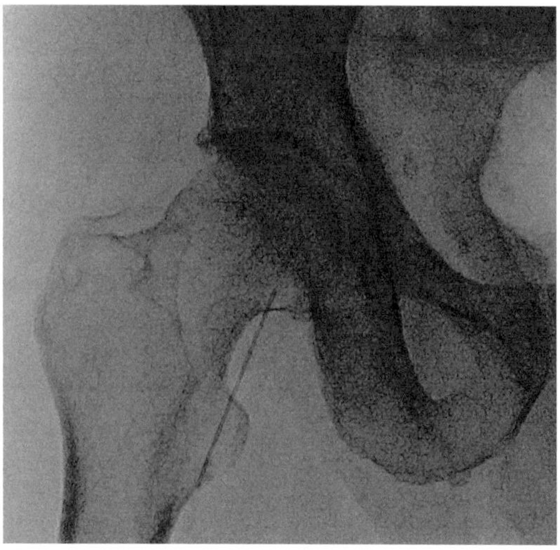

Fig. 13.1 Puncture at the level of the femoral head

S. Finitsis (✉)
Department of Diagnostic and Neurointerventional Radiology, AHEPA University Hospital, Aristotle University of Thessaloniki, Thessaloniki, Greece

A. Delantoni, K. Orhan (eds.), *Atlas of Dentomaxillofacial Anatomical Imaging*,
https://doi.org/10.1007/978-3-030-96840-3_13

ier manual compression and is thus less likely to local complications like hematomas. Practically it is used only in the case of impossible femoral access. Nowadays, the radial approach is gaining popularity for diagnostic and interventional DSA as it allows easy compression and control of the puncture site and may be performed on a day care basis.

13.1.1.3 Direct Carotid Puncture

It consists of the direct puncture of the common carotid artery. It is rarely used and may constitute an alternative under challenging catheterizations of the common carotid artery (for example, tight loops or right aortic arch).

13.1.2 Complications

These are rare but may be potentially serious (death, persistent neurological deficits). For this reason, the indication for cervical angiography has to be carefully contemplated and should always be substituted by non-invasive imaging, if possible.

13.1.2.1 Neurological Complications

These are the gravest and occur in 2.6% of cases, more commonly in the context of severe atherosclerosis. They may consist in a transient (2.5%) or permanent neurological deficit (0.14%). The most common mechanism is either distal migration of a fragment of an atheromatous plaque or a thrombus during catheterization or an air bubble during the injection of contrast.

Another rarer complication is the dissection of the vessel wall that may occur during catheterization or injection of contrast material at a high rate (Fig. 13.2).

13.1.2.2 Local Complications

More frequent (4%) but less grave, they consist in the formation of a hematoma at the puncture site (Fig. 13.3) with or without retroperitoneal extension, pseudoaneurysms, or dissection. These complications are by no means trivial; a hematoma, for example, may rapidly expand and lead to hypovolemic shock.

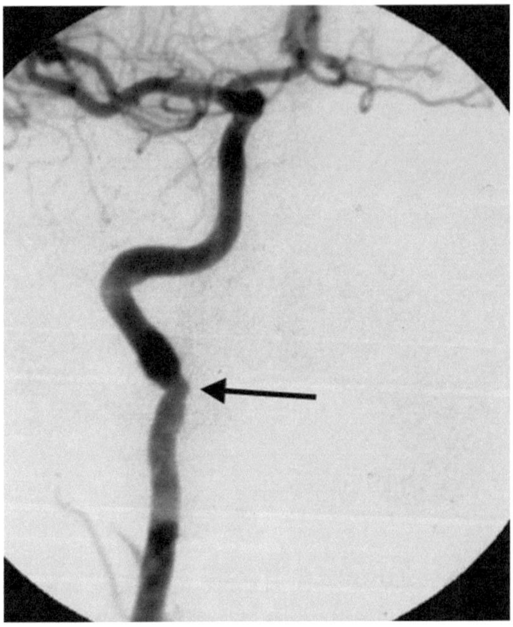

Fig. 13.2 Internal carotid artery dissection secondary to catheter high-flow contrast injection seen as an irregularity of the vessel wall

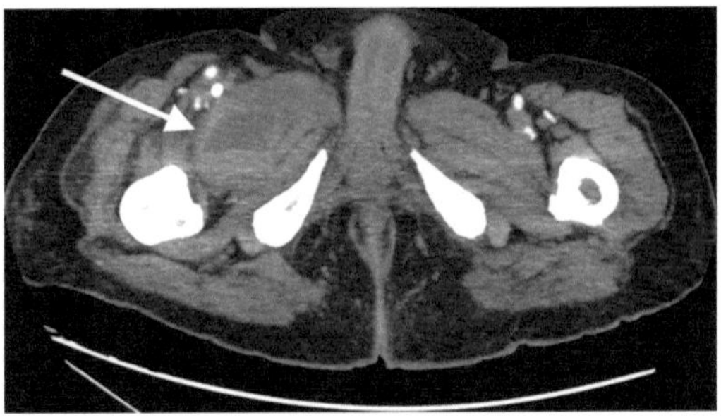

Fig. 13.3 Post-angiography right groin hematoma

13.1.3 Angiography of the Supra-Aortic Trunks

Today, there is practically no indication for invasive angiography of the supra-aortic trunks (SAT) except in the setting of a pre-therapeutic evaluation (for example, before implanting a carotid stent). Non-invasive angiography is preferred whenever possible and includes Doppler ultrasonography, MRI angiography (MRA) (Fig. 13.4), and mostly CT angiography. The last technique offers morphological information for the lumen and the wall of the arteries with a satisfactory spatial resolution.

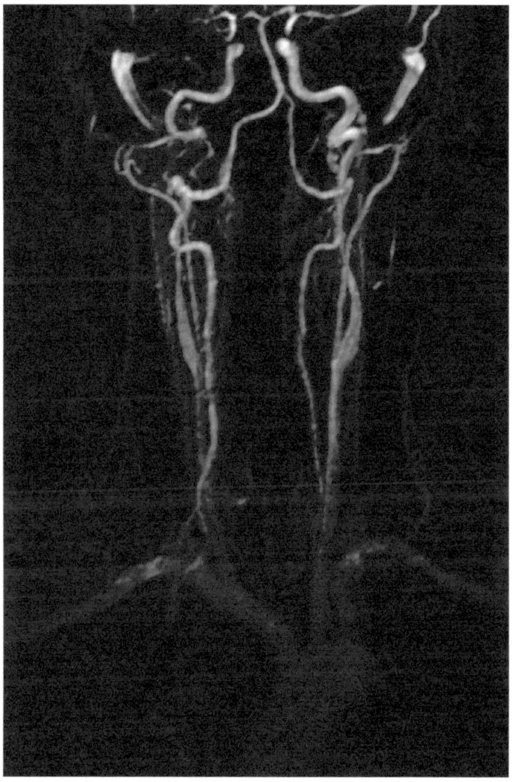

Fig. 13.4 Magnetic Resonance Angiography (MRA) of the aortic arch

13.1.4 Methods of Exploration

Angiography of the SAT is realized either with a global, high-rate aortic arch injection through a pigtail diagnostic catheter or after selective catheterization of the SATs. However, in severe atheromatous lesions, selective catheterization of the SATs entails the risk of dislodgment of an atheromatous plaque and subsequent ischemic stroke.

13.1.5 Radiologic Anatomy

The aortic arch is the origin of three arterial trunks that vascularize the neck and the head. At the proximal part of the aortic arch originates the arterial brachiocephalic trunk (ABCT). It gives off the proximal right common carotid artery (R CCA) and the right subclavian artery (RSA). After the origin of the ABCT follows the origin

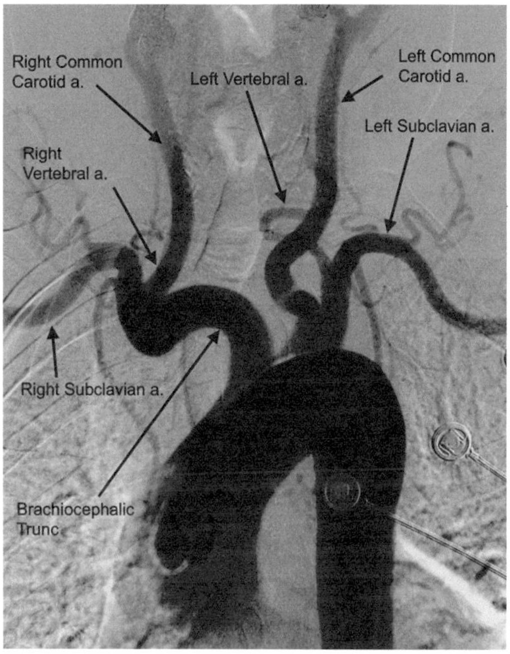

Fig. 13.5 Two-dimensional global aortic arch injection

of the left common carotid artery (L CCA) and the left subclavian artery (LSA) (Fig. 13.5).

13.1.6 Anatomic Variations

According to Lippert (Fig. 13.6), the anatomy is modal in 77% of cases (the ABCT is the origin of the R CCA and the RSA, while the origins of the L CCA are located more distally on the aortic arch). Variations of the origins of the SATs occur in 23% of patients. The most frequent is the origin of the left common carotid artery from the proximal part of the arterial brachiocephalic trunk (13%) or directly from the arterial brachiocephalic (9%). A direct origin of the left common carotid artery from the arterial brachiocephalic trunk is commonly referred to as a "bovine" origin.

Another common variation is the origin of the right subclavian artery directly from the aortic arch distally on the left, after the origin of the left subclavian artery and not from the arterial brachiocephalic trunk. In this case, the right subclavian artery is referred to as "arteria lusoria" and courses behind the esophagus before following

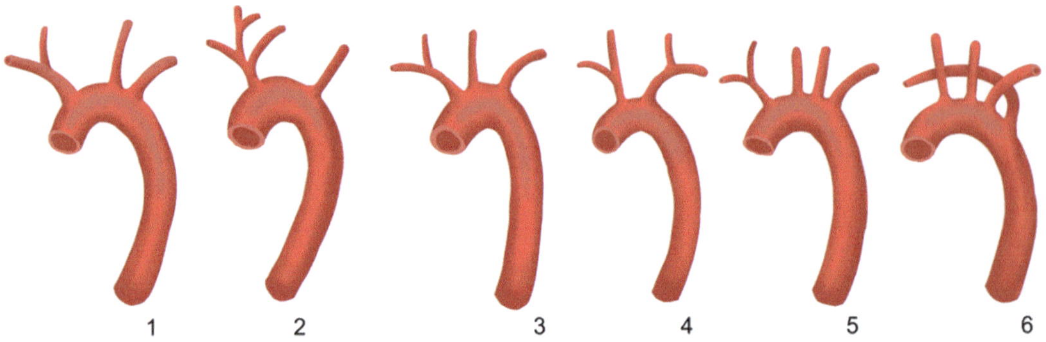

Fig. 13.6 Aortic arch variations (according to Lippert). (1) Normal (77%); (2) Origin of the left common carotid artery (LCCA) at the origin of the brachiocephalic trunk (BCT) (13%); (3) Origin of the LCCA directly from the BCT (9%); (4) Origin of the LCCA and of the left subclavian artery from a common trunk; (5) Origin of the right subclavian artery directly from the aortic arch; (6) Origin of the right subclavian artery distally on the aortic arch which then takes a retro-oesophageal course (arteria lusoria)

its usual course and may provoke dysphagia. This variation is the result of an abnormal fourth right aortic arch during fetal life.

Finally, a not uncommon variation is the direct origin of the left vertebral artery from the aortic arch (4%) between the origins of the left common carotid artery and the left subclavian artery.

13.1.7 Common Carotid Artery

It originates from the arterial brachiocephalic trunk on the right and the aortic arch on the left. It courses in the carotid sulcus medially to the internal jugular vein and the sternocleidomastoid muscle. Its terminal portion usually resides at the level of the body of the C4 vertebra and gives rise to the internal carotid artery (which vascularizes intracranial structures) and to the external carotid artery (which vascularizes the cervical facial area). However, the upper part of the common carotid may variate between C6 and the angle of the mandible.

13.1.8 External Carotid Artery

Among others, it vascularizes the face and the meninges and the extracranial portion of the cranial nerves.

Classical angiography of the external carotid artery is obtained only for vascular malformations and head and neck tumors. It arises from the carotid bifurcation.

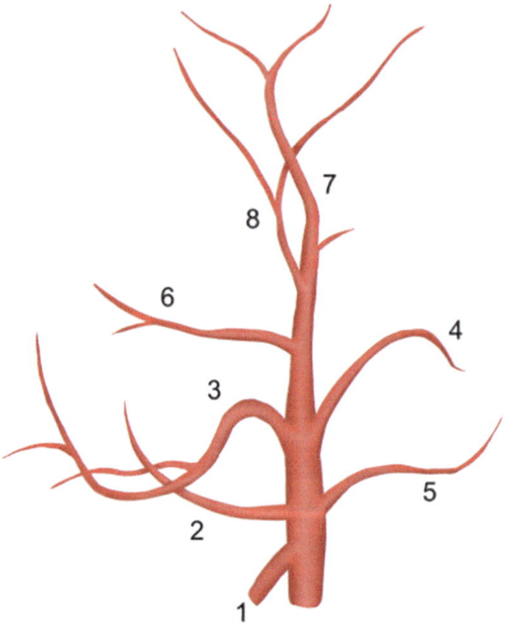

Fig. 13.7 The external carotid artery and its main branches; (1) Superior thyroidal artery; (2) Lingual artery; (3) Facial artery; (4) Auricular artery; (5) Occipital artery; (6) Internal maxillary artery; (7) Superficial temporal artery; (8) Middle meningeal artery. The ascending pharyngeal artery (not shown) is a small vessel that courses parallel to the main ECA trunk

13.1.8.1 The External Carotid Artery

It originates from the bifurcation of the common carotid artery (Fig. 13.7). In an anteroposterior view, the external carotid artery courses usually slightly mediately to the internal carotid artery. Another element that allows making the

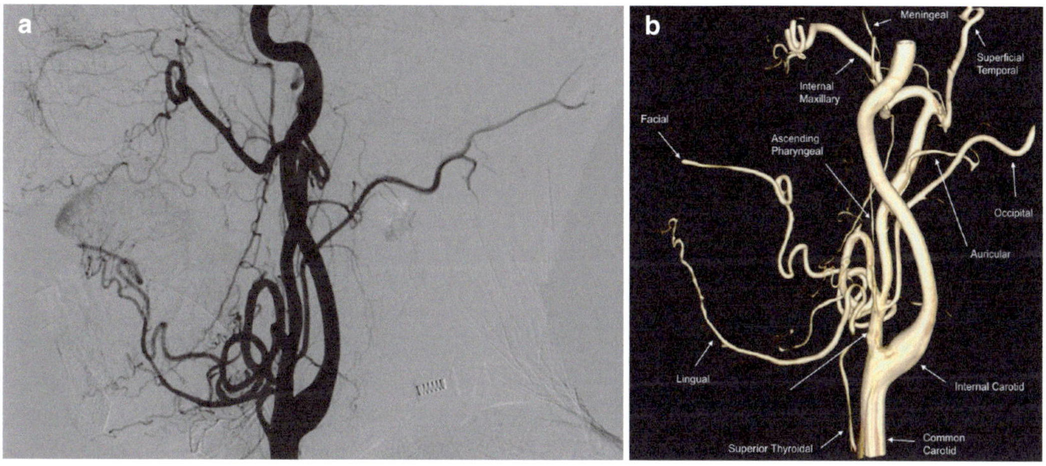

Fig. 13.8 Global injection of the common carotid artery, lateral view (**a**) two-dimensional angiography and (**b**) annotated three-dimensional angiography

distinction from the internal carotid artery is the presence of multiple branches, while the internal carotid artery has none at the level of the neck.

These branches, from proximal to distal, all the following (Fig. 13.8a, b):

The Superior Thyroidal artery.
The Lingual artery.
The Facial artery.
The Ascending Pharyngeal artery.
The Occipital artery.
The Auricular artery.
The Superficial Temporal artery.
The Internal Maxillary artery.

13.1.8.2 The Ascending Pharyngeal Artery

The ascending pharyngeal artery vascularizes the posterior portion of the pharynx, the medial part of the cranial base, the petrous bone, and the posterior part of the posterior foramen lacerum. It also gives a meningeal branch for the vascularization of the posterior fossa.

13.1.8.3 The Occipital Artery

The occipital artery vascularizes the posterior neck as well as the occipital region. It almost constantly gives a meningeal branch that courses under the lateral sinus and vascularizes to the meninges of the posterior fossa. Usually, it also presents one or two anastomoses with the homolateral vertebral artery.

13.1.8.4 The Internal Maxillary Artery

The internal maxillary artery vascularizes the nasal fossa, the sphenoid sinus, the orbital walls, and the anterior and middle cranial fossa (Fig. 13.9). It gives off three segments:

Mandibular Segment (Proximal)

This segment is the origin of a significant vessel:

The middle meningeal artery (MMA) is the first and the largest branch of the internal maxillary artery. The MMA courses superiorly. It traverses the foreman spinosum and is visualized as a sharp anterior curve on lateral angiography before entering the cranium. The accessory meningeal artery is another smaller branch with a more anterior origin of the mandibular segment of the internal Maxillary artery. It also has an ascending course and penetrates the cranial vault through the foramen ovale. Sometimes it gives off small cavernous branches through the foramen of Vesalius.

Pterygoid Segment (Middle)

It is located in the subtemporal fossa and crosses towards the pterygopalatine fossa.

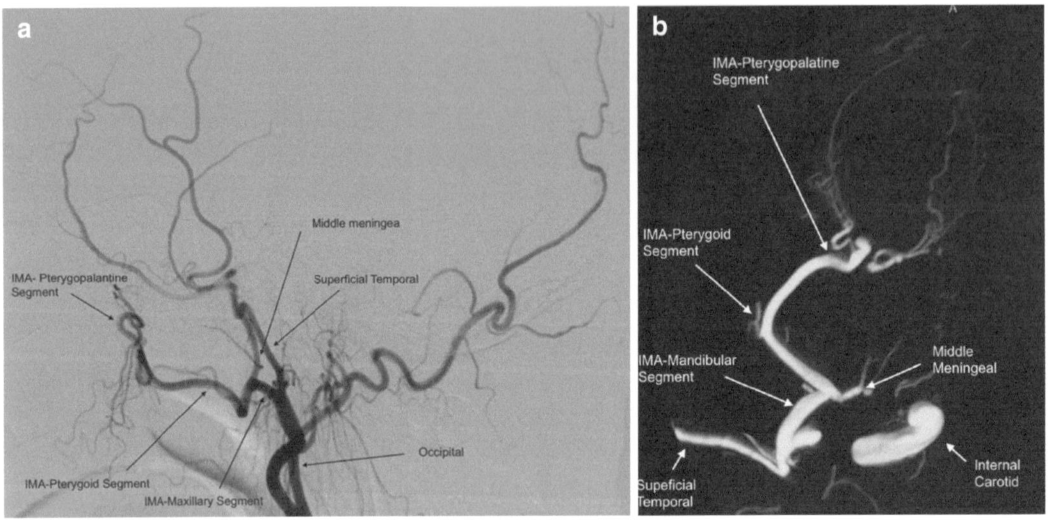

Fig. 13.9 (**a**) Selective external carotid injection, two-dimensional angiography, lateral view. (**b**) Axial reconstruction at the level of the infratemporal fossa

The main branches of this segment are the anterior and posterior deep temporal arteries, the masseteric and buccal arteries.

The Pterygopalatine (Distal) Segment

It makes a turn inside the pterygopalatine fossa anteriorly around the posterior wall of the maxillary sinus and posteriorly around the pterygoid process.

Its principal branches are (a) the superior alveolar artery (which originates before the pterygoid artery enters the pterygopalatine fossa), (b) the infra-orbital arteries (which course through the infra-orbital fissure), (c) the major palatine artery (which courses through the incisive canal), and (d) the sphenopalatine artery which is the terminal branch of the maxillary artery and courses medially through the sphenopalatine foramen to vascularize the nose.

The primary anastomoses between the ECA and the ICA are:

1. Between the angular artery (a branch of the facial artery) located near the inner canthus of the eye and branches of the ophthalmic artery.
2. Between the superficial temporal artery and the ICA through branches of the ophthalmic artery.
3. Between the internal maxillary artery and the ICA through the inferolateral trunk, through branches of the ophthalmic artery, or the vidian artery.
4. Between the ascending pharyngeal artery and the ICA, through the inferno lateral trunk, the vidian artery, and the caroticotympanic artery.

The anastomoses between the external carotid artery and the ophthalmic are a major collateral channel to the brain in the case of ICA occlusion.

13.1.9 Interior Carotid Artery (ICA)

Most of the time, on anteroposterior projections, the proximal ICA has a more lateral trajectory than the ECA.

The ICA (Fig. 13.10) has four segments: the cervical segment, the petrous segment, the intracavernous segment, and the supra-cavernous segment.

The first segment courses in the maxillopharyngeal space, along with the internal jugular vein. It then penetrates the petrous bone, courses in the carotid canal with a proximal vertical course and a distal horizontal course. The ICA enters the cranium through the foramen lacerum.

It then courses inside the cavernous sinus to penetrate in the subarachnoid spaces in its supra-clinoid portion (Fig. 13.11). It has an anterior portion which gives of the ophthalmic artery and a posterior portion, a few millimeters proximally to the posterior communicating artery and the anterior choroidal artery. Finally, it bifurcates into the anterior and the middle cerebral artery.

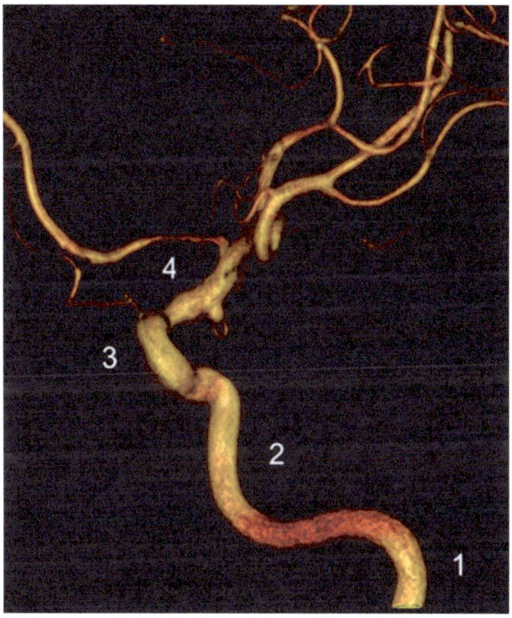

Fig. 13.10 The internal carotid artery has four segments; (1) Cervical segment; (2) Petrous segment; (3) Intracavernous segment; (4) Supra-cavernous segment

In its intracavernous course, the ICA presents several curves that form an italic "S" shape, open superiorly. This curved portion represents the carotid siphon. According to Fischer, the carotid siphon has five segments, with the most proximal named C5 and the most distal C1 (Fig. 13.11).

The segments C4 and C3 are intracavernous and the C1 and C2 segment supra-cavernous.

The C5 segment gives the meningohypophyseal trunk, which vascularizes the hypophysis and the adjacent dura mater.

The C4 segment has an anterior horizontal orientation. Its main collaterals are the capsular arteries that vascularize the sellar diaphragm and the inferolateral trunk. The inferolateral trunk gives off three branches: superior, anterior, and posterior, and vascularizes the roof of the cavernous sinus and the occult motor nerves.

The C3 segment is curved anteriorly.

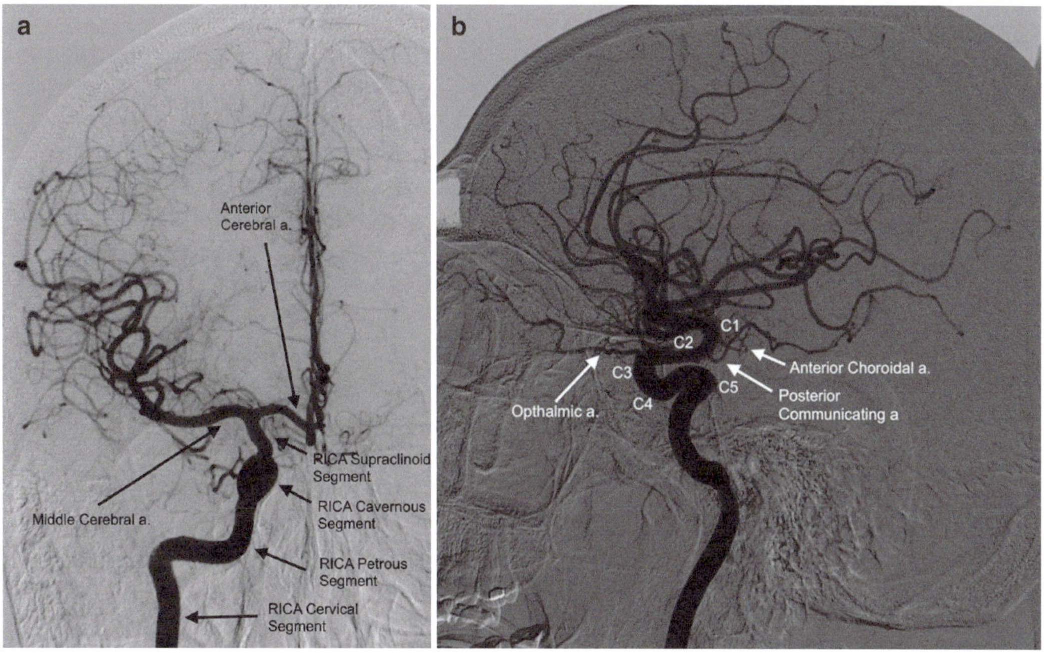

Fig. 13.11 Right internal carotid artery selective injection. (**a**) anteroposterior and (**b**) lateral view

The C2 segment is supracavernous and infraclinoidal and courses posteriorly horizontally or slightly superiorly. It gives off the superior hypophyses arteries that vascularize the anterior portion of the hypophysis.

The ophthalmic artery originates from the anterior portion of the superior C2 segment.

It is usually located in the subarachnoid space and more rarely intradural and courses anteriorly inside the optical canal, inferolateral to the optic nerve.

Finally, the C1 segment is supracavernous and supraclinoidal.

The ICA's supraclinoid portion gives four branches: the posterior communicating, the anterior choroidal, the anterior cerebral, and the middle cerebral artery.

13.2 Conclusion

Classical maxillofacial angiography is nowadays performed by non-invasive means, mainly CT or MR Angiography. It is indicated only for the assessment of lesions before endovascular embolization. Knowledge of normal anatomy and extracranial to intracranial anastomoses is paramount for preventing embolic complications during therapeutic embolization.

Further Reading

Bracard S, Roland J, Picard L. Les vaisseaux du névraxe: anatomie et pathologie. Variations des artères de l'encéphale. [thèse]. CHU de Nancy; 1984.

Djindjan R, Merlan JJ. Super-selective angiography of the external carotid artery. Heidelberg: Springer-Verlag; 1978.

Kaufmann TJ, Huston J, Mandrekar JN, Schleck CD, Thielen KR, Kallmes DF. Complications of diagnostic cerebral angiography: evaluation of 19,826 consecutive patients. Radiology. 2007;243:812–9.

Lasjaunias P, Berenstein A. Functional vascular anatomy of brain, spinal cord and spine. In: Surgical neuroangiography. Berlin: Springer-Verlag; 1990.

Osborn AG. Diagnostic cerebral angiography. Baltimore: Lippincott-Williams and Wilkins; 1999.

Salomon G. Atlas de la vascularisation artérielle du cerveau chez l'homme. Paris: Sandoz; 1971.

14 Imaging of the Most Common Dental Pathologies

Kaan Orhan, Berkan Celikten, and Aysenur Oncu

14.1 Commonly Used Radiography Techniques in Dentistry

The most commonly used radiography techniques in dentistry are 2D imaging as well as Computed Tomography (CT), Cone Beam Computed Tomography (CBCT), Magnetic Resonance Imaging (MRI), and Ultrasound have entered into the scope of dentistry, enabling us to obtain three-dimensional images [1–3] of anatomical structures of maxillofacial region (Table 14.1).

14.1.1 Intraoral Radiography

1. Periapical Radiography Techniques.
   (a) Bi-secting Angle technique (short cone).
   (b) Long cone paralleling technique.
2. Bitewing radiography technique.
3. Occlusal radiography technique.
   (a) Periapical type occlusal radiography technique.
      a_1. Maxillary anterior occlusal.
      a_2. Maxillary lateral occlusal.
      a_3. Mandibular anterior occlusal
   (b) Cross-sectional Occlusal Radiography Technique.
      b_1. Maxillary Cross-sectional Occlusal (vertex)
      b_2. Mandibular Cross-sectional Occlusal (standard)
      - Anterior.
      - Posterior (lateral).

K. Orhan (✉)
Department of DentoMaxillofacial Radiology, Faculty of Dentistry, Ankara University, Ankara, Turkey
e-mail: knorhan@dentistry.ankara.edu.tr

B. Celikten · A. Oncu
Department of Endodontics, Faculty of Dentistry, Ankara University, Ankara, Turkey

Table 14.1 Anatomical structures

Maxilla	Nasal fossa, incisive foramen, lateral fossa, maxillary sinus, recess of the sinus
Mandible	Mental fossa, mental foramen, mandibular canal

14.1.1.1 Periapical Radiography Techniques

Bi-Secting Technique (Short Cone)
Short cone is used in this technique. In the bisecting technique, it is ensured that the angle between the central beam film plane and the long axis of the tooth is perpendicular to the bisector. The image of the object is obtained in the same size as the object thanks to the central beam coming to this area. If the central beam is perpendicular to the long axis of the tooth, the resulting image is larger than the object; if the central beam is perpendicular to the film axis, the resulting image will be smaller than

A. Delantoni, K. Orhan (eds.), *Atlas of Dentomaxillofacial Anatomical Imaging*,
https://doi.org/10.1007/978-3-030-96840-3_14

the object. This technique is frequently used in the endodontic practice due to its rapid and easy nature, and ability to provide sufficient information. However, difficulties are encountered in obtaining the real dimensions of the objects in this technique, because it is very difficult to achieve the radiation of the central beam on the desired area. Therefore, it has been reported that this technique should not be used in the follow-up of the teeth with periapical lesions healing after endodontic treatment [4, 5]. The patient is positioned ensuring that the occlusal plane is parallel to the ground. The film is adjusted so that the bump on the film faces the occlusal of the tooth and the tube. The periapical film is placed in the mouth of the patient with the help of the physician, and the patient is asked to support the film using his/her thumb. Next, the radiation is performed by adjusting the cone at the determined angles [6] (Tables 14.2 and 14.3).

Parallel Technique

In this technique, the central beam falls perpendicular to both the film and the object since the object and the film are positioned parallel to each other. Hence, distortions are prevented according to bisecting technique. Contrary to the bisecting technique, long cones are used in the parallel technique. The sizes of these cones vary between 36 and 46 cm. In addition, attention should be paid to ensure that the distance to the object and the film is very short, and the focal spot should be small to avoid a shadow called penumbra in radiographs. This technique has advantages over other techniques in terms of patient follow-up and diagnosis, which includes obtaining better results regarding the clarity of the details.

In this technique, the film is placed distant to the crown parts of the teeth to ensure parallel positioning. Film holders are used to ensure the parallel position. When a film holder is not used, a cotton roll is placed between the tooth and the film, bringing the film and the tooth to be radiographed to a parallel position; and radiation is performed using long cones [5].

Table 14.2 Radiation angles of the lower jaw

Lower jaw	Central area	−15° vertical film
	Canine area	−20° vertical film
	Premolar area	−10° horizontal film
	Molar area	−5° horizontal film

Table 14.3 Radiation angles of the upper jaw

Upper jaw	Central area	+40° vertical film
	Canine area	+45° vertical film
	Premolar area	+30° horizontal film
	Molar area	+20° horizontal film

14.1.1.2 Bitewing Radiography Technique

This technique is used in endodontics to evaluate the presence of overflow fillers, detection of interface caries, evaluation of the relationship of interface or occlusal caries with pulp, diagnosis of secondary caries, presence of pulp stones, and pulp chamber calcifications. In addition to endodontics, alveolar crest height, the level of resorption in the interdental alveolar crests, and the presence of tartar are also evaluated.

While performing bitewing radiography, the patient is positioned with his/her occlusal plane parallel to the ground. The bite tab on the film is placed between the teeth of the patient, and the patient is asked to bite. Next, the central beam is adjusted to fall on the junction of the bite tab and the film, forming an angle of +8°, +10° with the bite tab. The disadvantage of this technique compared to other techniques is the inability to provide the imaging of the apex areas of the teeth [6].

14.1.1.3 Occlusal Radiography Technique

This technique is applied in two ways. Occlusal films can be in screen or non-screen type. Their size is bigger compared to the periapical film. They are 5.5 × 7.5 cm in size. They are used in palatine and alveolar process fractures, in embedded teeth, in the detection of foreign bodies in the jaws, especially in locations of salivary gland stones (sialolithiasis) in the lower jaw, in the detection of supernumerary or partial anodontia, in the surgical or orthodontic examination of the hard and soft palate defects, and the examination of the torus. They have two types as cross-sectional and topographic. In the cross-sectional technique, the occlusal faces of all teeth are visible; however, their apex is not visible. It is aimed to ensure that the central beam falls perpendicular to the film, approximately at the level of the anterior teeth. There is an angle of ~90°. It is aimed that the central beam is parallel to the long axis of the teeth. To perform the cross-section in the lower jaw, the head of the patient is tilted. In the topographic technique, it is ensured that the sagittal plane is perpendicular to the ground, and the horizontal plane is parallel to the ground. The central beam is radiated perpendicular to the bisector of the angle between the long axis of the teeth and the film plane. For the upper jaw, it is performed over the nose arch at an angle of +60°. The patient is asked to bite the film. If the patient does not have teeth, the thumb is pressed on the upper jaw, the index finger is pressed on the lower jaw, or finger rolls are placed at the crest level, and the patient is asked to bite. It is radiated through the symphysis in the lower jaw at an angle of −55°, and the patient's head is slightly bent backward.

In the topographic technique, teeth are visible with their apex, and there are superpositions in the posterior teeth in the lower jaw. With one of the modifications of the occlusal technique, the image of the maxillary sinus is obtained by radiating from a 5 cm distance to the ala naris.

14.1.2 Other Radiography Techniques

14.1.2.1 Digital Subtraction Radiography (DSR)

It is not possible to detect the minimal changes in the bone using radiography. Various subtraction software have been developed to detect the minimal changes in the bone. Bone loss, which occurs in the early stages of periodontal disease, should be diagnosed clinically. Subtraction software is one of the techniques that increase the detectability of existing bone changes by eliminating the structural deterioration observed on the radiograph by overlapping the images in the radiographs performed at periodic intervals [7–10]. This technique, which was first introduced by the German radiologist Ziedses des Plantes in 1934, started to be used in the field of dentistry by Gröndahl et al. in 1983. Digital subtraction radiography software is used in areas such as diagnosis of alveolar bone loss encountered in periodontal diseases, evaluation of the results of the treatment, evaluation of the results of implant treatments, and osteointegration, due to its high sensitivity and precision [8, 9, 11]. In digital subtraction imaging, both images must have the same standardized imaging technique and radiographic contrast. On the other hand, subtraction software developed in recent years eliminate certain angulation errors and contrast differences. In a conventional technique, a mineralization change of 30–60% per unit volume is required to determine a change in bone tissue by an experienced radiologist. Ortman et al. demonstrated that in cases where standardization can be achieved, a mineral loss of 5% can be monitored by using DSR [12].

In a conventional technique, a mineralization change of 30–60% per unit volume is required to determine a change in bone tissue by an experienced radiologist. Ortman et al. demonstrated that in cases where standardization can be achieved, a mineral loss of 5% can be monitored by using DSR [12]. In the digital subtraction technique, digital imaging systems should be preferred to increase sensitivity. The data loss experienced during the transfer of the films obtained using the conventional technique to the computer decreases the sensitivity in the subtraction technique.

14.1.2.2 Tuned Aperture Computed Tomography (TACT)

TACT technique (tuned aperture computed tomography) is a synthesized tomographic imaging system developed in recent years, which uses a flat panel detector extremely sensitive to X-rays with a low-frequency noise feature. TACT is an imaging system with an algorithm that can create a 3-dimensional image, which can be used with almost all imaging systems providing digitalized output. This system can generate real 3D data by using the numerical data of two-dimensional projections.

It was first developed in the USA in 1990. Theoretically, the main algorithm of TACT is the algorithm of digital monographs. Intraoral radiography is performed based on the acquisition of intraoral radiographs from different angles by placing a small flat panel detector into the oral cavity. The images consist of a combination of projections, which constitute the main images of TACT. Images are obtained four or six times from different angles. The operating software of TACT stores these generated images and reconstructs these marked images as cross-sectional multi-planar images by placing specific markers on each image. Blurring is eliminated and a sharp image is obtained by creating reconstructed pseudo-holograms. Albeit their limited use in endodontics, it has been reported that they have significantly good performances in terms of the examination of the root fractures, particularly the vertical root fractures [13, 14].

14.1.3 Panoramic Radiography

The idea of displaying all dental arches on a single film was put forward by Bouchacourt in 1904. Bouchacourt planned to record the image of the arches on a film located outside the mouth by radiating from an X-ray source placed inside the mouth. Later, the panoramic radiography technique was developed in 1949 upon the studies conducted by Prof. Panoramic radiography technique has been developed with the studies of Dr. Yrjo V. Paatero. Panoramic Radiology is a technique that enables the imaging of a single tomographic image belonging to both dental arches and adjacent anatomic structures, with minimal geometric distortion and superposition. Panoramic radiography is a technique that displays all teeth and jaws, maxillary area up to 1/3 upper part of the eye socket, maxillary sinuses, mandible, and temporomandibular joint together.

Major advantages of panoramic imaging include:

- Comprehensive imaging of facial bones and teeth,
- Exposure of the patient to minimal radiation dose,
- Ease of positioning the patient,
- Facilitating the examination of the patient,
- Ease of obtaining the film in patients with restricted mouth opening,
- Short duration,
- Being useful in informing the patients since they can easily understand the panoramic film.

Major disadvantages of panoramic imaging include:

- Difficulty in diagnosing small carious lesions due to poor image quality compared to intraoral radiographs,
- Inability to display the locations that need to be screened as they may be hidden due to the shadows created by the soft tissues and the airway,
- Ghost images and artifacts,
- Distortion and magnification,
- Inability to perform in children below 5 years of age and the disabled individuals due to the long exposure period.

The endodontic indication of panoramic radiography is limited. However, it can be used to examine cystic and parodontitis lesions in the periapical area. In addition, panoramic radiography can also be used for diagnosing dentition anomalies. Cases with hypodontia, hyperdontia, gemination or fusion in deciduous dentition, and anomaly in permanent dentition belong to the high-risk group. Due to this close relationship between deciduous dentition and permanent dentition, early diagnosis of anomalies helps the physician to examine for predicting the future, and determine the best treatment plan at the earliest stage.

Panoramic radiography has a very important place in the identification, localization, and surgical removal of supernumerary teeth. In addition, anomalies In addition, anomalies of the permanent dentition observed in cases of cleidocranial dysplasia, supernumerary teeth, and morphological anomalies of maxilla and mandible are diagnosed using panoramic radiography. Gardner syndrome, which accompanies multiple embedded supernumerary teeth, osteomas in the skull and jaws in long bones, multiple polyps in the intestines, and epidermoid or dermoid cysts, can be diagnosed by using panoramic radiography. When there are osteomas and multiple supernumerary teeth that are observed in panoramic radiography, early diagnosis of Gardner syndrome can also be made. It has an important place in the early diagnosis of macrodontia in terms of the planning of orthodontic treatment. Panoramic radiography helps also early diagnosis if there is macrodontia and tooth development delay. Taurodontism is an inherited morphological anomaly seen in multi-root teeth due to invagination error of the Hertwig epithelial root sheath. Taurodontism is the enlargement of the pulp chamber resulting from the displacement of the pulp base and bifurcation towards the apical. Taurodontism is usually seen as symmetrical and bilateral. Rarely, a single tooth may also be affected. No anomalies are encountered in the relevant teeth during a clinical examination. Taurodontism is diagnosed using radiography. Panoramic radiography is reliable for the diagnosis of taurodontism. Since the anomalies of dentition development may affect the aesthetics and self-worth perceptions of the patients, early diagnosis of dental anomalies enables us to make the necessary treatment planning. In addition to clinical examinations, panoramic radiography is very effective and useful in diagnosing dental anomalies. Early diagnosis of dental anomalies enables early intervention. The treatment of anomalies that are not diagnosed early is more difficult, and the prognosis is poor. Panoramic radiography is generally not suitable for diagnosing endodontic diseases (Fig. 14.1).

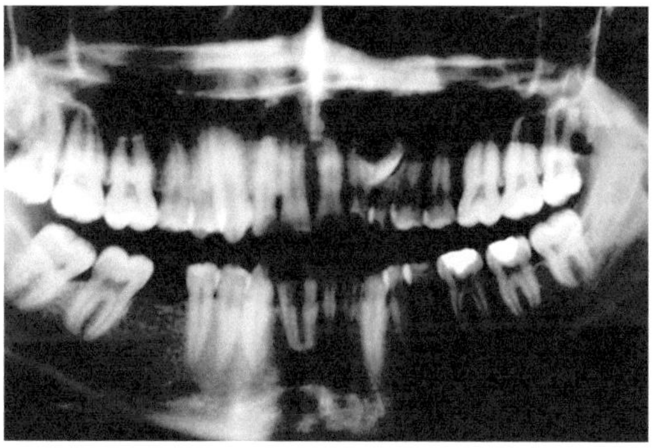

Fig. 14.1 Pre-eruptive intracoronal resorption in the embedded canine tooth in panoramic radiography. (From the archive of Dr. Kaan Orhan)

14.1.4 CBCT

It can be used in the diagnosis of endodontic diseases, examination of canal morphologies, detection of non-endodontic pathologies, evaluation of TYPE C and traumas, analysis of external and internal root resorption, and invasive cervical resorption, planning before endodontic surgery, and planning endodontic implants. Recent studies have demonstrated that CBCT is more useful in determining both horizontal and vertical root fractures compared to conventional periapical radiographs. In addition, studies have been carried out recently on the usefulness of CBCT in the examination of the fractures after root canal treatment or for fractures after post-core application. The photo displays a case with a fracture formed after the post-core application. However, no fracture was found as a result of the examination of the case, which had been performed CBCT. Therefore, it is recommended to be careful in examining broken instruments and such fractures, especially after canal filling sealant, which may cause errors in the examination of the structures around the radio-opaque material in the CBCT. However, CBCT can also be used in endodontic cases of apical surgery. Especially for endodontic surgical procedures to be performed in the molar area, it is important to know the thickness of the labial cortex for the buccal or anterior area to access the area. Since there are problems in accessing palatal roots, especially in the molar area, it is necessary to utilize CBCT in infected cases, and cases where apical surgery is considered. Another benefit of this can be expressed as preventing damage to the complex anatomical structure in these areas [15–21].

14.2 Uses of Radiographs in General Dental Practice

The usage areas of radiographs in endodontics can be briefly summarized as follows:

14.2.1 Before Treatment

14.2.1.1 Identification of the Dental Diseases

Evaluation of the Relationship Between Deep Caries and Pulp

Radiographs are widely used for detecting carious lesions in the tooth, and to evaluate the relationship between caries and pulp. Generally, bitewing, periapical, and panoramic radiographs are used for this purpose (Figs. 14.2 and 14.3).

It should be remembered that the size of caries detected on the radiographs is generally not the same as the size observed after the cleaning of the teeth clinically. The size of caries detected in radiographs is usually smaller compared to the size detected in the clinical examination due to the presence of decalcified carious tooth tissue. On the other hand, there may be cases with contrary conditions. Caries may be perceived as enlarged to areas where there are intact tooth tissue, and areas that are not carious.

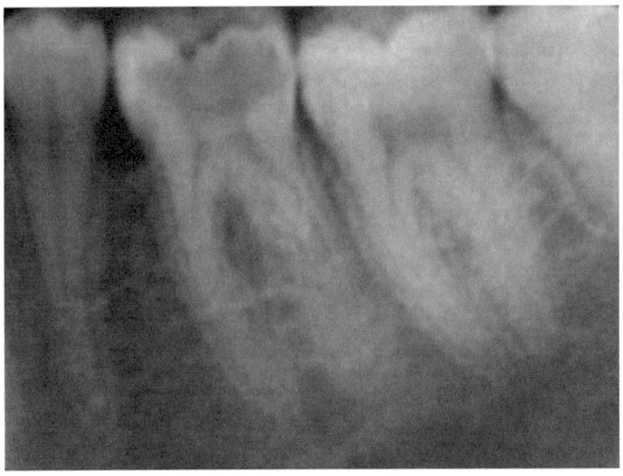

Fig. 14.2 Periapical radiography of the lower-left sixth tooth. Occlusal caries combined with the pulp chamber of the tooth are observed

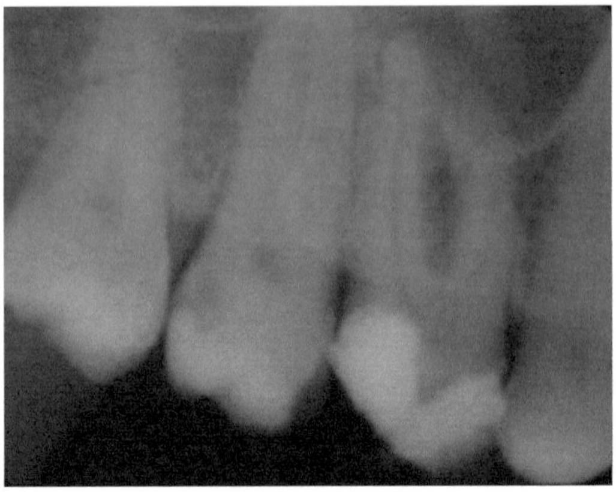

Fig. 14.3 Periapical radiography of the right upper seventh tooth. Deep dentin caries are observed relatively far from the pulp chamber of the tooth

In such cases, caries may be perceived as larger than their actual size [22].

Such visual misconceptions may occur based on them:

1. The amount of decalcification in the carious lesion,
2. Incorrect angulation of the X-ray beam,
3. Complete elimination of caries through clinical intervention.

In addition, in the radiographic evaluation of caries, non-carious structures can be perceived as caries due to factors such as "cervical burnout and optical illusion, Mach band effect, radiolucent restorations, dental anomalies, radiation errors, and projection errors." Therefore, the clinical examination should be performed together with the radiographic examination.

When dental caries reach the pulp tissue, the pulp connective tissue starts to respond against irritants, which can be observed in clinical examination, leading to the development of irreversible pulpitis. In the radiographic evaluation of irreversible pulpitis, only a deep restoration is observed where the pulp chamber meets the carious cavity or is located close to the pulp chamber. In addition, a slight enlargement of the periodontal space can be detected in the advanced stages of irreversible pulpitis.

Identification of Periapical Diseases

Although the diagnosis of periapical diseases is determined histologically, some lesions may show specific radiographic signs.

In endodontics, periapical diseases can be classified into five main categories:

1. Acute Apical Periodontitis,
2. Acute Apical Abscess,
3. Chronic Apical Periodontitis (periapical granuloma and periapical cyst),
4. Chronic Apical Abscess,
5. Condensing Osteitis.

If *Acute Apical Periodontitis* has developed after pulpitis, it cannot be visible in the radiograph. On the other hand, in the presence of an Acute Apical Periodontitis that has developed as a result of gangrene or necrosis in the pulp, an enlargement is observed in the periodontal space.

There may be differences in the radiographic image of *Acute Apical Abscess.* If Acute Apical Abscess occurs as a result of Acute Apical Periodontitis, an enlarged apical periodontal gap is observed on radiographs. In Acute Apical Abscess that occurs in the presence of Acute Chronic Apical Periodontitis, a distinct local apical radiolucent image is observed.

Chronic Apical Abscess is radiographically observed as a dark and diffuse lesion. However, this image should not be confused with cystic lesions. In these types of lesions, the radiographic image is more rounded and more prominent compared to the chronic apical abscess.

Chronic Apical Periodontitis (periapical granuloma and periapical cyst) appears on radiographs in the form of radiolucent areas in different sizes in the apical area of the root. A periapical cyst is usually visible when the size of the lesion is greater than 200 mm^2.

Asymptomatic focal osteosclerotic lesions such as *Condensing Osteitis* are frequently encountered on radiographs. These radiopacities, which are referred to by different names in the literature, are generally observed as distinctly limited, nonexpansile, uniform radiopaque masses that may differ according to size, shape, and relationship with the apical of the tooth roots in the area. If this radiopaque area in the jawbones cannot be explained due to any reason, it is called "idiopathic osteosclerosis"; if it accompanies an inflammation, it is called "condensing osteitis." Idiopathic osteosclerosis is radiographically observed as non-expanding radiopaque areas with smooth or irregular borders that can be easily differentiated from the surrounding normal bone. On the other hand, condensing osteitis can be observed as a well-circumscribed or diffuse radiopacity, or a sclerosed bone surrounding an enlarged periodontal ligament.

Radiographic images cannot be used alone in the diagnosis of periapical diseases. They can only help with the preliminary diagnosis. The definitive diagnosis can only be determined by histological and clinical examination (Figs. 14.4, 14.5, 14.6, and 14.7).

Determination of Internal or External Root Resorptions

Internal root resorption is radiographically observed as a well-circumscribed radiolucent circle within the root canal or pulp chamber. This radiolucency has the same intensity, and

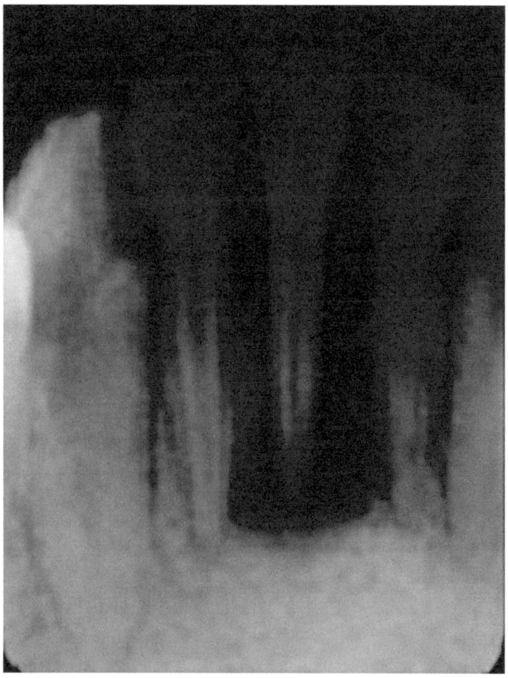

Fig. 14.4 Pathology found in the periapical of the lower right central tooth

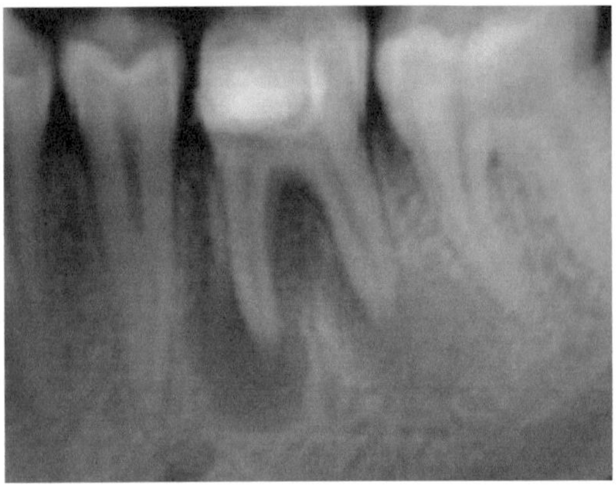

Fig. 14.5 Pathology in the periapical of the lower-left sixth tooth

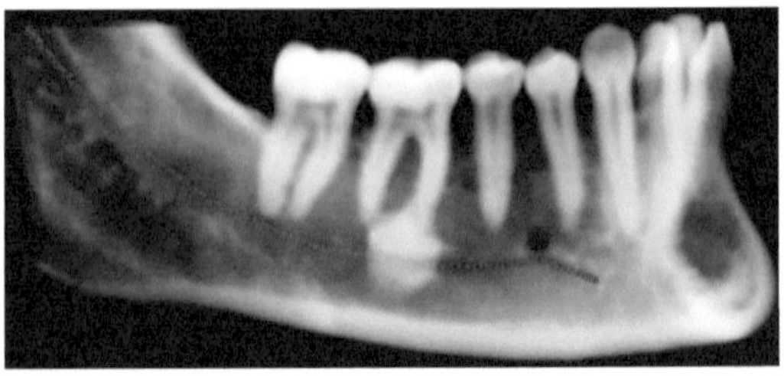

Fig. 14.7 Condensing osteitis CBCT image

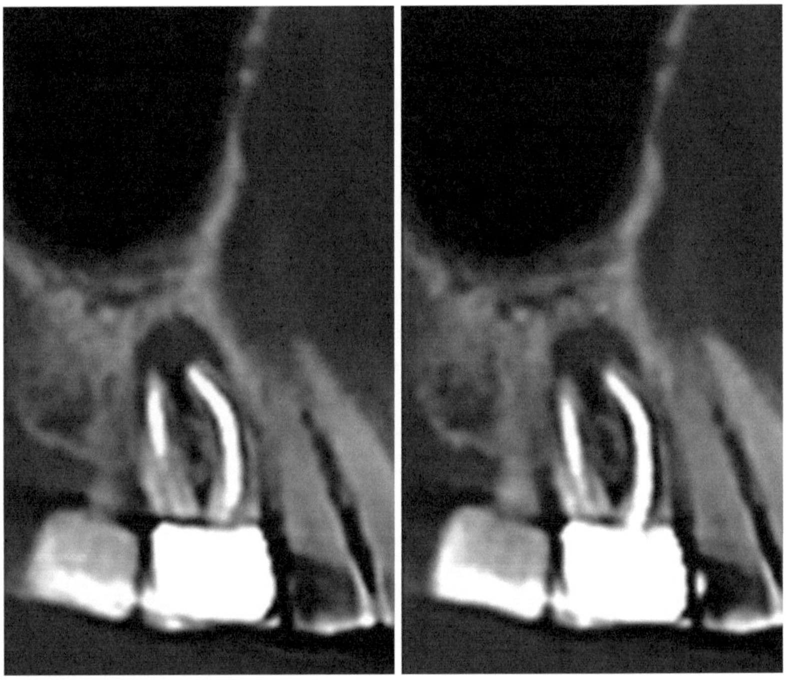

Fig. 14.6 Chronic apical periodontitis CBCT image

the course of the root canal cannot be observed within this area. In addition, the location of the radiolucent area does not change as a result of the radiographs performed from different angles (Figs. 14.8a, b, 14.9a, b, 14.10, and 14.11).

On the other hand, external root resorption is observed radiographically, not in a round and well-circumscribed appearance unlike internal root resorption; on the contrary, it is observed with an indented protrusion. Differences are observed in the radiopacity of the radiolucent part. In addition, a superposition into the root canal at the resorption area is observed there is a superposition into the root canal at the resorption area, following the course of the root canal. With the radiographs from different angles, the change in the position of the lesion is determined.

Identification of Dental Anomalies

Since the anatomical structures of such teeth are different from the known structures, some difficulties are encountered during endodontic treatments. In this group, important diseases in terms of endodon-

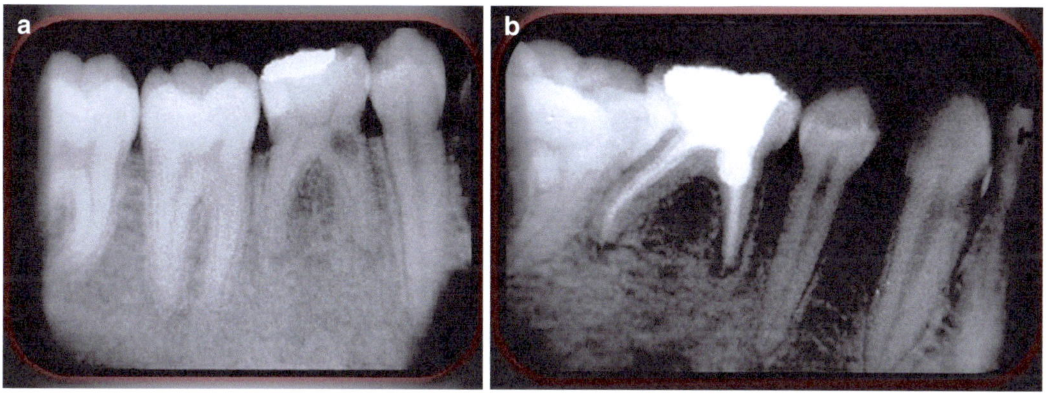

Fig. 14.8 (**a**) Internal root resorption in the coronal root pulp of the lower right sixth tooth. (**b**) Treatment of internal resorption in the coronal root pulp of the right lower sixth tooth

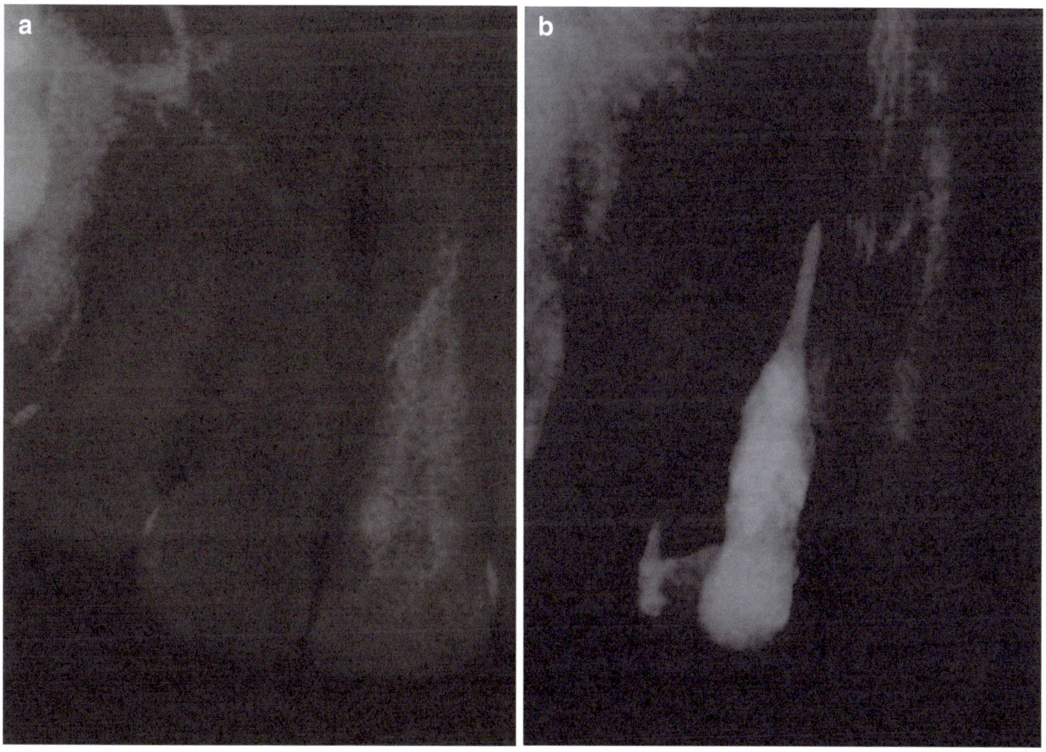

Fig. 14.9 (**a**) Internal resorption in the crown and root of the upper right first tooth. (**b**) Endodontic treatment of the upper right first tooth

tics include Dens invaginatus, Dens invaginatus, fusion, gemination, C-shaped root canals, taurodontism, dilaceration, and palatal groove.

Dens invaginatus is a developmental dental anomaly caused by the inward folding of the epithelium during the formation of the hard tissues of the tooth. The invagination zone constitutes an important potential site for caries and plaque formation.

Dens Evaginatus is a developmental anomaly resulting from the coronal enamel and dentine folding outward together with the pulp. It can be

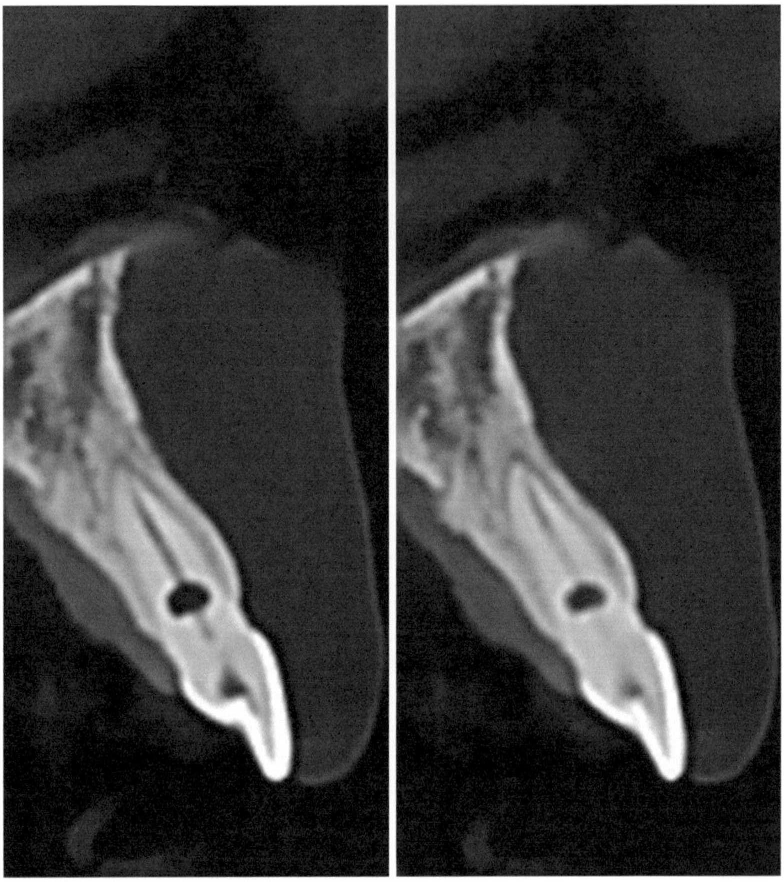

Fig. 14.10 Internal root resorption on cross-sectional CBCT iamges

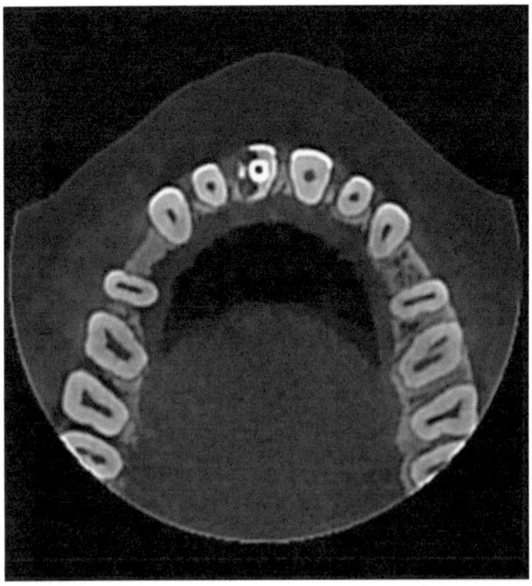

Fig. 14.11 The image of an external root resorption on axial CBCT images

expressed in terms such as tubercle cusp, accessory tubercle, premolar occlusal tubercle, occlusal pearl, or talon tubercle. Its importance in terms of endodontics is that the extra tubercle of the teeth with this type of structure can easily be broken, causing the pulp of the tooth to open into the mouth environment; and as a result of this, an infection may develop in the tooth. In addition, if it is observed in the upper incisors, it may affect occlusal closure.

Fusion results from the union of two tooth buds at the embryological stage. The pulp chamber and root canals can be positioned as separate or together according to the union during the development of the tooth.

Gemination is the formation of a partially or completely divided dental crown on a single root resulting from the change of a single tooth germ. Shortly, it occurs as a result of the splitting of a single tooth bud.

The C-shaped root canal is an anomaly caused by the merging of the lingual or buccal surfaces of mesial and distal roots. When viewed from the occlusal surface of the tooth, the root canal appears like the letter C. It is believed to occur as a result of the accumulation of cementum between the roots or because the Hertwig epithelial root sheath is not fully decomposed at the bifurcation point. C-shaped root canal anatomy is an anomaly that makes endodontic treatment difficult.

Taurodontism occurs as a result of the pulp chamber expanding towards the root apex. Taurodontism is observed on radiographs as the long teeth with enlarged pulp chambers and short roots. The etiology of taurodontism is not fully known; however, it is believed to occur when the Hertwing epithelial sheath does not invaginate properly (Fig. 14.12a, b).

Dilacerations of the root are examined in two planes, which are mesiodistal or buccolingual. Angulations of 90° and above 90° are defined as dilacerations (Fig. 14.13a–c).

The exact etiology of *the palatal groove* is not fully known; however, it is assumed that the tooth is involved in the invagination of the Hertwing epithelial sheath or enamel organ at the stage of odontogenesis. Dental caries and periodontal diseases may occur due to the effect of plaques accumulated in the palatal groove. Chronic pulpitis or pulp necrosis may occur due to advanced caries and periodontal diseases [23, 24].

Evaluation of Traumatized Teeth

Radiographic examination is also important in addition to the oral examination of a traumatized patient. Unlike other conditions, intraoral films may be insufficient alone. Extraoral films of the patient should also be obtained.

Extraoral films are generally used in the diagnosis of alveoli, jaw, and joint fractures in complex facial traumas, detecting the displacement of teeth exposed to trauma and detecting teeth and foreign bodies embedded in soft tissues such as lips as a result of trauma.

Intraoral radiographs are also used in the detection of hard tissue and periodontal tissue injuries of the tooth. These include;

Hard Tissue Injuries of the Tooth

1. Enamel fractures and cracks: Includes fractures, and cracks involving only the enamel.
2. Uncomplicated crown fracture: Enamel-dentin fracture not involving the pulp.
3. Complicated crown fracture: Enamel-dentine fracture involving the pulp.
4. Root fractures (horizontal and vertical).
5. Crown root fracture without involving the pulp.
6. Fracture of the crown root involving the pulp.

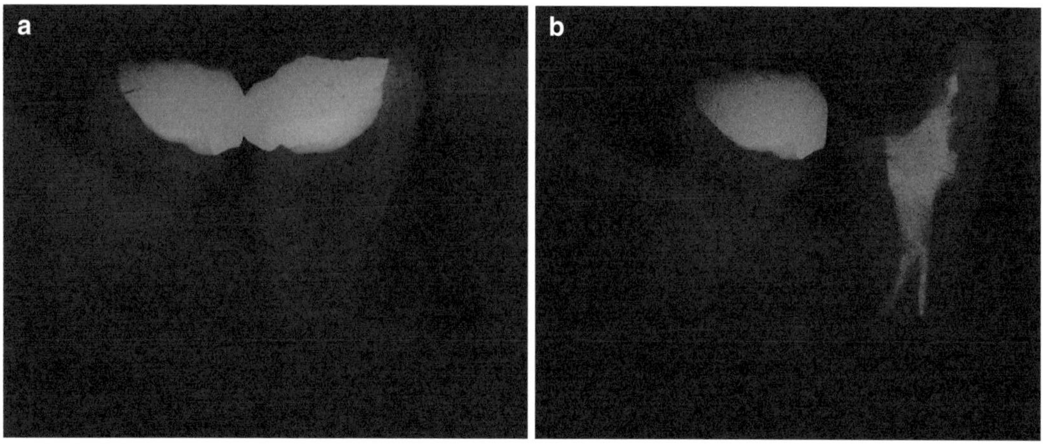

Fig. 14.12 (**a**) Hypertaurodontism was found in the right lower sixth tooth due to the displacement of the pulp base towards the apical. (**b**) Treatment of the lower right sixth tooth

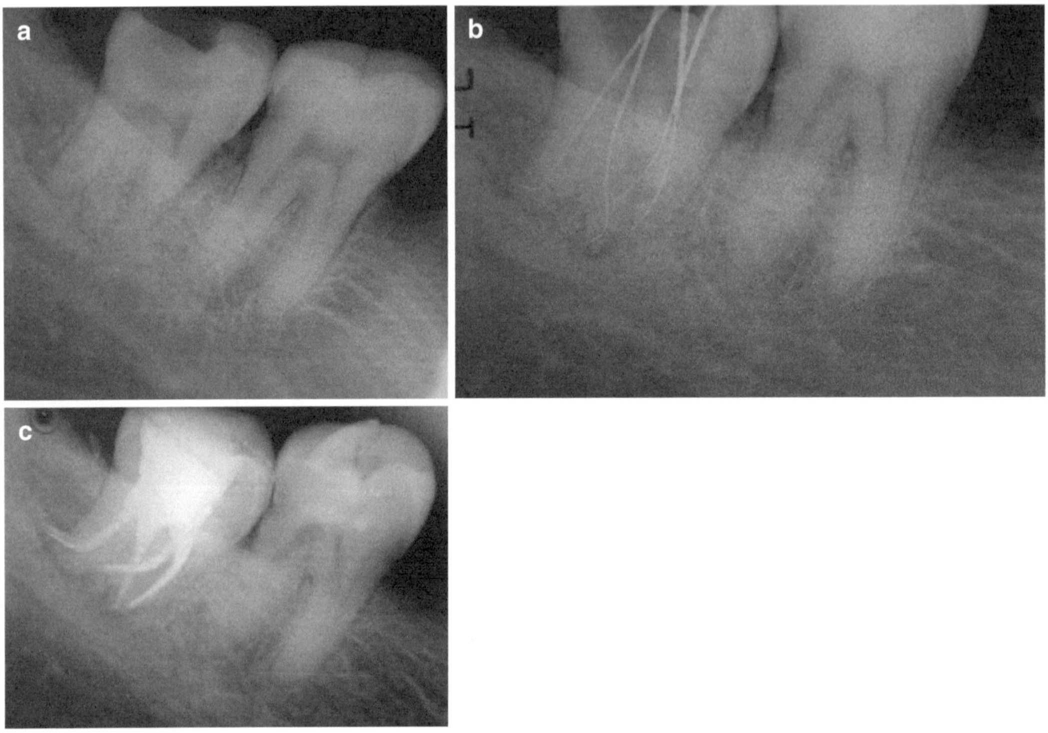

Fig. 14.13 (**a**) It was determined that the lower right third molar tooth has four roots and four canals, and the distobuccal canal is dilated. (**b**) Determination of the working length of the lower right third molar tooth. (**c**) Completing the endodontic treatment of the lower right third molar tooth

Periodontal Tissue Injuries

1. *Concussion*: There is sensitivity in percussion without too much mobilization and displacement in the tooth. As long as the tooth maintains its vitality, no radiographic finding is observed.
2. *Subluxation*: It is a condition of loosening of the tooth and surrounding tissues without a clinical or radiographic displacement of the tooth.
3. *Intrusive luxation*: It is the dislocation of the tooth into the alveolar bone.
4. *Extrusive luxation*: It is the dislocation of the tooth towards the outside of the alveolar socket.
5. *Lateral luxation*: It is the eccentric dislocation of the tooth.
6. *Avulsion*: It is the complete dislocation of a tooth from its socket in the alveolar bone.

Identification of Calcified Root Canals

In calcific degeneration, some or almost all of the pulp tissue is replaced by calcific material. Root canal calcifications can be detected on radiographs, and usually, it is not possible to enter the root canal (Fig. 14.14).

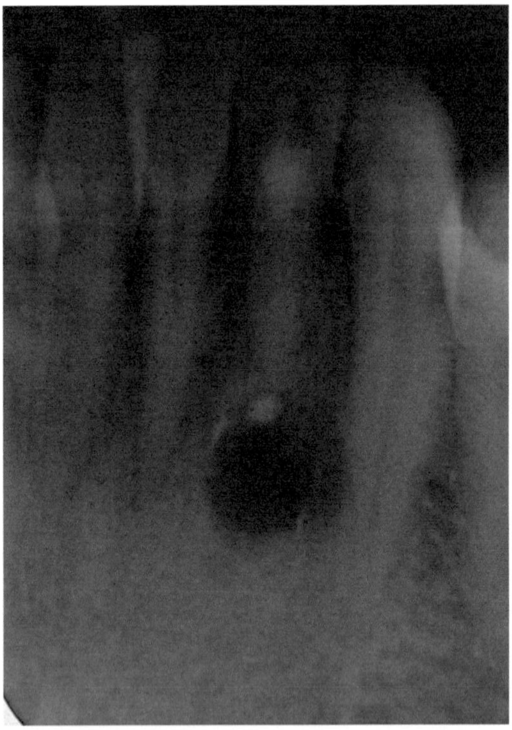

Fig. 14.14 Appearance of the root canal of the lower-left first tooth calcified

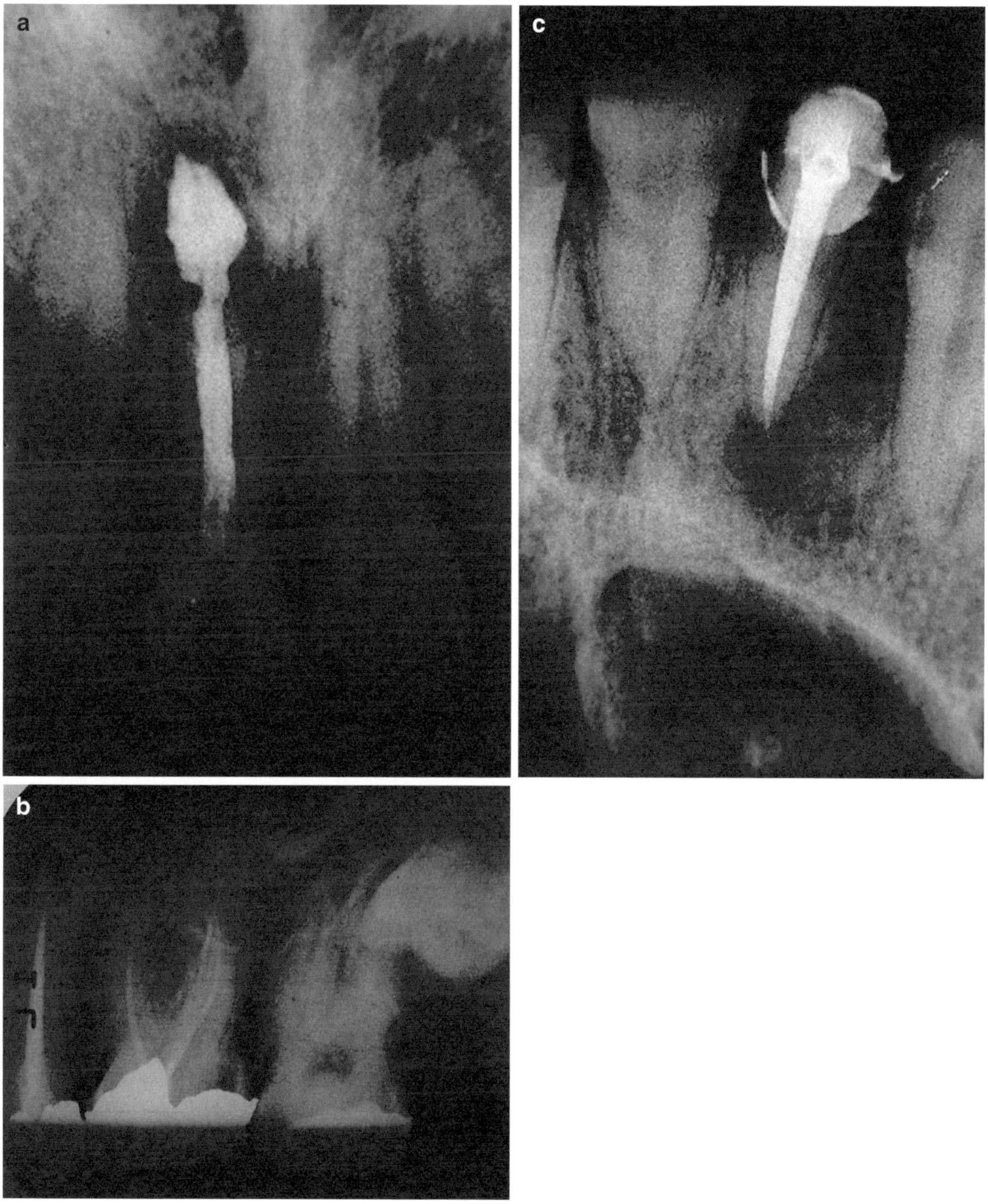

Fig. 14.15 (**a**) Root canal filling emerging from the apex of the root canal of the upper right first tooth. (**b**) Insufficient endodontic treatment of upper left sixth tooth. (**c**) Radiographically successful endodontic treatment of upper right second tooth

I. *Evaluation of root canal filling quality and apical position of endodontically treated teeth*

The quality of root canal filling of endodontically treated teeth can be examined on radiographs (Fig. 14.15a–c). Radiographs provide us with information about missing or overflowing root canal fillings. In this way, the physician may decide whether the endodontic treatment of a tooth should be renewed (Fig. 14.16a, b) or the tooth should be extracted.

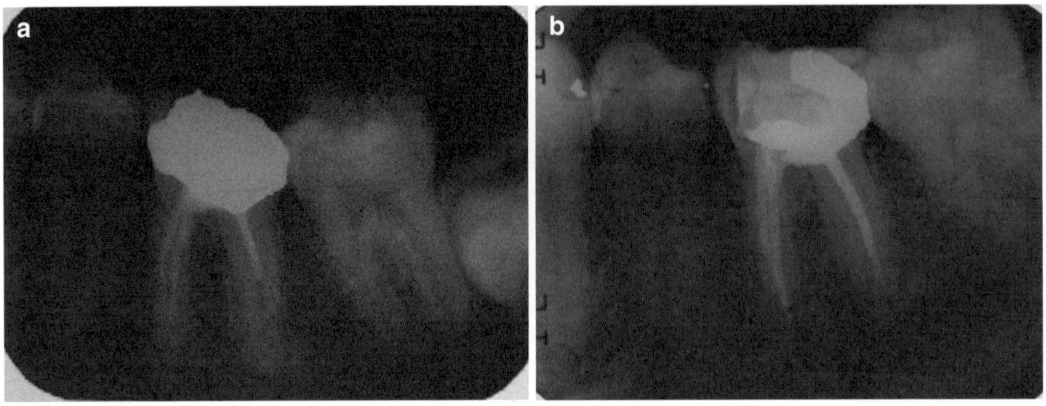

Fig. 14.16 (**a**) Root canal filling previously applied to the lower left tooth sixth and missing in the apical region. (**b**) Retreatment of the root canal treatment of the lower-left sixth tooth

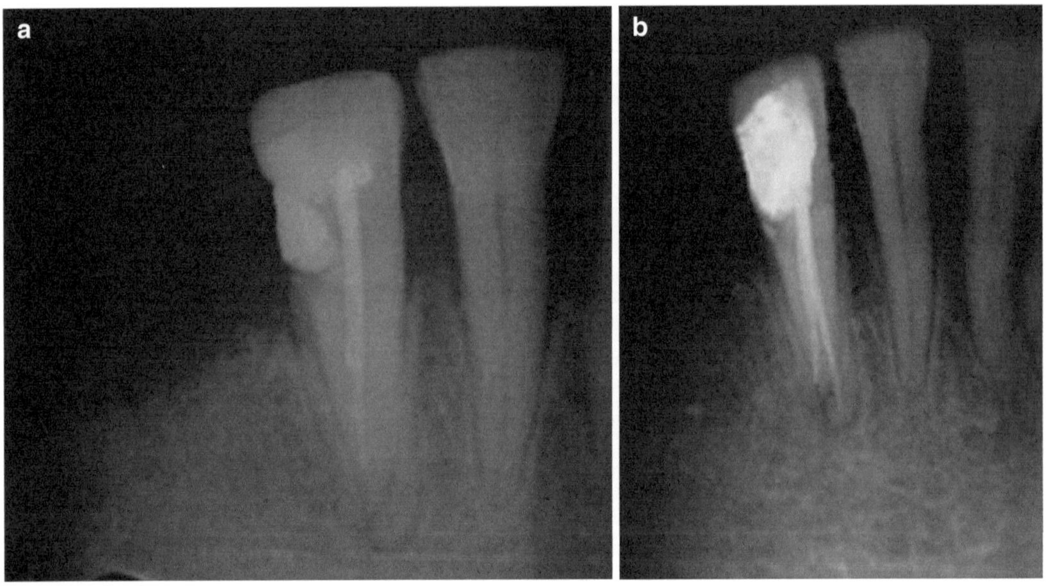

Fig. 14.17 (**a**) It seems that the upper right lateral tooth has two roots and one root is not endodontic. (**b**) Noticing the other root as a result of careful examination and completing the patient's treatment

II. *Determination of root canal anatomy before endodontic treatment; determination of the number, shape, size, and direction of roots and canals*

Radiographs taken before endodontic treatment constitute an important place for the success of endodontic treatment. Thanks to these radiographs, root canal anatomy can be examined, diseased structures can be detected and structures with unknown morphology can be diagnosed. Root pulp may have different morphologies, contrary to what is known. As a result of this, if a careful radiographic examination is not performed, excessive root or canals can be overlooked, and this may lead to the failure of the endodontic treatment (Figs. 14.17a, b, 14.18a, b, and 14.19a, b).

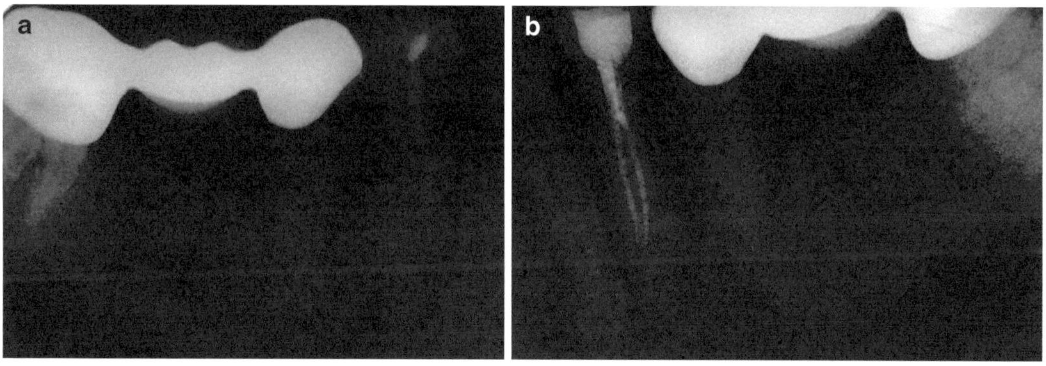

Fig. 14.18 (**a**) It seems that the lower-left first premolar tooth has two canals and one canal does not have endodontic treatment. (**b**) Noticing the other root as a result of careful examination and completing the patient's treatment

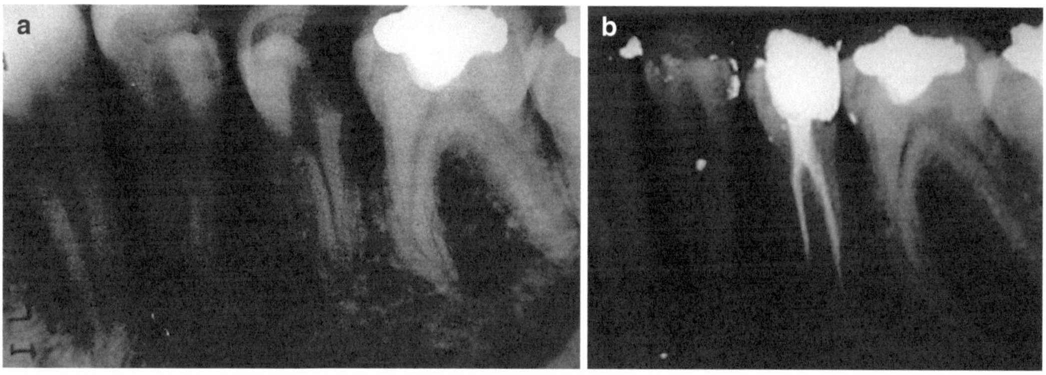

Fig. 14.19 (**a**) It seems that the lower-left second premolar tooth has canals and one canal does not have endodontic treatment. (**b**) Noticing the other root as a result of careful examination and completing the patient's treatment

14.2.2 Using Radiography During Endodontic Treatment

(a) To determine the working length (Fig. 14.20a, b).
(b) Controlling the shaping made in the root canal before root canal filling with the main cone,
(c) Identifying complications such as furcation and lateral perforations in the crown or canal during endodontic treatment (Figs. 14.21 and 14.22),
(d) Determining and viewing the location of the instrument fractures.

Instrument fracture is a complication that can occur during endodontic treatment, affecting the course of the treatment (Figs. 14.23 and 14.24). The prognosis of the tooth is affected by the location where the fracture of the instrument occurs, the stage of the endodontic treatment when the fracture occurs, and the previous condition of the tooth.

14.2.3 After Treatment

(a) For evaluation of the quality of root canal filling and the apical position immediately after treatment,
(b) Follow-up of the root canal fillings (Fig. 14.25a, b),
(c) Controlling adaptation of retrograde fillings after endodontic surgery, and removal of roots after hemisection (Fig. 14.26),
(d) Controlling the closure of root ends after the apexification procedure.

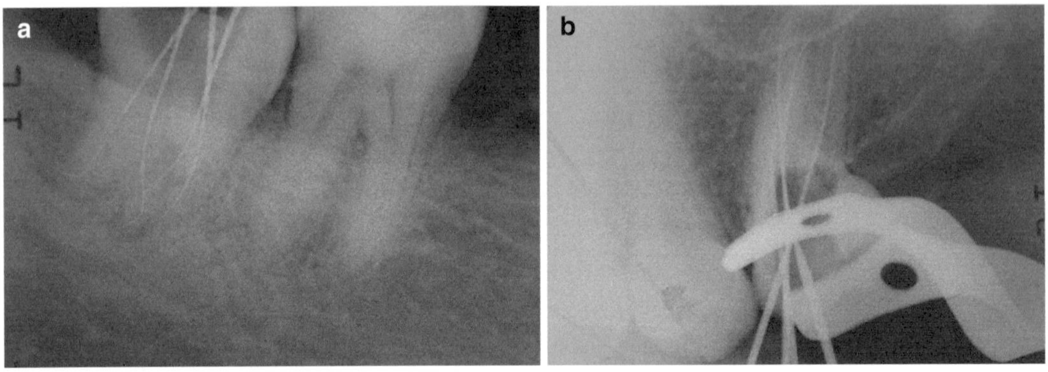

Fig. 14.20 (**a**) Determination of the working length of the lower right third molar tooth with K-type files. (**b**) Determination of the working length of the upper left second molar tooth with K-type files

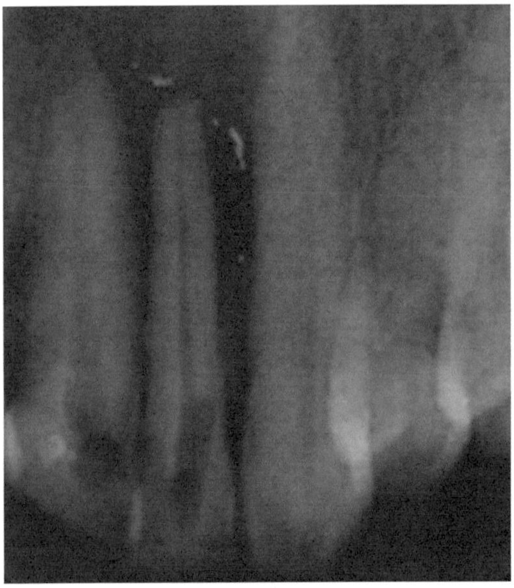

Fig. 14.21 In the upper right lateral tooth, the fissure was opened with a bur and moved in a different direction from the course of the root canal

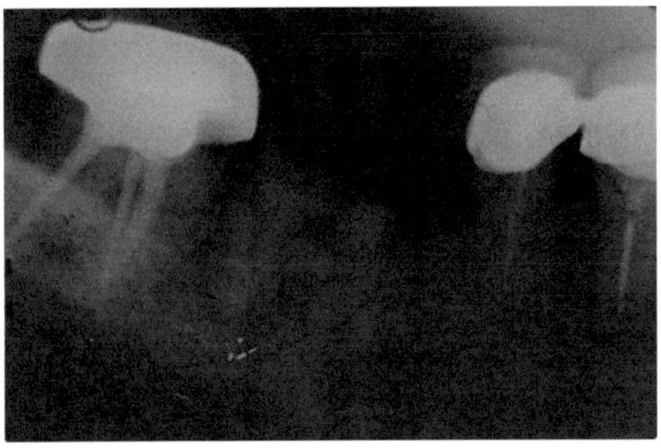

Fig. 14.22 Radiography of an accidental furcation perforation while searching the root canals of the lower right one molar tooth

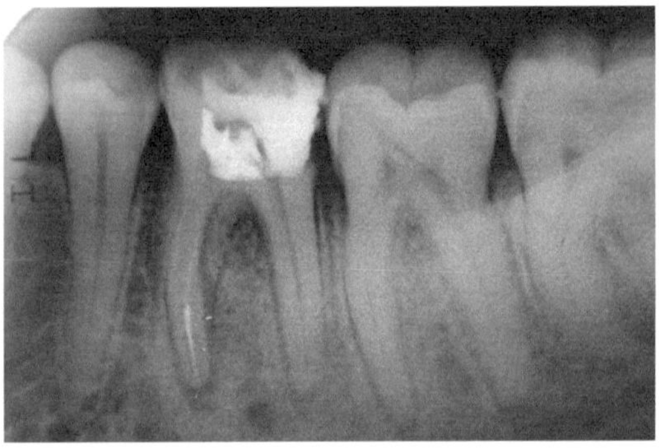

Fig. 14.23 Endodontic instrument fractured in the apical trio of the lower right first molar tooth

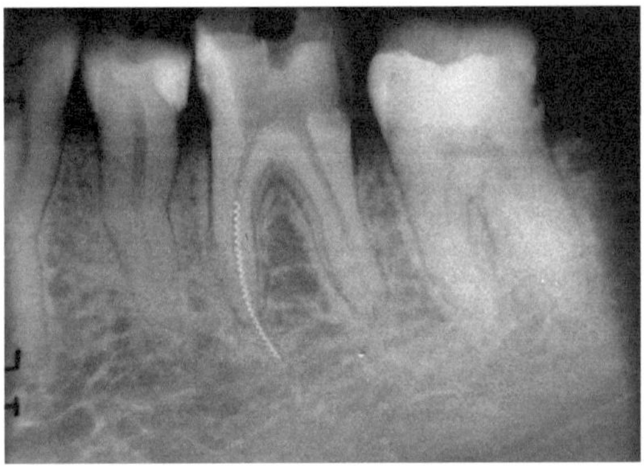

Fig. 14.24 Broken endodontic instrument by removing the lower left first molar from its apical

As explained above, intraoral radiography is frequently used in endodontics. Therefore, intraoral radiographs should be interpreted carefully.

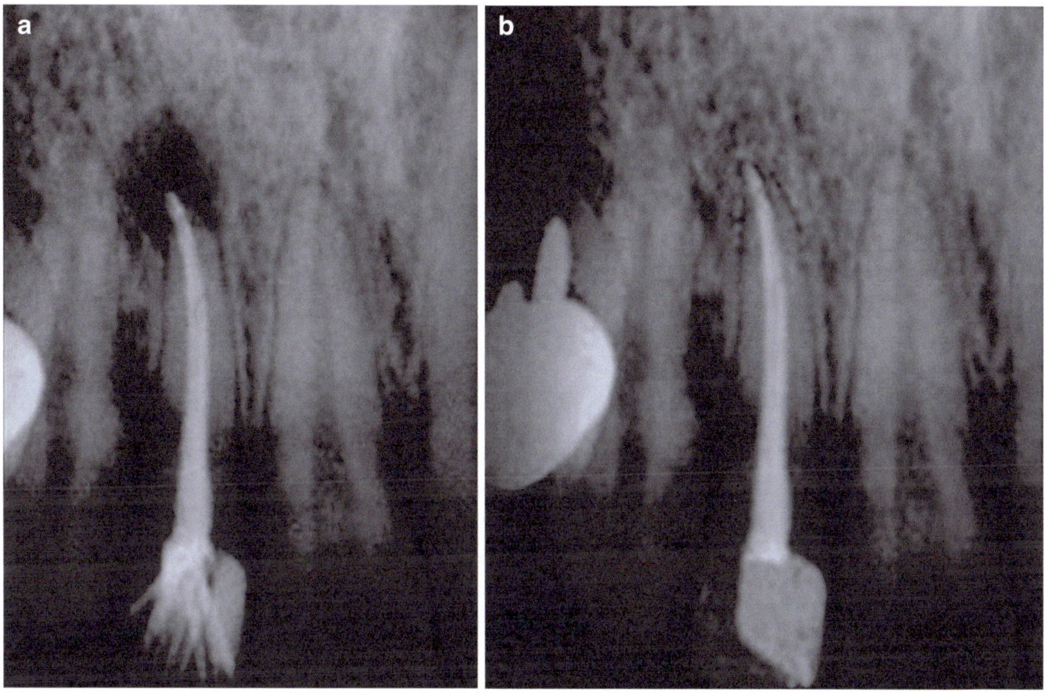

Fig. 14.25 (**a**) Radiolucent lesion at the apical of the upper right lateral tooth. (**b**) It is observed that the radiolucent lesion at the apical of the upper right lateral tooth completely healed after 6 months

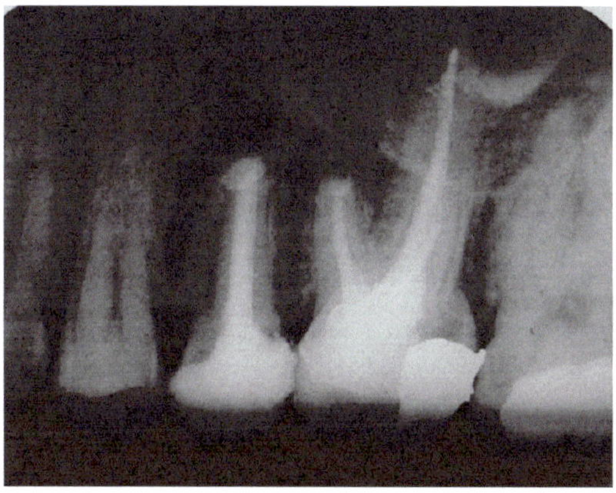

Fig. 14.26 Control of retrograde fillings by radiography after apical resection of upper right first molar

14.3 Imaging Other Common Pathologies of the Oral Cavity

14.3.1 Identification of Periodontal Diseases

If gingivitis is not treated, it can progress with the destruction of supporting tissues, and cause periodontitis. Periodontitis is characterized by a chronic inflammation produced in response to multiple types of the bacterial population, and bone resorption associated with periodontal disease in the subgingival area [25]. For the diagnosis of periodontal diseases, radiography is used to evaluate bone levels, in addition to periodontal probing and clinical examination [26]. The amount of bone present, the condition of the alveolar crests, the furcation areas of the teeth, the areas with bone resorption, and the periodontal interval can be examined with radiography. Periapical and bitewing radiographs are widely used today in determining the level and type of alveolar bone resorption due to its advantages such as relatively low cost and low radiation dose. In addition, panoramic radiography allows examining the entire dentition including the lower and upper jaw, and aid in the differential diagnosis of localized or generalized periodontitis. However, these two-dimensional imaging methods are insufficient in detecting intra-osseous defects with a three-dimensional configuration due to the superposition of intact

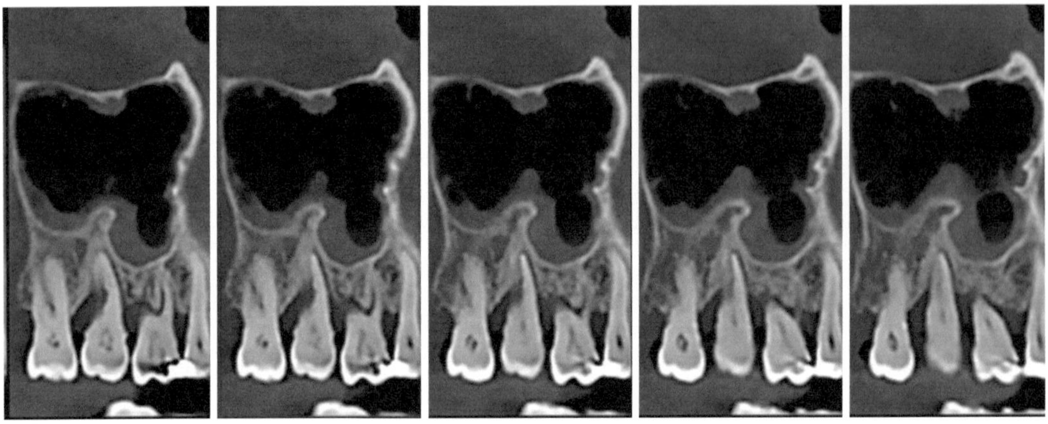

Fig. 14.27 The CBCT images showing periodontal bone destruction with sinus mucosal thickening

bone walls over the resorption areas. It is not possible to detect the buccal and lingual bone levels and the morphology of bone deformities. On the other hand, CBCT, which is an advanced imaging technique that provides cross-sectional and three-dimensional analysis of bone structures in the area, allows the visualization of the defects in the teeth and periodontal bone [27] (Fig. 14.27).

Cases of chronic periodontitis are usually seen with periodontal resorption associated with high amounts of plaque and calculus. Clinical symptoms are considered to be the direct effects of inflammation, pocket formation, loss of attachments and bone loss, and subgingival plaque deposition to the area. Aggressive periodontitis has a rapid progression rate and is seen mostly at early ages. When permanent teeth are affected, it is characterized by vertical directional bone defects and rapid bone resorption around the first molar and incisor teeth [28].

14.3.2 Endodontic-Periodontal Lesions

These lesions also develop when an endodontically induced periapical lesion is present in a tooth affected by periodontitis. Interpretation of individual periapical or lateral lesions is of clinical importance in determining the cause of the lesion and recommending appropriate diagnostic procedures to be followed to confirm this affecting factor. The initial phases of periradicular bone resorption of endodontic origin are usually limited only to the cancellous bone. Therefore, it cannot be detected on radiographs unless the cortical bone is also affected [29].

14.3.3 Imaging of Impacted Third Molar Teeth

Panoramic tomography and CBCT are used to evaluate the anatomy and position of the third molar teeth before treatment, to view the pathologies associated with the teeth, and to determine the age in forensic dentistry. Embedded third molars can be classified according to their inclination to the long axis of the second molar (for instance; mesioangular, distoangular, or horizontal) based on the Archer classification for maxillary third molars. Embedded third mandibular molar teeth are classified as vertical, mesioangular, horizontal, and distoangular according to Winter's classification based on the angle between the second molar tooth. The mesioangular position is the most common position among these positions [30]. The third molar teeth trigger resorption in the distal surface of the second molar teeth, and inflammation at the interface, leading to marginal bone loss. This may cause necrosis and tooth loss in the second molar teeth in the future. Intraoral radiographs taken from the area contribute to the observation of the amount of bone tissue surrounding the tooth, the location and configuration of the neighboring tooth,

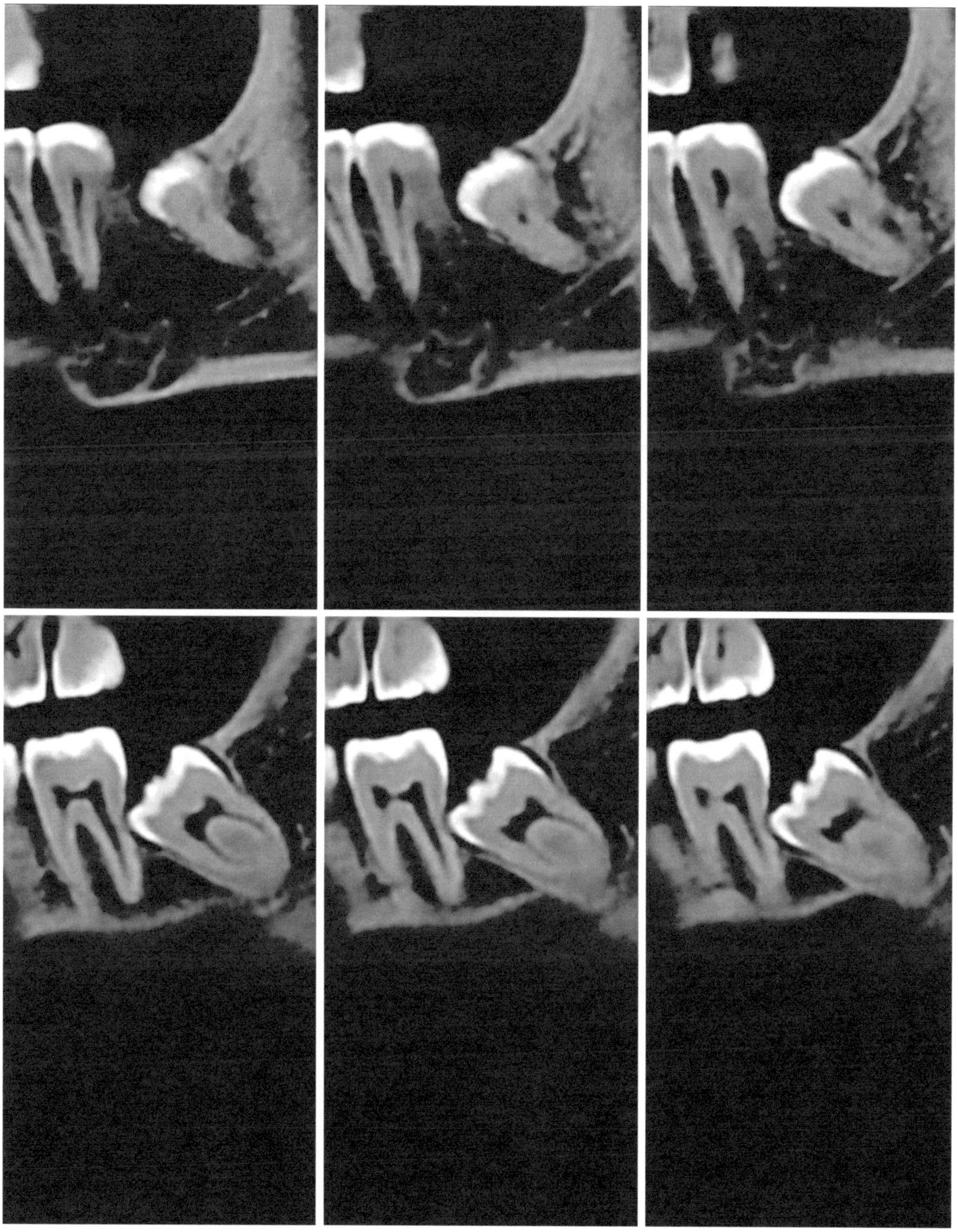

Fig. 14.28 Lower impacted third molar tooth and its relationship with the neighboring tooth

and early diagnosis [31–33]. On the other hand, periapical radiography has limitations such as the inability to clearly define the proximity to the mandibular canal, the area being too large to be viewed with periapical radiography, and the effect on the perceived position in the radiography due to the angulation of the film. Therefore, panoramic radiography is mostly preferred as an imaging technique for appropriate surgical operation planning [34] (Fig. 14.28).

14.3.4 Evaluation of the Relationship Between Lower Molar Teeth and Inferior Alveolar Nerve Canal

The apex of the lower molar roots or the embedded third molar teeth may be in close relationship with the inferior alveolar nerve canal. The inferior alveolar canal should be viewed comprehensively and its location should be determined to avoid possible nerve damage before planned surgical operations, implant placement, and root canal treatment [35].

Panoramic radiography is used as a useful scanning tool to evaluate the anatomical relationship between the teeth and the inferior alveolar nerve canal, which has advantages such as relatively low radiation dose, wide representation of oral structures, and easy accessibility for clinicians. On the other hand, it is insufficient to understand the buccal, lingual, or inter-root position of the roots due to the lower image resolution, the superposition of the anatomical structures, and the two-dimensional information [36]. In cases where the lower molar teeth are in close relationship with the inferior alveolar canal, CBCT should be used to examine the area in detail before the surgical operation of extraction [37] (Fig. 14.29).

14.3.5 Relationship of Upper Molar Teeth and Periapical Lesions with Maxillary Sinus

The maxillary sinus located in the maxillary bone is the largest paranasal sinus. The maxillary sinus has a pyramid shape with its base adjacent to the nasal cavity and its apex pointing towards the zygoma. The inner surface of the sinus cavity is adhered to the periosteum and is covered by a thin respiratory mucosa with a thickness of approximately 1 mm. This soft tissue is not visible on radiographs under normal conditions. However, thickening may occur due to an infectious disease, an allergic process, or a pathological factor; and as a result, a change in the sinus is observed in the radiography. The lower border of the maxillary sinus cavity is closely related to the alveolar crest and upper molar tooth roots. This anatomical proximity of the root apices with the sinus causes periapical lesions to affect the sinus. On the other hand, complications such as perforation of the sinus floor and dislocation of the tooth into the sinus cavity may occur during the surgical extraction of the upper third molar teeth. CBCT helps to evaluate the preoperative and postoperative status of the maxillary sinuses and to resolve the etiology of the relationship between the periapical lesion and the sinus [38–41] (Fig. 14.30a, b).

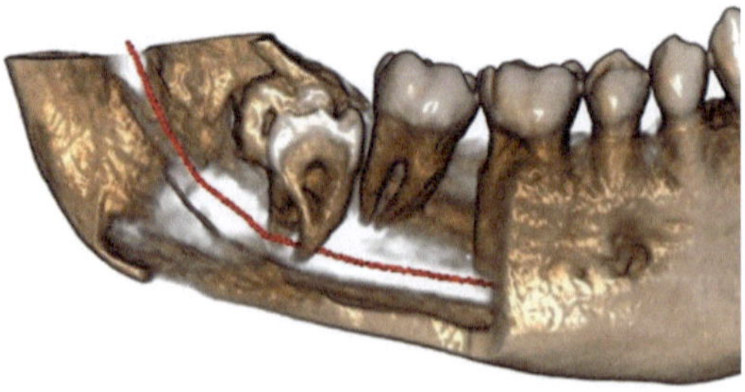

Fig. 14.29 Reconstruction of roots associated with the inferior alveolar canal

14.3.6 Radicular Cyst

Radicular cysts are one of the most common odontogenic lesions developing in the maxillofacial area. They are caused by inflammation due to epithelial debris or necrotic pulp in the periodontal space. Since it is mostly observed at the apex of the relevant tooth, it can also be called a periapical cyst. It is not possible to detect the lesion with clinical examination when it is small and there is no pain; however, it is identified as an incidental finding on radiographic examination. It is more common in the anterior maxillary region. Unless it is infected, it can progress slowly and asymptomatically, and expand. Radicular cysts are difficult to distinguish from a pre-existing chronic apical periodontitis lesion in the radiography. While small cystic lesions can often heal with endodontic treatment, a surgical operation is also necessary for the treatment of larger lesions. Both periapical radiography and panoramic radiography can be used in the diagnosis of these

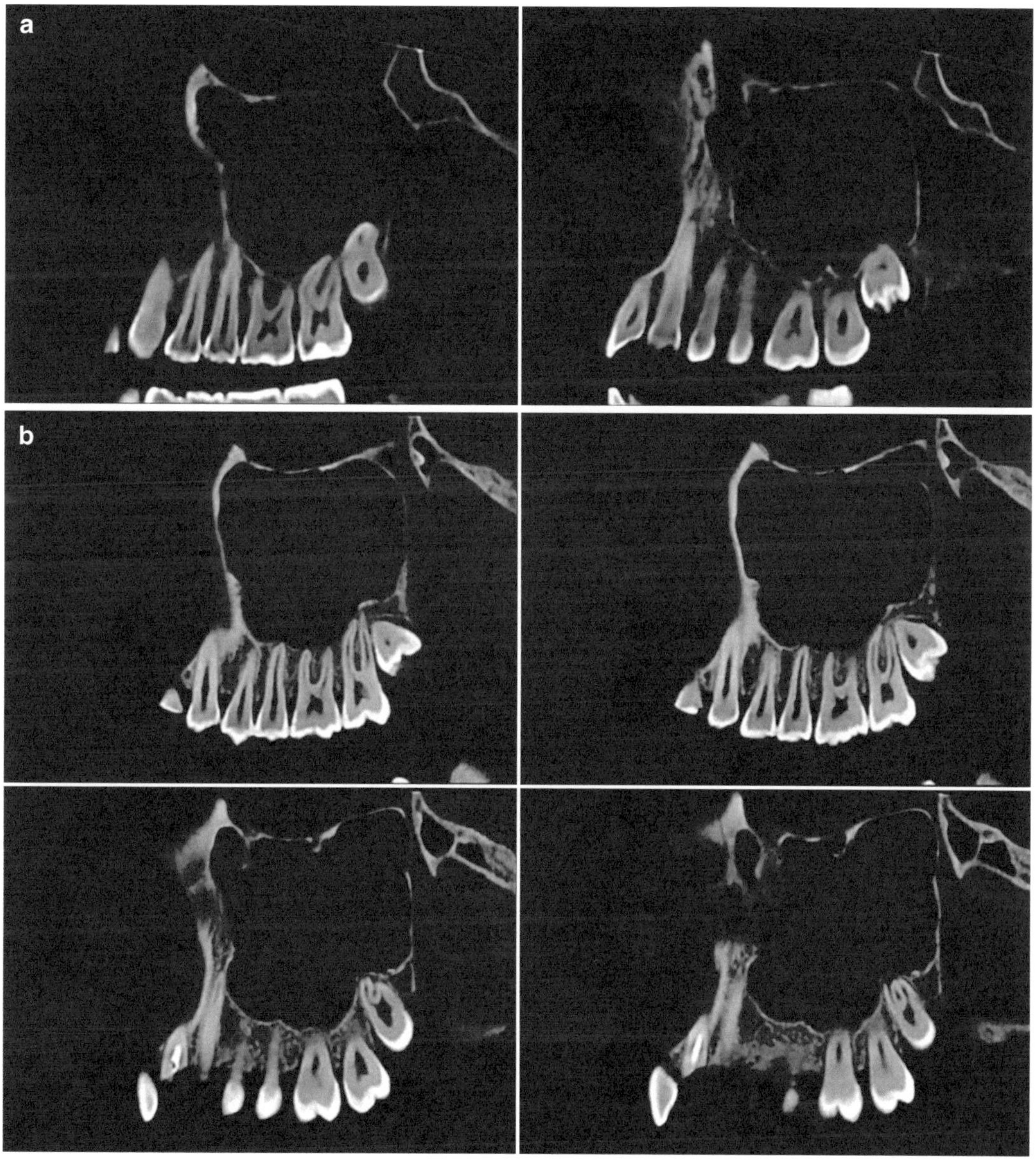

Fig. 14.30 (**a**) Sinus mucosal thickening on CBCT, (**b**) Maxillary third molar psoitions on CBCT

lesions, and the postoperative follow-up process. If the margins of the lesion involve anatomical formations, or if they are near, CBCT imaging should be used as a support [42, 43] (Fig. 14.31).

14.3.7 Dentigerous Cyst

A dentigerous cyst is a developmental-odontogenic cyst usually observed adjacent to the crown of an embedded or unerupted tooth. It is the second most common type of cyst among odontogenic cysts observed in the oral area. It is believed to occur due to the accumulation of fluid between the thinned enamel epithelium and the crown of the tooth. Dentigerous cysts are usually asymptomatic and are detected incidentally during the evaluation of an unerupted tooth. They are mostly observed in mandibular molar teeth, maxillary canines, and mandibular premolar teeth. In

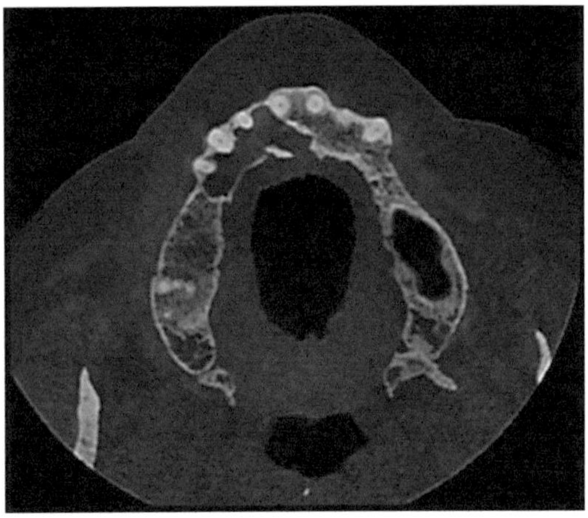

Fig. 14.31 A large radicular lesion on axial CBCT

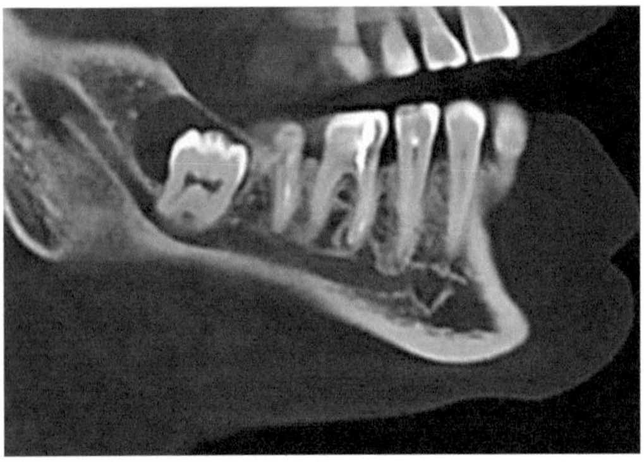

Fig. 14.32 Dentigerous cyst

the panoramic radiography, a unilocular radiolucent lesion is observed around the embedded tooth crown surrounded by a thin sclerotic band. Root resorption can be observed in other teeth adjacent to the lesion [44, 45] (Fig. 14.32).

14.3.8 Lateral Periodontal Cyst

The lateral periodontal cyst is a developmental odontological type of cyst with a low incidence. They are intraosseous lesions located adjacent to the root of a vital tooth and are generally asymptomatic. They are usually seen in the mandibular canine-premolar teeth region. Radiologically, they are defined as a well-circumscribed round or oval radiolucent area less than 1 cm in diameter with sclerotic edges [46, 47].

14.3.9 Odontogenic Keratocyst

Odontogenic keratocyst with aggressive clinical features and high recurrence potential is observed in the mandibular corpus and ramus area, maxillary canine, and third molar teeth. It originates from dental lamina debris and accounts for 10% of developmental odontogenic cysts. No symptoms appear until bone expansion occurs or becomes infected. It is observed as a well-defined, unilocular radiolucent lesion on radiography; however, it can also be observed as multilocular. Satellite cysts may accompany the fibrous wall of the cyst [48–50].

14.3.10 Nasopalatine Duct Cyst

Nasopalatine duct cyst arising from embryogenic epithelial residues in the nasopalatine canal is one of the most common nonodontogenic cysts in the oral cavity. It may also be called an incisive duct cyst. This cyst, which constitutes 1% of the cysts observed in the maxilla, is located intraosseous in the midline of the anterior palate. In addition to its spontaneous proliferation, it can also be stimulated by factors such as local trauma and infection. This cyst creates a heart-shaped image at the apex of the upper anterior tooth roots on the periapical radiography. Cone-beam computed tomography helps detailed evaluation of the nasopalatine area with its three-dimensional CT-based surgical planning and measurement potential [51, 52] (Fig. 14.33).

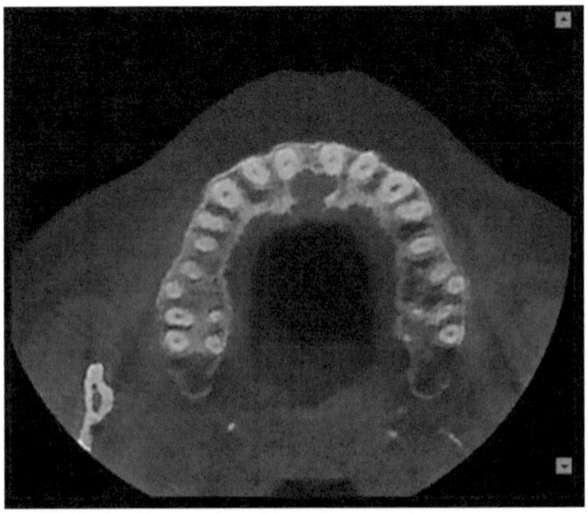

Fig. 14.33 Nasopalatine duct cyst

References

1. Gröndahl HG, Huumonen S. Radiographic manifestations of periapical inflammatory lesions: how new radiological techniques may improve endodontic diagnosis and treatment planning. Endod Top. 2004;8(1):55–67.
2. Deepak B, Subash T, Narmatha V, Anamika T, Snehil T, Nandini D. Imaging techniques in endodontics: an overview. J Clin Imag Sci. 2012;2:13.
3. Venskutonis T, Plotino G, Juodzbalys G, Mickevičienė L. The importance of cone-beam computed tomography in the management of endodontic problems: a review of the literature. J Endod. 2014;40(12):1895–901.
4. White SCPM. Oral radiology, intraoral radiographic examinations. Principles and Interpretation. 5th ed. Amsterdam: Elsevier; 2004.
5. Basrani B. Endodontic radiology. Hoboken, NJ: Wiley; 2012.
6. Langland O, Langlais R. Principles of dental imaging. 1st ed. Baltimore: Lippincott Williams; 1997.
7. Gröndahl HG, Gröndahl K. Subtraction radiography for the diagnosis of periodontal bone lesions. Oral Surg Oral Med Oral Pathol. 1983;55(2):208–13.
8. Reddy MS, Jeffcoat MK. Digital subtraction radiography. Dent Clin N Am. 1993;37(4):553–65.
9. Ellwood RP, Davies RM, Worthington HV. Evaluation of a dental subtraction radiography system. J Periodontal Res. 1997;32(2):241–8.
10. Mol A, Dunn SM. The performance of projective standardization for digital subtraction radiography. Oral Surg Oral Med Oral Pathol Oral Radiol Endod. 2003;96(3):373–82.
11. Lehmann T, Gröndahl H-G, Benn D. Computer-based registration for digital subtraction in dental radiology. Dentomaxillofac Radiol. 2000;29(6):323–46.
12. Dubrez B, Jacot-Descombes S, Cimasoni G. Reliability of a paralleling instrument for dental radiographs. Oral Surg Oral Med Oral Pathol Oral Radiol Endod. 1995;80(3):358–64.
13. Gray CF, Redpath TW, Smith FW, Staff RT. Advanced imaging: magnetic resonance imaging in implant dentistry: a review. Clin Oral Implants Res. 2003;14(1):18–27.
14. Hayakawa Y, Yamamoto K, Kousuge Y, Kobayashi N, Wakoh M, Sekiguchi H, et al. Clinical validity of the interactive and low-dose three-dimensional dentoalveolar imaging system, tuned-aperture computed tomography. Bull Tokyo Dent Coll. 2003;44(3):159–67.
15. Patel S, Dawood A, Ford TP, Whaites E. The potential applications of cone-beam computed tomography in the management of endodontic problems. Int Endod J. 2007;40(10):818–30.
16. Vandenberghe B, Jacobs R, Yang J. Detection of periodontal bone loss using digital intraoral and cone-beam computed tomography images: an in vitro assessment of bony and/or infrabony defects. Dentomaxillofac Radiol. 2008;37(5):252–60.
17. Tyndall DA, Rathore S. Cone-beam CT diagnostic applications: caries, periodontal bone assessment, and endodontic applications. Dent Clin N Am. 2008;52(4):825–41.
18. Orhan K, Aksoy U, Kalender A. Cone-beam computed tomographic evaluation of spontaneously healed root fracture. J Endod. 2010;36(9):1584–7.
19. Scarfe WC, Farman AG. What is cone-beam CT and how does it work? Dent Clin N Am. 2008;52(4):707–30.
20. Krennmair G, Ulm C, Lugmayr H. Maxillary sinus septa: incidence, morphology and clinical implications. J Cranio Maxillofac Surg. 1997;25(5):261–5.
21. Pauwels R, Beinsberger J, Collaert B, Theodorakou C, Rogers J, Walker A, et al. Effective dose range for dental cone beam computed tomography scanners. Eur J Radiol. 2012;81(2):267–71.
22. A W. Dental caries: The C.V. Mosby Company; 2004.
23. Sisman Y, Uysal T, Gelgors IE. Hypodontia. Does the prevalence and distribution pattern differ in orthodontic patient Eur J Dent. 2007;1(3):167–73.
24. Sener 1 S, Unlu N, Basciftci FA, Bozdag G. Bilateral geminated teeth with talon cusps: A case report Eur J Dent. 2012;6(4):440–4.
25. Hoare A, Soto C, Rojas-Celis V, Bravo D. Chronic inflammation as a link between periodontitis and carcinogenesis. Med Inform. 2019;2019:1029857.
26. Gasner NS, Schure RS. Periodontal disease. In: StatPearls [Internet]. Treasure Island, FL: StatPearls; 2020.
27. Suphanantachat S, Tantikul K, Tamsailom S, Kosalagood P, Nisapakultorn K, Tavedhikul K. Comparison of clinical values between cone-beam computed tomography and conventional intraoral radiography in periodontal and infrabony defect assessment. Dentomaxillofac Radiol. 2017;46(6):20160461.
28. Miller K, Treloar T, Guelmann M, Rody WJ Jr, Shaddox LM. Clinical characteristics of localized aggressive periodontitis in the primary dentition. J Clin Pediatr Dent. 2018;42(2):95–102.
29. Shenoy N, Shenoy A. Endo-perio lesions: diagnosis and clinical considerations. Indian J Dent Res. 2010;21(4):579.
30. Khojastepour L, Khaghaninejad MS, Hasanshahi R, Forghani M, Ahrari F. Does the Winter or Pell and Gregory classification system indicate the apical position of impacted mandibular third molars. J Oral Maxillofac Surg. 2019;77(11):2222.e1–9.
31. Matzen LH, Schropp L, Spin-Neto R, Wenzel A. Radiographic signs of pathology determining removal of an impacted mandibular third molar assessed in a panoramic image or CBCT. Dentomaxillofac Radiol. 2017;46(1):20160330.
32. Loureiro R, Sumi D, Tames H, Ribeiro S, Soares C, Gomes R, et al. Cross-sectional imaging of third molar–related abnormalities. Am J Neuroradiol. 2020;41(11):1966–74.
33. Franco A, Vetter F, de Fátima CE, Fernandes Â, Thevissen P. Comparing third molar root development

staging in panoramic radiography, extracted teeth, and cone-beam computed tomography. Int J Leg Med. 2020;134(1):347–53.
34. Juodzbalys G, Daugela P. Mandibular third molar impaction: a review of the literature and a proposal of a classification. J Oral Maxillofac Res. 2013;4(2):e1.
35. Patil V, Pai KM, Vineetha R, Rajagopal K, Dkhar W. Comparison of conventional techniques and higher imaging modalities in the evaluation of the relation between the third molar and inferior alveolar nerve canal: a pilot study. Contemp Clin Dent. 2019;10(1):93.
36. Patel PS, Shah JS, Dudhia BB, Butala PB, Jani YV, Macwan RS. Comparison of panoramic radiograph and cone-beam computed tomography findings for impacted mandibular third molar root and inferior alveolar nerve canal relation. Ind J Dent Res. 2020;31(1):91.
37. Saraydar-Baser R, Dehghani-Tafti M, Navab-Azam A, Ezoddini-Ardakani F, Nayer S, Safi Y, et al. Comparison of the diagnostic value of CBCT and Digital Panoramic Radiography with surgical findings to determine the proximity of an impacted third mandibular molar to the inferior alveolar nerve canal. J Med Life. 2015;8(Spec Issue 3):83.
38. Whyte A, Boeddinghaus R. The maxillary sinus: physiology, development and imaging anatomy. Dentomaxillofac Radiol. 2019;48(8):20190205.
39. Jung Y-H, Cho B-H. Assessment of maxillary third molars with panoramic radiography and cone-beam computed tomography. Imag Sci Dent. 2015;45(4):233.
40. Goller-Bulut D, Sekerci A-E, Köse E, Sisman Y. Cone-beam computed tomographic analysis of maxillary premolars and molars to detect the relationship between periapical and marginal bone loss and mucosal thickness of maxillary sinus. Med Oral Patol Oral Cir Bucal. 2015;20(5):e572.
41. Chavez-Lazo YE, Arriola-Guillén LE, Rodríguez-Cárdenas YA, Ruiz-Mora GA, Guerrero ME. Morphological variations of the maxillary sinus floor adjacent to periapical chronic injuries. Ind J Dent Res. 2019;30(3):381.
42. Bava FA, Umar D, Bahseer B, Baroudi K. Bilateral radicular cyst in the mandible: an unusual case report. J Int Oral Health. 2015;7(2):61.
43. Bahadure RN, Khubchandani M, Thosar NR, Singh RK. Radicular cyst of primary tooth associated with maxillary sinus. BMJ Case Rep. 2013;2013:bcr2013009146.
44. Borrás-Ferreres J, Sánchez-Torres A, Aguirre-Urizar J-M, Gay-Escoda C. Dentigerous cyst with parietal and intracystic calcifications: a case report and literature review. J Clin Exp Dent. 2018;10(3):e296.
45. Vasiapphan H, Christopher PJ, Kengasubbiah S, Shenoy V, Kumar S, Paranthaman A. Bilateral dentigerous cyst in impacted mandibular third molars: a case report. Cureus. 2018;10(12):e3691.
46. Carvalho LFC, Lima CF, LAG C, AAH B, Almeida JD. Lateral periodontal cyst: a case report and literature review. J Oral Maxillofac Res. 2011;1:e5.
47. Ramesh R, Sadasivan A. Lateral periodontal cyst—a diagnostic dilemma: report of a rare case with CBCT and histological findings. Int J Surg Case Rep. 2020;75:454–7.
48. Shastry SP, Pandeshwar P, Padmashree S, Kumar NN, Garg S, Sanjay C. Imaging characteristic of 11 lesions of odontogenic keratocyst in the Indian subpopulation: a cone-beam computed tomography experience. Contemp Clin Dent. 2020;11(1):20.
49. Arshad F. Syndromic odontogenic keratocyst: a case report and review of the literature. J Int Soc Prevent Commun Dent. 2016;6(1):84.
50. Bruno-Teixeira-Gonçalves Rodrigues M-S, Israel K-L-MM, Giulianna-Lima Pinheiro RC. Peripheral odontogenic keratocyst: report of two new cases and review of the literature. J Clin Exp Dent. 2020;12(10):e1005.
51. Dedhia P, Dedhia S, Dhokar A, Desai A. Nasopalatine duct cyst. Case Rep Dent. 2013;2013:869516.
52. Al-Shamiri HM, Elfaki S, Al-Maweri SA, Alaizari NA, Tarakji B. Development of nasopalatine duct cyst to dental implant placement. N Am J Med Sci. 2016;8(1):13.

15 Micro-CT in Dentistry

Kaan Orhan, Bora Akat, and Berkan Celikten

15.1 General Introduction of Micro-CT and Nano-CT in Dentistry

Traditionally, the histology has long been a popular approach in dentistry research for resolving the interior microstructure of teeth and alveolar bone samples. It is feasible to get a two-dimensional resolution at the micron level by histological preparation of the materials, such as tissue cutting and chemical staining, but this is destructive and time-consuming. The biological sample cannot usually be utilized for further tests after the permanent changes that occur during histological preparation, such as serial sections, transparency, and dye penetration. As a result, researchers would benefit from an alternate technology that allows three-dimensional studies, such as X-ray microtomography (XMT, commonly known as micro-CT), to examine the internal structure of oral tissues without destroying or shrinking the samples [1, 2].

Radiology has made a breakthrough in the last 50 years, especially with computerized tomography (CT) and the later discovered magnetic resonance imaging (MRI) technique. CT, was discovered in 1972 and is being used routinely today. CT allows visualization of normal and abnormal soft tissue and bone tissues. It is also an ideal method for the determination of calcifications. CT applications in the head and neck region allow the evaluation of inflammation, cysts, benign and malignant tumors. It provides detailed visualization of the nasal cavity, lateral nasal wall, osteomeatal unit, and sinuses before functional endoscopic sinus surgery. Apart from this, it is useful in maxillofacial, reconstructive and orthognathic pre-surgery planning, dental implant applications, trauma, and temporomandibular joint (TMJ) diseases. Compared to conventional imaging methods of CT, it allows visualization of the structure desired to be examined without superposition of the surrounding tissues, high contrast resolution enabling two tissues with different physical densities to be separated from each other more easily, allowing tissue to be visualized in axial, coronal, and sagittal planes, absence of distortion and magnification. It has many advantages such as allowing determination of whether these lesions have a solid or liquid structure by density measurements in the presence of cysts or

K. Orhan (✉)
Department of DentoMaxillofacial Radiology, Faculty of Dentistry, Ankara University, Ankara, Turkey
e-mail: knorhan@dentistry.ankara.edu.tr

B. Akat
Department of Prosthodontics, Faculty of Dentistry, Ankara University, Ankara, Turkey

B. Celikten
Department of Endodontics, Faculty of Dentistry, Ankara University, Ankara, Turkey

A. Delantoni, K. Orhan (eds.), *Atlas of Dentomaxillofacial Anatomical Imaging*,
https://doi.org/10.1007/978-3-030-96840-3_15

tumors. In addition, there are also disadvantages such as the need for contrast agent for imaging soft tissues, giving more radiation than conventional methods, and deterioration of image quality due to scattering of metallic objects in the image.

Computed microtomography (Micro-CT) devices can select the field of view (FOV) according to the size of the area to be examined, and in this way, higher resolution images can be obtained when working in smaller areas. Currently, in vitro and in vivo micro-CT devices are available, and the varying FOV ratios in these devices determine the area to be examined and the resolution to be obtained. Micro-CT systems use microfocal X-ray source and high resolution detectors to create 3D reconstructions of samples. The main parts of the device are the X-ray tube, a computer-controlled stepping motor that rotates the sample fixed on it at certain intervals, an image intensifier that concentrates the X-ray in the environment on the camera sensor, a CCD camera that converts the X-rays falling on it into image data, an image collector and a computer to control all the system.

The scanned object rotates on a bed while the system takes multiple X-ray shadow transition images from different angles. Using these shadow images, the reconstruction of the cross-sectional images of the object is processed and a three-dimensional model of the internal microstructure and density in the selected height range is created in the transition images. With reconstruction (reconstruction), internal morphological parameters can also be calculated. Traditional medical CT scanners allow three-dimensional imaging. The three-dimensional imaging of anatomical landmarks can be meaured without using sample preparation steps. The spatial resolution (resolution) of Medical Computed Tomographs (CT) is 1–2 mm, which corresponds to 1–10 mm^3 voxel (three-dimensional pixel) size. Micro-CT, on the other hand, enable spatial resolution of less than 10 μm, reaching 1×10^{-6} mm^3 voxel size. Micro-CT is currently used in biomedical research, materials science, pharmaceutical drug development and production, composites, dental research, electronic components, geology, zoology, botany, construction materials, paper production, and many other fields.

15.2 The Application of Micro-CT in Dentistry

In dentistry, there are a variety of samples that can be evaluated directly utilizing micro-CT. Mineralized tissues with a greater attenuation coefficient, such as teeth and bone, polymers, biomaterial scaffolds, and even high-density materials like metal implants and ceramics, are common examples of these samples. Micro-CT imaging can now be performed on soft tissues such as periodontal blood vessels that have been perfused with a contrast agent, as long as the contrast agent has a higher density than the surrounding tissue. With the rapid advancement of micro-CT systems over the last decade, the latest generation of systems, such as SkyScan nano-CT® and Phoenix nanotom®, now allow for even higher spatial resolution at the submicron level. Furthermore, in vivo imaging of small live animals has become available for long-term investigation of developmental deformities or pathology of the jaw.

15.2.1 Gap Formations for Dental Materials

Gaps and bubbles are imperfections in dental materials that impair their mechanical qualities. The gaps can be assessed for root canal therapy, but they can also be analyzed in dental composite replacement materials.

Although the composite structure has adequate mechanical properties at first, gaps can impair the repairs' performance under fatigue loading. Internal gaps can impair the composite's durability, which can lead to fracture and clinical failure in restorations. Furthermore, an increase in gaps in the composite mass, as well as further staining of the restoration, can result in higher water absorption (Fig. 15.1).

For prosthodontic restorations, the internal gap between restoration and abutment tooth is significant. Also, the gap on the finish line is a

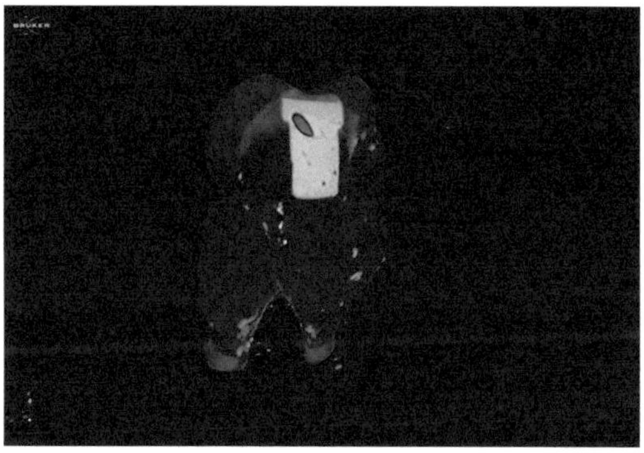

Fig. 15.1 Gap (void) formation in restorative researches

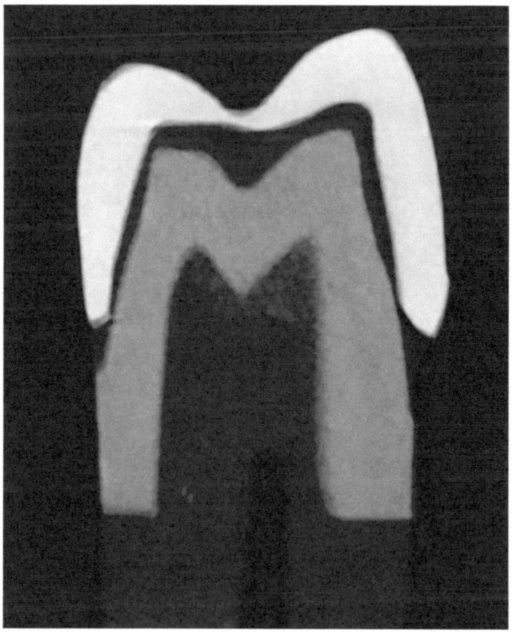

Fig. 15.2 Gap (void) between crown and abutment tooth

subject that has been widely evaluated. Due to the thickness of the gap between restoration and tooth, the strain of the cement is affected. And the improper thickness of cement gap may cause decementation, micro-leakage, and carious formation (Fig. 15.2).

Micro-organisms from gutta and outer coverings, or directly from the dentin can be important factors in root canal treatment and healing (Fig. 15.3). These factors have led and also demnaded for micro-leakage studies in endodontics (Figs. 15.4 and 15.5) [3, 4].

15.2.2 Evaluations in Implantology

Dental implants' evaluations are another key application of micro-CT in dental research. A high-resolution 3D model of peri-implant bone created using micro-CT scanning could be used to assess treatment choices such as implant insertion techniques, antibiotics, antibacterial coatings, and anti-resorbing coatings on peri-implant bone remodeling and adaption (Fig. 15.6). Furthermore, in vivo micro-CT (e.g. SkyScan 1276) gives tiny animals a minimal radiation dosage with implant therapy, allowing for numerous scans in longitudinal preclinical research without the possibility of undesirable radiation-induced side effects.

The region of interest where the bone-implant contact remains has gotten a lot of attention from researchers. It used to be a 2D histological investigation (Fig. 15.7), but it has now evolved into a 3D non-invasive method. Here is a diagram of how to choose 3D volumes of interest for morphometric analysis in the peri-implant bone region.

The 3D VOIs were mostly made up of trabecular bone, which was chosen using interpolated cross-sections and proprietary processing. In each section, irregular anatomic regions of interest (ROIs) can be created, excluding cortical bone in the ring-shaped ROIs and retaining only trabecular features for assessment. Following the recommendations of the American Society of Bone and Mineral Metabolism and Parfitt's system, standard three-dimensional structural parameters of trabecular bone architecture could be estimated using CTAn on these VOIs [3–5].

Metal artefacts, which usually appear as strong streaks surrounding metallic objects, remain a barrier during imaging acquisition and segmentation, despite the numerous applications in the dental implant area. Examples of typical metal artifacts from screw-shaped Ti metal alloy implants include halo, shadow, and blurring effects generated by the material's composition, the implant's sharp-edged or perpendicular shape, and projection images from a single optical axis (Fig. 15.8a, b) [6].

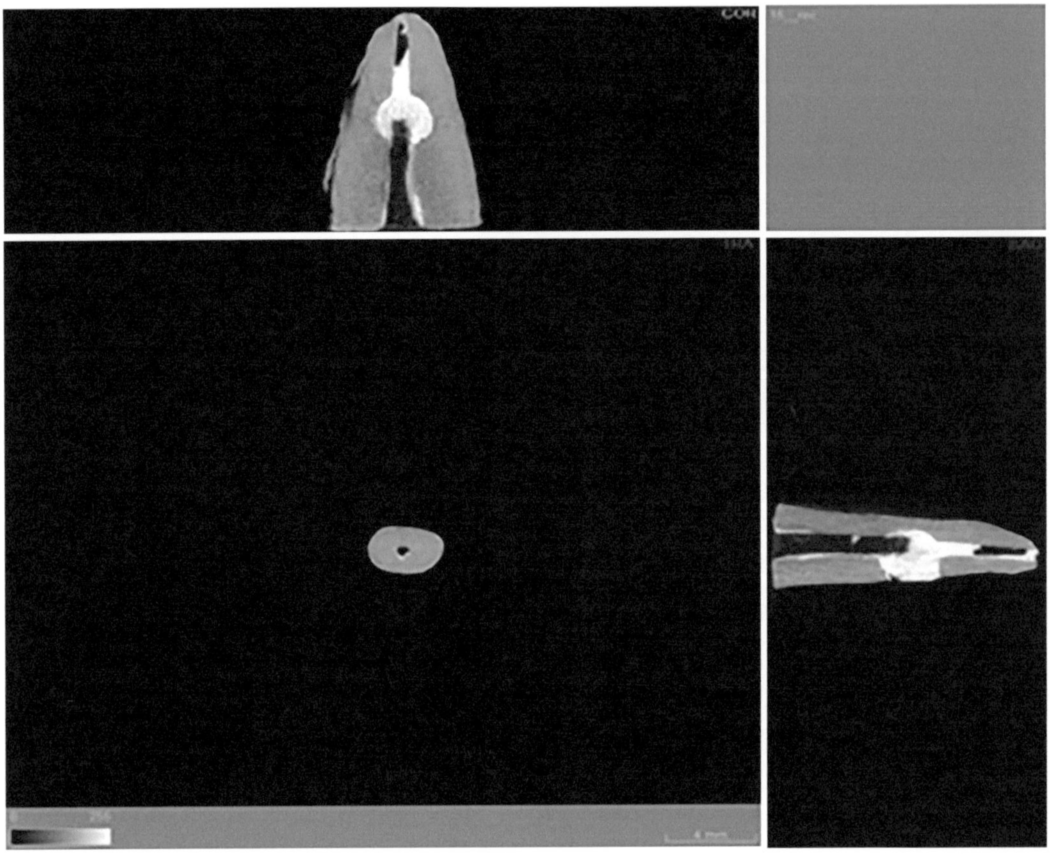

Fig. 15.3 Observation of root canal dressings

Metal artefacts are caused by beam hardening, photon scattering, and photon starvation. According to the authors, implant materials made of pure Ti (titanium), biodegradable PLA (polylactic-coglycolic acid) collagen, or Mg can have relatively favorable imaging results, whereas heavy materials like Zr and Pt, which have higher atomic numbers and higher attenuation coefficients than body tissues, can cause serious imaging artifacts. As a result, obtaining high-contrast pictures is challenging, making it difficult to distinguish bone from implants (Fig. 15.9).

It is always recommended to scan the sample with metal implants at a high voltage, high filtering, a small rotation step, a high frame averaging value, and 360° full scan, round scanning to minimize metal artifacts. Furthermore, according to the current study, an optical axis method of spiral scanning with a unique optical axis will aid in the removal of these artefacts. Metal artifacts, it is also expected, will be decreased to a limited extent as a result of the current development of reconstruction algorism [7, 8].

15.2.3 Carious Formations

Micro-CT has been authorized and widely regarded as a more precise and dependable method of measurement than direct measurement, 3D scanning, or photography. As a result, when measuring the distance between internal and external structures in teeth, such as the crown, enamel, dentin, and pulp chamber, this imaging technique might be recognized as an accurate and valuable tool (Fig. 15.10). However, because of partial volume effects, a lower resolution micro-CT scanning with a pixel size of

10 m is not capable of resolving very thin enamel thicknesses of less than 100 m. As a result, it is usually best to choose a suitable pixel size for the evaluated objects before beginning the study project, which should be 10 times less than the true structure thickness [9].

Furthermore, micro-CT and associated data analysis tools may generate volume information more correctly and reliably. With this quantitative data, it is simple to examine the changes or differences that occurred before and after a specific therapy, such as caries excavation.

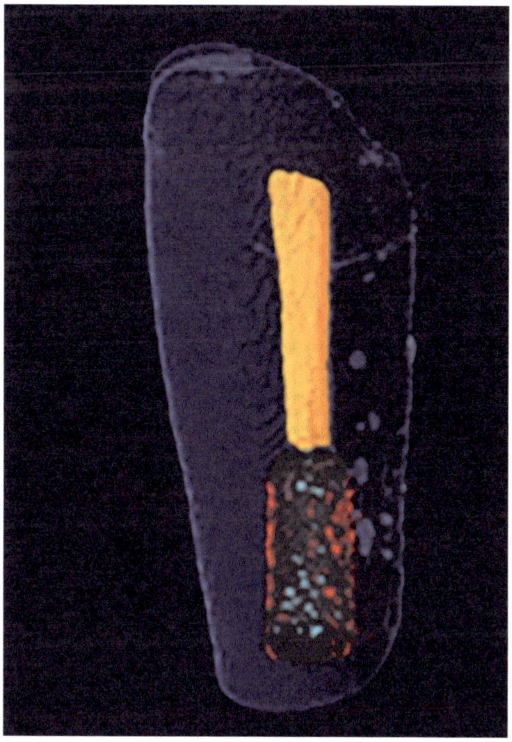

Fig. 15.4 Different root canal sealer materials are filled in one root canal

Another fascinating application is molar incisor hypomineralization (MIH), a structural aberration that affects the quality of tooth enamel and has far-reaching implications for the entire oral health system. Although the ethological elements are still unknown. The use of micro-CT to identify hypo-mineralized enamel in a non-destructive manner has been validated for onset of MIH, which will aid in understanding the pathology and clinical management of MIH lesions. If a density calibration technique is performed, Micro-CT can be used to quantify mineral density of enamel white spot lesions and dentin caries, either using default Hounsfield units or utilizing homogeneous porous hydroxyapatite (HA) phantoms with varying densities (Fig. 15.11).

15.2.4 Tooth Resorption

Micro-CT, in comparison to clinical cone beam CT, can not only give non-invasive 3D imaging of teeth, but also more exact measurements and higher contrast on the devoted anatomical components of teeth, which is especially important when investigating tooth internal/external resorption (Fig. 15.12). A study found that by comparing the morphological characteristics of the pulp cavity, the volume ratio at the horn, floor, and overall regions of the pulp chamber, and the diameters of the buccal and lingual orifices of the root canals between different study groups, it is possible to identify the morphological characteristics of the pulp cavity, the volume ratio at the horn, floor, and overall regions of the pulp chamber, and the

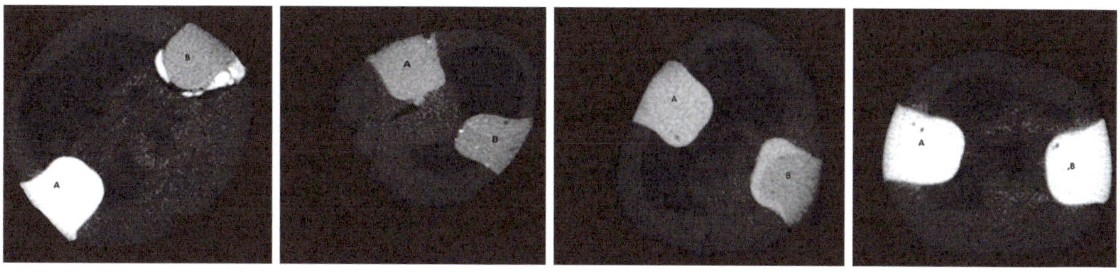

Fig. 15.5 Figures showing voids under and inside the different composite materials

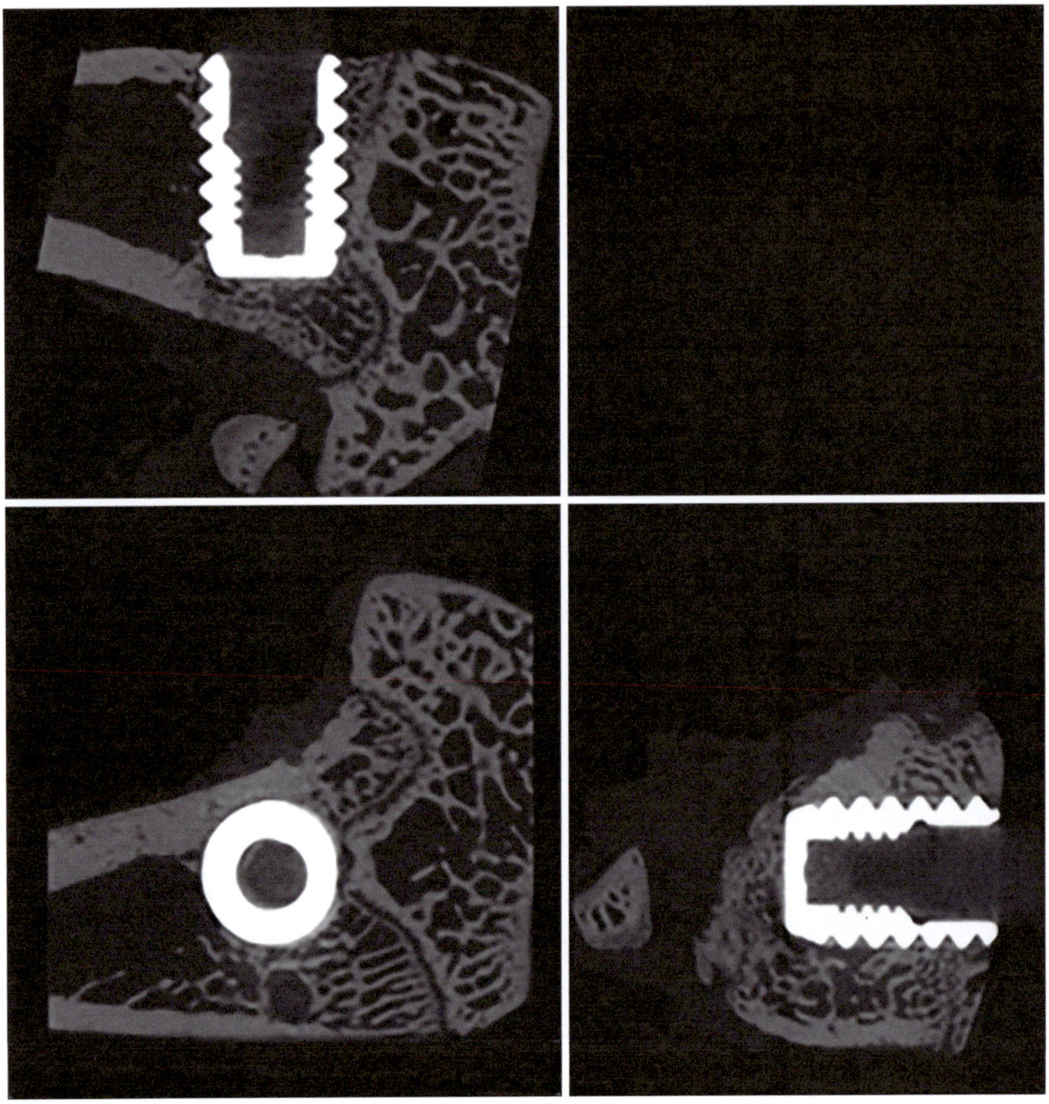

Fig. 15.6 The implant in relation to bone using micro-CT imaging

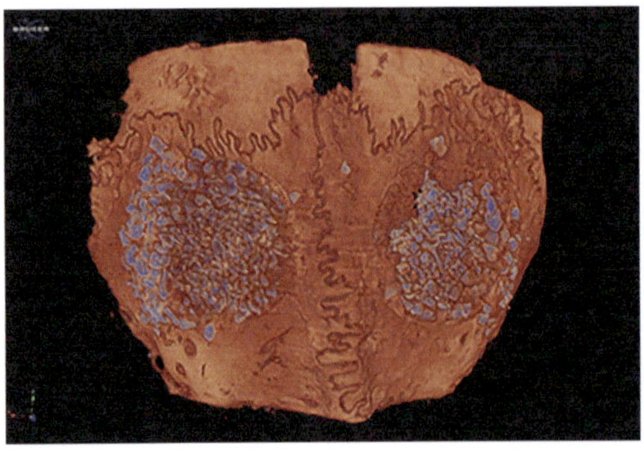

Fig. 15.7 Observation of surgical graft

diameters of the buccal and lingual orifices of the root canals.

It is worth noting that using higher image resolution allows you to see more features within and outside the tooth. This will inevitably result in unnecessary scanning time and resources being wasted. Despite this, the lack of consistency in scanning techniques may result in inconsistent outcomes. As a result, comparing micro-CT and Nano-CT images to identify the cut-off voxel size value for assessing root canal filling gaps is required. A voxel

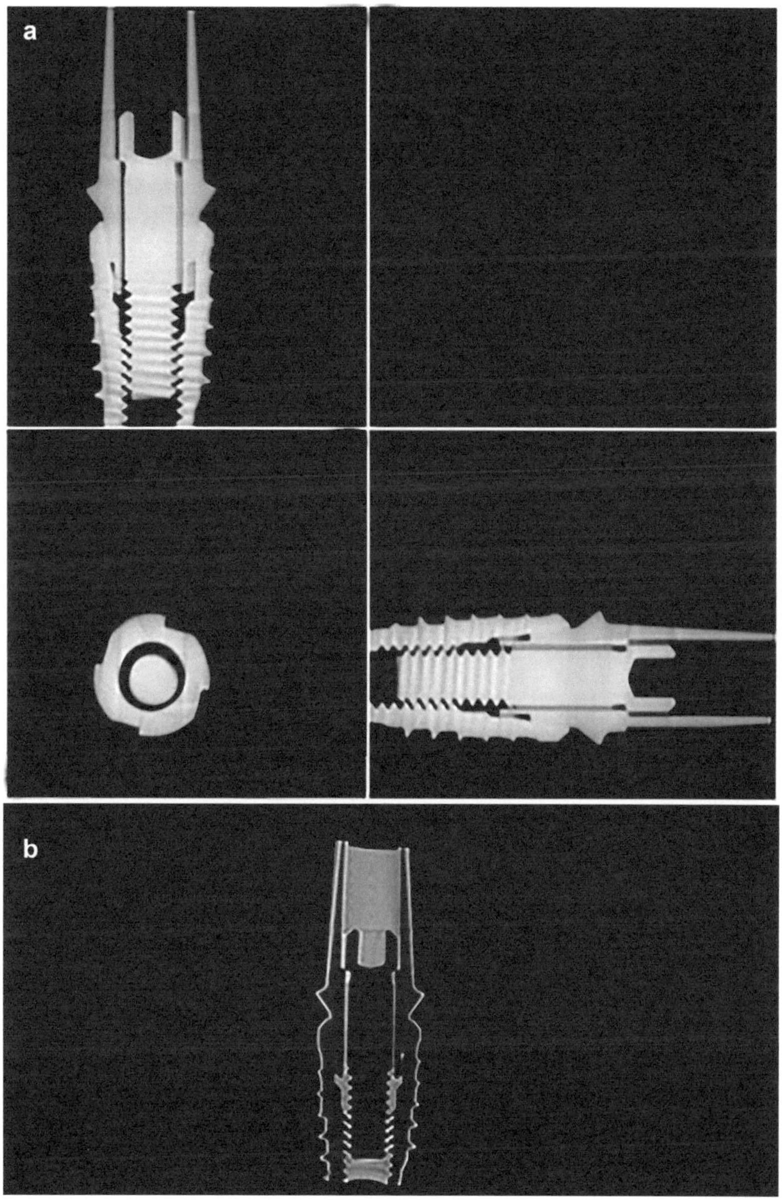

Fig. 15.8 (**a**) Adaptation of implant screw in 2D view. (**b**) Adaptation of implant screw in 3D view

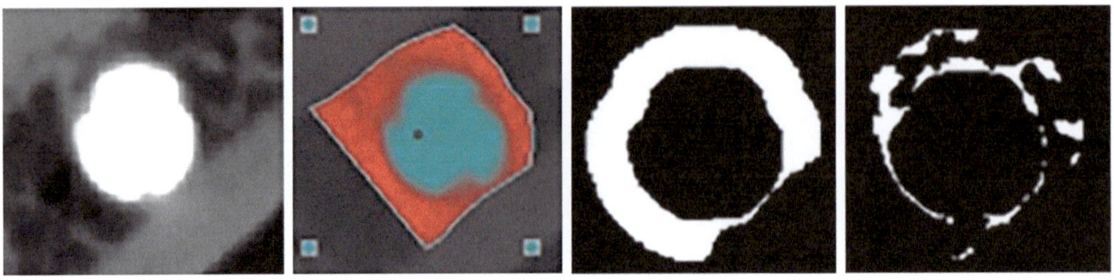

Fig. 15.9 A morphometric quantification of peri-implant bone quality. From left to right, original cross-sectional gray image; manually rough selection of the ROI; binary ROI automatically generated by a custom processing algorithm based on thresholding segmentation for the implant protocols, excluding implant and cortical bone; binary segmentation of trabecular bone in this ROI, from which trabecular morphometric parameters were calculated

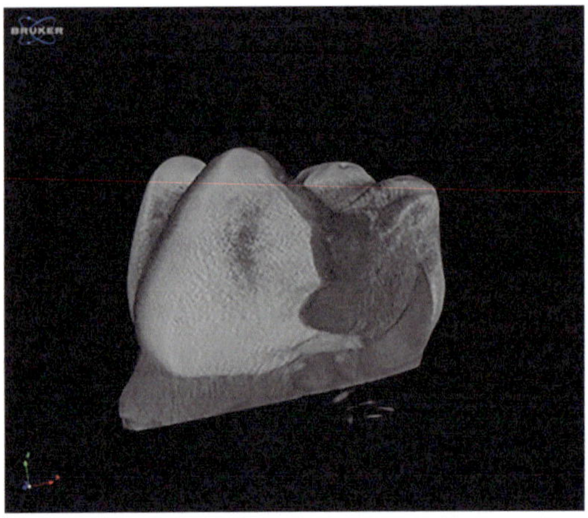

Fig. 15.10 Carious formation in primary tooth

resolution of 11.2 m was defined as a cut-off value in micro-CT imaging for the evaluation of root canal filling gaps, according to a recent study [10].

15.3 Micro-CT Combination with Other Techniques

Due to the poor absorption contrast, it is difficult to visualize the soft tissues, including as blood vessels, periodontal ligaments, and nerve fibers, which is one of the main limitation of the micro CT technique. Contrast-enhanced micro-CT imaging has a growing demand and interest especially for invivo imaging. Superior imaging and quantification of 3D soft tissue under micro CT is now available because to these contrast enhanced agents. An example of such a contrast agent is Angiofil [11].

The virtual finite element analysis allows compression, bending, and screw pull-out tests to be performed directly from the 3D micro-CT dataset. With varying loadings or restorative materials, detailed and valid three-dimensional finite element models of tooth, implant, and peri-implant bone can be created. When this technology can able to process data more rapidily, there will be additions applictions for dental research [4, 12, 13] (Fig. 15.13).

Dual-energy CT is also described as an imaging technique that describes the major contrast changes caused by the staining period, the staining agent utilized, and the organ investigated. Two separate X-ray energy spectra (usually one high and one low energy) will be employed to gain further quantitative information on the accumulation of staining agents within the soft-tissue samples in 3D. For mouse heart and lung ex vivo, it showed shorter staining periods (many hours) and higher resolution contrast (Fig. 15.14).

By obtaining a resonance signal from the hydrogen nucleus, such as water in the bodily tissue, MRI investigates the target region. This

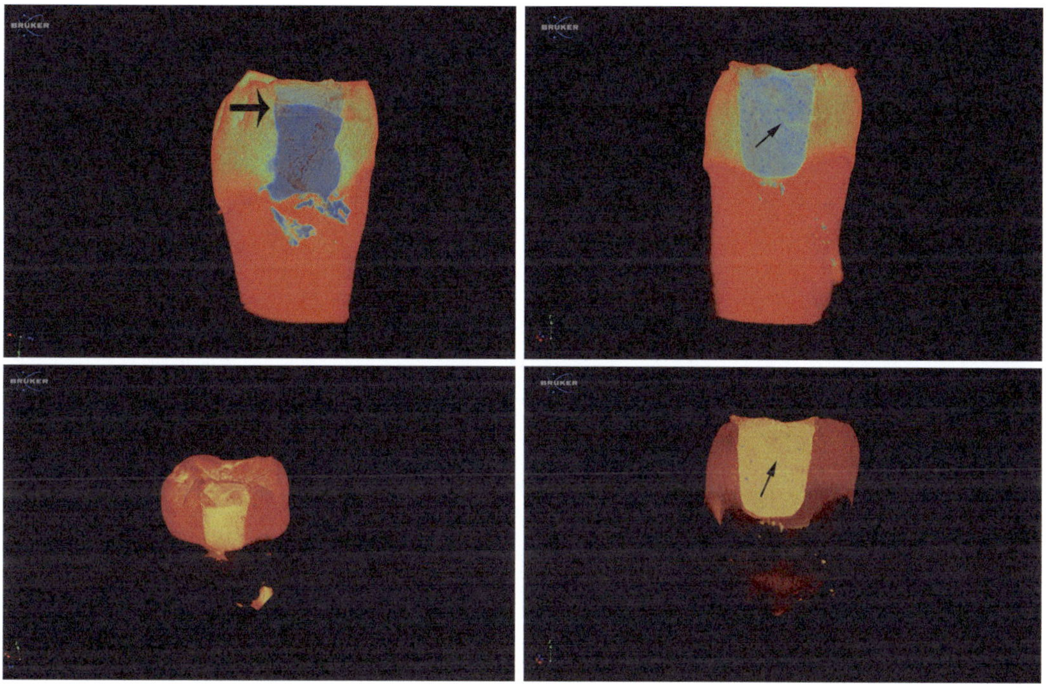

Fig. 15.11 Micro-CT images showing different composites. Bold arrow indicates the layer separation of composites, small arrows indicates voids inside dental composites

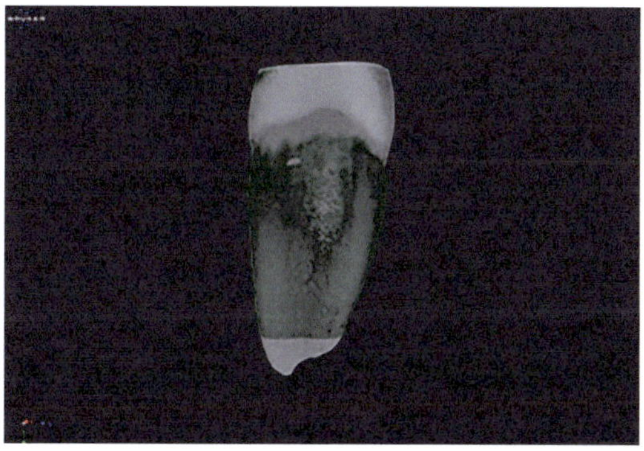

Fig. 15.12 Micro-CT image of dentine resorption

imaging approach excels at resolving soft tissues and inflammatory processes without the use of a contrast agent. It is the ideal alternative for the research of TMJ location and morphology, skeletal physiology, tumors, and the healing of grafts, regardless of cost or availability Combining MRI and micro-CT to analyze the trabecular structure of human bone specimens and comparing it to bone mineral density in the prediction of bone strength is also achievable [14–16].

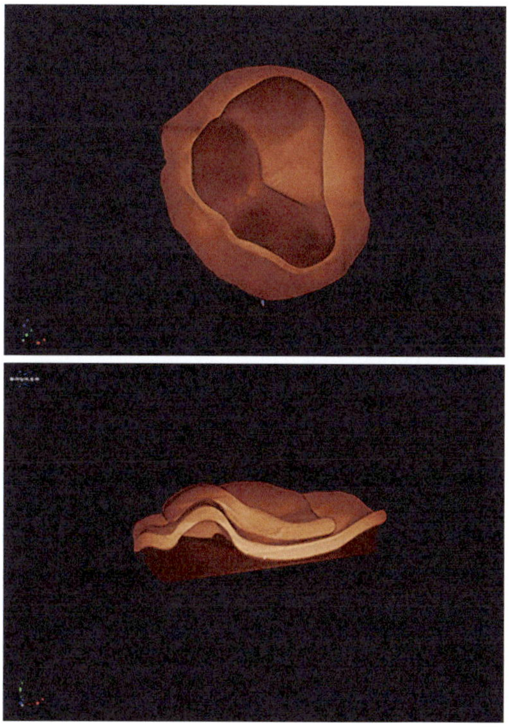

Fig. 15.13 Micro-CT evaluation of a occlusal splint that is being used for cleft palate surgery. Note that Micro-CT can accurately measure the gap between the bone and splint

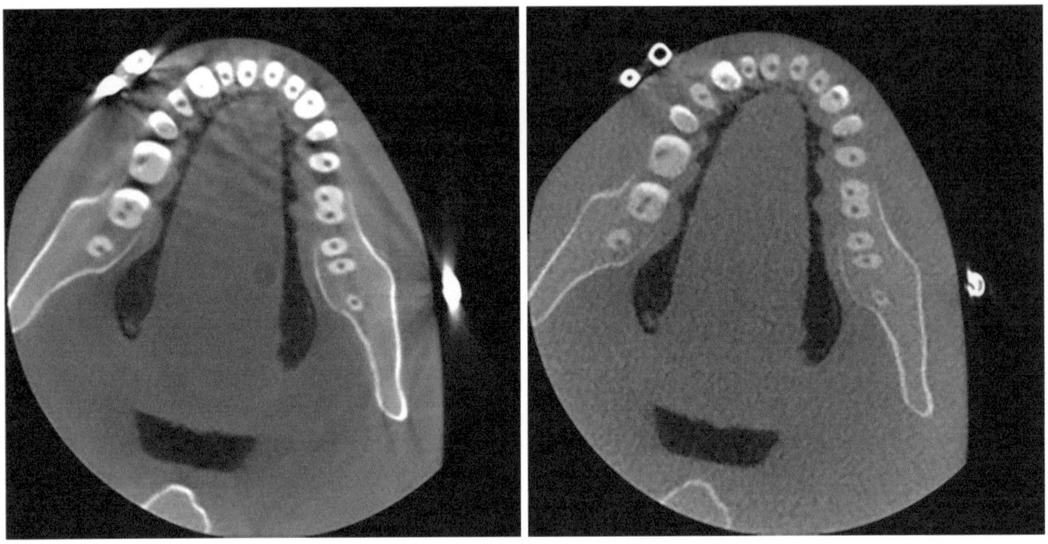

Fig. 15.14 A comparison of image quality from normal CT (left) and dual-energy CT (right)

15.4 Future Projection for Micro-CT

Micro-CT, which was once a costly and unknown imaging tool, has now become a practical and routine application, particularly in the dentistry scientific field. Given that micro-CT can resolve a lot of fine structures of teeth and periodontal tissues in a non-invasive manner, it is a viable alternative to many traditional dental research methods. As a result, micro-CT data could be used to further investigate root canal anatomy in experimental endodontics, preclinical training in fundamental endodontic procedures, periapical and periodontal pathology, craniofacial skeletal structure and development, and peri-implant osseointegration, as well as a valuable mathematical modeling of tooth morphology in both healthy and pathological states.

However, it can only be used in in vitro human investigations and in vivo animal studies right now. With the development of micro-CT techniques, additional micro/nano-CT applications will be broadening the dental research, from millimeters to nanometers, from biological samples to material samples, from the lab bench to the chairside, for both research and industrial applications, without destroying dental samples.

References

1. Davis GR, Elliott JC. High definition X-ray microtomography using a conventional impact X-ray source. J Phys IV. 2003;104:131–4.
2. Davis G, Evershed A, Elliott J, Mills D. Quantitative X-ray microtomography with a conventional source. Dev X-Ray Tomogr. 2010;7:7804.
3. Parfitt AM, Drezner MK, Glorieux FH, et al. Bone histomorphometry: standardization of nomenclature, symbols, and units. Report of the ASBMR Histomorphometry nomenclature committee. J Bone Miner Res. 1987;2:595–610.
4. Magne P. Efficient 3D finite element analysis of dental restorative procedures using micro-CT data. Dent Mater. 2007;23(5):539–48.
5. Bouxsein ML, Boyd SK, Christiansen BA, Guldberg RE, Jepsen KJ, Müller R. Guidelines for assessment of bone microstructure in rodents using micro-computed tomography. J Bone Miner Res. 2010;25:1468–86.
6. Huang Y, Van Dessel J, Liang X, Depypere M, Zhong W, Ma G, Lambrichts I, Maes F, Jacobs R. Effects of immediate and delayed loading on peri-implant trabecular structures: a cone beam CT evaluation. Clin Implant Dent Relat Res. 2014;16(6):873–83.
7. Alghamdi HS, Bosco R, van den Beucken JJJP, Walboomers XF, Jansen JA. Osteogenicity of titanium implants coated with calcium phosphate or

collagen type-I in osteoporotic rats. Biomaterials. 2013;34(15):3747–57.
8. Bissinger O, Probst FA, Wolff K-D, Jeschke A, Weitz J, Deppe H, Kolk A. Comparative 3D micro-CT and 2D histomorphometry analysis of dental implant osseointegration in the maxilla of minipigs. J Clin Periodontol. 2017;44(4):418–27.
9. Olejniczak AJ, Grine F. Assessment of the accuracy of dental enamel thickness measurements using micro-focal X-ray computed tomography. Anat Rec Pt A. 2006;288A:263–75.
10. Oi T, Saka H, Ide Y. Three-dimensional observation of pulp cavities in the maxillary first premolar tooth using micro-CT. Int Endod J. 2002;37(1):46–51.
11. Hlushchuk R, Zubler C, Barre S, Shokiche CC, Schaad L, Röthlisberger R, Wnuk M, Daniel C, Khoma O, Tschanz SA, Reyes M, Djonov V. Cutting-edge microangio-CT: new dimensions in vascular imaging and kidney morphometry. Am J Physiol Renal Physiol. 2018;314(3):F493–9.
12. Bona AD, Borba M, Benetti P, Duan Y, Griggs JA. Three-dimensional finite element modelling of all-ceramic restorations based on micro-CT. J Dent. 2013;41(5):412–9.
13. Almedia EO, Rocha EP, Junior ACF, Anchetia RB, Poveda R, Gupta N, Coelho PG. Tilted and short implants supporting fixed prosthesis in an atrophic maxilla: a 3D-FEA biomechanical evaluation. Clin Implant Dent Relat Res. 2015;17(Suppl 1):e332–42.
14. De Souza e Silva JM, Utsch J, Kimm MA, Allner S, Epple MF, Achterhold K, Pfeiffer F. Dual-energy micro-CT for quantifying the time-course and staining characteristics of ex-vivo animal organs treated with iodine- and gadolinium-based contrast agents. Sci Rep. 2017;7:17387.
15. Karatas OH, Toy E. Three-dimensional imaging techniques: a literature review. Eur J Dent. 2014;8(1):132–40.
16. Link TM, Majumdar S, Lin JC, Newitt D, Augat P, Ouyang X, Mathur A, Genant HK. Comparative study of trabecular bone properties in the spine and femur using high resolution MRI and CT. J Bone Miner Res. 1998;13(1):122–32.

MIX
Papier aus verantwortungsvollen Quellen
Paper from responsible sources
FSC® C105338

If you have any concerns about our products,
you can contact us on
ProductSafety@springernature.com

In case Publisher is established outside the EU,
the EU authorized representative is:
Springer Nature Customer Service Center GmbH
Europaplatz 3, 69115 Heidelberg, Germany

Printed by Libri Plureos GmbH
in Hamburg, Germany